# Sleep and Neurorehabilitation

*Editors*

**RICHARD J. CASTRIOTTA**
**MARK C. WILDE**

# SLEEP MEDICINE CLINICS

www.sleep.theclinics.com

December 2012 • Volume 7 • Number 4

**ELSEVIER**

1600 John F. Kennedy Boulevard • Suite 1800 • Philadelphia, Pennsylvania, 19103-2899

http://www.theclinics.com

**SLEEP MEDICINE CLINICS Volume 7, Number 4**
**December 2012, ISSN 1556-407X, ISBN-13: 978-1-4557-5842-5**

Editor: Katie Saunders
Developmental Editor: Donald E. Mumford

*Sleep Medicine Clinics* (ISSN 1556-407X) is published quarterly by Elsevier Inc., 360 Park Avenue South, New York, NY 10010-1710. Months of issue are March, June, September and December. Business and Editorial Offices: 1600 John F. Kennedy Blvd., Ste. 1800, Philadelphia, PA 19103-2899. Customer Service Office: 3251 Riverport Lane, Maryland Heights, MO 63043. Periodicals postage paid at New York, NY and additional mailing offices. Subscription prices are $174.00 per year (US individuals), $86.00 (US residents), $368.00 (US institutions), $214.00 (foreign individuals), $120.00 (foreign residents), and $406.00 (foreign institutions). Foreign air speed delivery is included in all *Clinics* subscription prices. All prices are subject to change without notice. **POSTMASTER:** Send change of address to *Sleep Medicine Clinics*, Elsevier Health Sciences Division, Subscription Customer Service, 3251 Riverport Lane, Maryland Heights, MO 63043. Customer Service: **Tel: 1-800-654-2452 (U.S. and Canada); 314-447-8871 (outside U.S. and Canada). Fax: 314-447-8029. E-mail: journalscustomerservice-usa@elsevier.com (for print support); journalsonlinesupport-usa@elsevier.com (for online support).**

*Reprints.* For copies of 100 or more of articles in this publication, please contact the Commercial Reprints Department, Elsevier Inc., 360 Park Avenue South, New York, NY 10010-1710. Tel.: 212-633-3812; Fax: 212-462-1935; E-mail: reprints@elsevier.com.

Printed and bound by CPI Group (UK) Ltd, Croydon, CR0 4YY

Transferred to digital print 2012

## GOAL STATEMENT
The goal of *Sleep Clinics of North America* is to keep practicing physicians up to date with current clinical practice by providing timely articles reviewing the state of the art in patient care.

## ACCREDITATION
The *Sleep Clinics of North America* is planned and implemented in accordance with the Essential Areas and Policies of the Accreditation Council for Continuing Medical Education (ACCME) through the joint sponsorship of the University of Virginia School of Medicine and Elsevier. The University of Virginia School of Medicine is accredited by the ACCME to provide continuing medical education for physicians.

The University of Virginia School of Medicine designates this enduring material activity for a maximum of 15 *AMA PRA Category 1 Credit(s)*™ for each issue, 60 credits per year. Physicians should only claim credit commensurate with the extent of their participation in the activity.

The American Medical Association has determined that physicians not licensed in the US who participate in this CME enduring material activity are eligible for a maximum of 15 *AMA PRA Category 1* Credit(s)™ for each issue, 60 credits per year.

Credit can be earned by reading the text material, taking the CME examination online at http://www.theclinics.com/home/cme, and completing the evaluation. After taking the test, you will be required to review any and all incorrect answers. Following completion of the test and evaluation, your credit will be awarded and you may print your certificate.

## FACULTY DISCLOSURE/CONFLICT OF INTEREST
The University of Virginia School of Medicine, as an ACCME accredited provider, endorses and strives to comply with the Accreditation Council for Continuing Medical Education (ACCME) Standards of Commercial Support, Commonwealth of Virginia statutes, University of Virginia policies and procedures, and associated federal and private regulations and guidelines on the need for disclosure and monitoring of proprietary and financial interests that may affect the scientific integrity and balance of content delivered in continuing medical education activities under our auspices.

The University of Virginia School of Medicine requires that all CME activities accredited through this institution be developed independently and be scientifically rigorous, balanced and objective in the presentation/discussion of its content, theories and practices.

All authors/editors participating in an accredited CME activity are expected to disclose to the readers relevant financial relationships with commercial entities occurring within the past 12 months (such as grants or research support, employee, consultant, stock holder, member of speakers bureau, etc.). The University of Virginia School of Medicine will employ appropriate mechanisms to resolve potential conflicts of interest to maintain the standards of fair and balanced education to the reader. Questions about specific strategies can be directed to the Office of Continuing Medical Education, University of Virginia School of Medicine, Charlottesville, Virginia.

The faculty and staff of the University of Virginia Office of Continuing Medical Education have no financial affiliations to disclose.

**The authors/editors listed below have identified no professional or financial affiliations for themselves or their spouse/partner:**
Stamatia Alexiou, MD; James A. Barker, MD, CPE, FCCP; Christian R. Baumann, MD; Carl D. Boethel, MD, FCCP; Lee J. Brooks, MD; Cynthia Brown, MD (Test Author); Richard J. Castriotta, MD (Guest Editor); Fabio Fabbian, MD; Madeleine M. Grigg-Damberger, MD; Katie Hartner, (Acquisitions Editor); Shirley F. Jones, MD, FCCP; Francesco Portaluppi, MD, PhD; Francoise J. Roux, MD, PhD; Sandeep Sahay, MD; Gilbert Seda, MD, PhD; Bernardo Selim, MD; Amir Sharafkhaneh, MD, PhD, DABSM; Sudha S. Tallavajhula, MD; Lana K. Wagner, MD; and Mark C. Wilde, Psy.D (Guest Editor).

**The authors/editors listed below identified the following professional or financial affiliations for themselves or their spouse/partner:**
**Lee K. Brown, MD** is a consultant for Considine and Associates Inc.
**John Harrington, MD** receives research support from Philip Respironics and Sleep Methods, Inc.
**Erhard Haus, MD** is employed by Regions Hospital, St. Paul, MN and University of MN, Mpls, MN, and is a consultant for Pharmasan Laboratories, Osceola, WI.
**Max Hirshkowitz, PhD, DABSM** is on the Speakers' Bureau for Cephalon.
**Eric B. Larson, PhD, ABPP** is employed by Rehabilitation Institute of Chicago, is on the Speakers' Bureau for the Feinberg School of Medicine, Northwestern University, and is a consultant for the National Football League Player Benefits.
**Teofilo Lee-Chiong, MD (Consulting Editor)** is employed by Respironics, and is an industry funded research/investigator for Respironics and Embla/Natus.
**Jeremy D. Slater, MD** is on the Speakers' Bureau for UCB, Lundbeck, and Cyberonics; receives research support from Lundbeck; and is a consultant for Lundbeck and Cyberonics.
**Michael H. Smolensky, PhD** is a consultant for Horizon Pharma.

***Disclosure of Discussion of Non-FDA Approved Uses for Pharmaceutical Products and/or Medical Devices.***
**The University of Virginia School of Medicine, as an ACCME provider, requires that all faculty presenters identify and disclose any off-label uses for pharmaceutical and medical device products. The University of Virginia School of Medicine recommends that each physician fully review all the available data on new products or procedures prior to clinical use.**

## TO ENROLL
To enroll in the Sleep Clinics of North America Continuing Medical Education program, call customer service at 1-800-654-2452 or visit us online at http://www.theclinics.com/home/cme. The CME program is available to subscribers for an additional fee of $114.00.

# SLEEP MEDICINE CLINICS

**NOW AVAILABLE FOR YOUR iPhone and iPad**

# Contributors

## CONSULTING EDITOR

**TEOFILO LEE-CHIONG Jr, MD**
Professor of Medicine and Chief, Division
of Sleep Medicine, National Jewish Health;
Associate Professor of Medicine, University
of Colorado Denver School of Medicine,
Denver, Colorado

## GUEST EDITORS

**RICHARD J. CASTRIOTTA, MD**
Professor and Director, Division of Pulmonary,
Critical Care and Sleep Medicine, University
of Texas Health Science Center at Houston;
Medical Director, Sleep Disorders Center,
Memorial Hermann Hospital–Texas Medical
Center, Houston, Texas

**MARK C. WILDE, PsyD**
Clinical Neuropsychologist, Department
of Physical Medicine and Rehabilitation,
University of Texas Medical School at Houston,
Houston, Texas

## AUTHORS

**STAMATIA ALEXIOU, MD**
Pediatric Pulmonology Fellow, Division of
Pediatric Pulmonology and Sleep Medicine,
Children's Hospital of Philadelphia,
Philadelphia, Pennsylvania

**JAMES A. BARKER, MD, CPE, FACP, FCCP,
FAASM**
Division Director, Pulmonary, Sleep, and
Critical Care, Scott and White Healthcare,
Professor of Medicine, Texas A&M HSC COM,
Temple, Texas

**CHRISTIAN R. BAUMANN, MD**
Department of Neurology, University Hospital
Zurich, Zurich, Switzerland

**CARL D. BOETHEL, MD, FCCP, FAASM**
Medical Director, Scott and White Sleep
Institute, Assistant Professor Texas A&M HSC
COM, Temple, Texas

**LEE J. BROOKS, MD**
Clinical Professor of Pediatrics, Division of
Pediatric Pulmonology and Sleep Medicine,

Children's Hospital of Philadelphia,
Philadelphia, Pennsylvania

**LEE K. BROWN, MD**
Professor of Internal Medicine and
Pediatrics; Executive Director,
University of New Mexico Sleep
Disorders Center; Division of Pulmonary,
Critical Care and Sleep Medicine,
University of New Mexico School of
Medicine, Albuquerque, New Mexico

**RICHARD J. CASTRIOTTA, MD**
Professor of Medicine and Director, Division
of Pulmonary and Sleep Medicine, University
of Texas Medical School at Houston,
Houston, Texas

**FABIO FABBIAN, MD**
Department of Clinical and Experimental
Medicine, Hypertension Center, University
Hospital S. Anna, University of Ferrara,
Ferrara, Italy

**MADELEINE M. GRIGG-DAMBERGER, MD**
Professor of Neurology and Medical Director of
Pediatric Sleep Medicine Services, University
of New Mexico Sleep Disorders Center;
Associate Director of Clinical Neurophysiology,
University of New Mexico Medical Center,
Albuquerque, New Mexico

**JOHN HARRINGTON, MD, MPH**
Associate Professor of Medicine, Division
of Pulmonary Sciences and Critical Care
Medicine, National Jewish Health, University
of Colorado, Denver, Colorado

**ERHARD HAUS, MD**
Department of Laboratory Medicine and
Pathology, HealthPartners Medical Group,
Regions Hospital, St. Paul, Minnesota

**MAX HIRSHKOWITZ, PhD, DABSM**
Associate Professor, Menninger Department of
Psychiatry, Baylor College of Medicine;
Department of Medicine, Baylor College of
Medicine; Department of Medicine, Michael E.
DeBakey Veterans Affairs Medical Center,
Houston, Texas

**SHIRLEY F. JONES, MD, FCCP, FAASM**
Medical Director, Scott and White Sleep
Center, Horseshoe Bay, Assistant Professor
Texas A&M HSC COM, Temple, Texas

**ERIC B. LARSON, PhD, ABPP**
Clinical Neuropsychologist, Rehabilitation
Institute of Chicago; Assistant Professor,
Department of Physical Medicine and
Rehabilitation, Feinberg School of Medicine,
Northwestern University, Chicago, Illinois

**TEOFILO LEE-CHIONG, MD**
Professor of Medicine, Division of Pulmonary
Sciences and Critical Care Medicine, National
Jewish Health, University of Colorado, Denver,
Colorado

**FRANCESCO PORTALUPPI, MD, PhD**
Department of Clinical and Experimental
Medicine, Hypertension Center, University
Hospital S. Anna, University of Ferrara,
Ferrara, Italy

**FRANCOISE J. ROUX, MD, PhD**
Associate Professor of Medicine, Section of
Pulmonary, Critical Care and Sleep Medicine,
Yale Sleep Center, Yale University School of
Medicine, New Haven, Connecticut

**SANDEEP SAHAY, MD**
Pulmonary/Critical Care Fellow, Division of
Pulmonary and Sleep Medicine, University of
Texas Medical School at Houston, Houston,
Texas

**GILBERT SEDA, MD, PhD**
Fellow, Sleep Medicine, Division of Pulmonary
Sciences and Critical Care Medicine, National
Jewish Health, University of Colorado, Denver,
Colorado

**BERNARDO SELIM, MD**
Assistant Professor of Medicine, Section of
Pulmonary, Critical Care and Sleep Medicine,
Mayo Clinic Sleep Center, Mayo Clinic,
Rochester, Minnesota

**AMIR SHARAFKHANEH, MD, PhD, DABSM**
Associate Professor, Menninger Department
of Psychiatry, Baylor College of Medicine;
Department of Medicine, Michael E. DeBakey
Veterans Affairs Medical Center, Houston,
Texas

**JEREMY D. SLATER, MD**
Associate Professor, Department of
Neurology, University of Texas Health
Sciences Center, Houston, Texas

**MICHAEL H. SMOLENSKY, PhD**
Department of Biomedical Engineering,
The University of Texas at Austin, Austin,
Texas

**SUDHA S. TALLAVAJHULA, MD**
Assistant Professor, Department of Neurology,
University of Texas Health Sciences Center,
Houston, Texas

**LANA K. WAGNER, MD**
Sleep Medicine Fellow and Associate
Professor of Family and Community
Medicine, Division of Pulmonary,
Critical Care and Sleep Medicine,
University of New Mexico School of
Medicine, Albuquerque, New Mexico

**MARK C. WILDE, PsyD**
Clinical Neuropsychologist and
Associate Professor, Department of
Physical Medicine and Rehabilitation,
University of Texas Medical School at
Houston, Houston, Texas

# Contents

> Sleep is essentially a restorative process. Research focused on the underlying biology finds sleep to be critical for both somatic and psychological restoration, as well as being responsive to changing demands placed on the body and mind. Sleep-related breathing disorders are especially relevant to rehabilitation. The sleep disturbances provoked by frequent awakening adversely affect all aspects of health. Sleep can also provide prognostic indications. Sudden adverse changes in sleep and sleep-related phenomena are seldom good omens. Sleep can be a sensitive marker because it is fragile but resilient. In a sense, sleep serves as a bellwether of overall health. Consequently, we regard sleep as a vital sign.

> Insomnia is a disorder that is defined by subjective complaint concerning the duration and quality of sleep. It is associated with numerous medical complications and poor rehabilitation outcome. Polysomnography and actigraphy provide objective measures of sleep duration, but assessment of subjective complaints concerning sleep relies on self-report measures. Psychotherapy Is an effective treatment of insomnia, although neurocognitive factors often interfere with participation. Short-term pharmacologic treatment Is effective, but further study of adverse effects in neurologic populations is needed. This article summarizes alternative treatments and recommendations for further research.

> There is compelling evidence that suggests an independent association, possibly causal in nature, between obstructive sleep apnea (OSA) and cerebrovascular diseases such as transient ischemic attack and stroke. OSA is a preventable and treatable risk factor for stroke. Stroke patients with OSA represent a population at higher risk for recurrent stroke, mortality, and poorer functional outcomes than stroke patients without OSA. Continuous positive airways pressure (CPAP) therapy provides short- and long-term benefits for these patients. Stroke patients should be screened for OSA and other sleep disorders to implement the appropriate treatment in the early phase of the cerebrovascular event.

> Traumatic brain injury (TBI) is a prevalent worldwide condition. There is growing evidence that many TBI patients suffer from chronic posttraumatic sleep-wake disorders (SWD). In the following article, the literature on posttraumatic SWD are

reviewed with the objective of providing the reader with a solid understanding of the current knowledge of the relationship between TBI and SWD.

## Sleep and Epilepsy

619

Sudha S. Tallavajhula and Jeremy D. Slater

The bidirectional nature of the interaction between epilepsy and sleep is revealed in multiple observations. Interictal epileptiform discharges and the timing of seizures in some epilepsy syndromes show patterns of temporal synchrony with the sleep-wake cycle. Sleep deprivation is associated with an increase in cortical excitability. Both seizures and epilepsy are capable of altering sleep microarchitechture and macroarchitecture, sleep-related behaviors, and subjective sleep quality. Because sleep disturbances have been found to be one of the main predictors in quality of life in epilepsy, and because there are effective treatments available, addressing these efficiently is integral to the management strategy.

## Sleep Movement Disorders and Neurologic Movement Disorders

631

Carl D. Boethel, Shirley F. Jones, and James A. Barker

Movement during sleep is both normal and abnormal. We are only beginning to understand the underlying pathophysiology of sleep movement disorders. Neurologic movement disorders are perhaps better understood and most have underlying genetic causes or predilections. Worsening of sleep and consequent daytime sleepiness with progression of these disorders is the rule rather than the exception. Medications for the primary disorders may worsen sleep or even induce sleep disorders. There is much to learn in the future. We are only scratching the surface of this fascinating field of medicine.

## Sleep Disorders in Spinal Cord Injury

643

Richard J. Castriotta, Mark C. Wilde, and Sandeep Sahay

Pathophysiological changes resulting from spinal cord injury (SCI) result in four groups of sleep-related problems: (1) sleep-disordered breathing with hypoventilation and obstructive sleep apnea; (2) circadian rhythm disorders with disruption of melatonin and body temperature rhythms; (3) sensorimotor problems with restless legs and periodic limb movements; and (4) insomnia with multifactorial causes, including pain, paresthesias, mood and anxiety disorders and voiding problems in addition to the above. Sleep disorders are under-recognized in patients with SCI because sleep-related respiratory problems may be asymptomatic, and thus are not investigated. In patients with SCI, sleep-disordered breathing leads to neurocognitive impairment adversely affecting neurorehabilitation.

## Relevance of Chronobiology to the Research and Clinical Practice of Neurorehabilitation

655

Francesco Portaluppi, Michael H. Smolensky, Erhard Haus, and Fabio Fabbian

Chronobiology is the study of endogenous biological rhythms and the mechanisms of biological time-keeping in health and disease. The spectrum of circadian periodicities and the phase relationships between them constitute the so-called circadian time structure (CTS), which is of great relevance to medicine. Integrity of the CTS is critical for efficient biological and cognitive functioning. The practical relevance of chronobiology to meeting patient goals and optimizing outcomes of neurorehabilitation has been little explored; nonetheless, such is warranted given the findings of an increasing number of clinical studies showing detrimental interferences of poorly timed interventions and disrupted CTS.

## Sleep Hypoventilation in Patients with Neuromuscular Diseases          667

Madeleine M. Grigg-Damberger, Lana K. Wagner, and Lee K. Brown

> Sleep-disordered breathing (SDB), especially sleep-related hypercapnic hypoventilation, is common in patients with neuromuscular disorders (NMD). Whether the NMD is acute and reversible or indolent and progressive, the accompanied respiratory muscle weakness predisposes to hypoventilation. Probably the 3 most common NMD referred to sleep medicine specialists are Duchenne muscular dystrophy, myotonic dystrophy type 1, and amyotrophic lateral sclerosis. Symptoms-based and physiologic predictors of sleep hypoventilation have been described for patients with NMD. Nocturnal polysomnography remains the gold standard for diagnosis of SDB in NMD and for titration of nocturnal positive pressure ventilation.

## Congenital Disorders Affecting Sleep          689

Stamatia Alexiou and Lee J. Brooks

> Breathing efforts and the success of such are affected by genetic factors. Factors that decrease the size and/or increase the floppiness of the upper airway increase the individual's risk of obstructive sleep apnea. Many genetic syndromes can therefore affect breathing during sleep, through anatomic abnormalities affecting central respiratory control, or anatomic and physiologic factors affecting the properties of the upper airway. Congenital disorders affecting breathing during sleep can be classified into 1 of 4 categories: micrognathia, midface hypoplasia, disorders of neuromuscular control, and miscellaneous disorders. Some of the more common syndromes with these features are reviewed here.

## Sleep Derangements in Central Nervous System Infections          703

Gilbert Seda, Teofilo Lee-Chiong, and John Harrington

> Significant disturbances of sleep architecture and sleep quality can develop in several central nervous system (CNS) infections. The changes in sleep differ among the various infectious agents. Some cases of narcolepsy are believed to be related to postinfectious autoimmune processes by the interaction between innate genetic susceptibility and exposure to specific pathogens. Infection with HIV can give rise to insomnia, daytime fatigue, and depression. Infections of the CNS can affect the brainstem respiratory centers resulting in abnormal breathing patterns during sleep. Parasomnias and alterations in circadian rhythms have been described in some CNS infections.

# Introduction
# Sleep Disorders in
# Neurorehabilitation

There is a strong link between sleep disorders and several neurologic disorders commonly encountered in routine neurorehabilitation practice.[1–3] Sleep disorders have an impact on daytime functioning, which in turn can have an effect on quality of life.[4] Indeed, several studies lend support to the idea that dually diagnosed patients with both a sleep disorder and a traumatic brain injury (TBI) have a less desirable outcome than those with TBI alone.[5,6] For this reason, the proper diagnosis and treatment of sleep disorders in a neurorehabilitation setting could be important to maximize outcome. In the following special issue of *Sleep Medicine Clinics*, there are 11 papers from distinguished experts in the field of sleep disorders. Each article provides a unique perspective on a different topic germane to neurorehabilitation and sleep. The first article is authored by Max Hirshkowitz, PhD, one of the world's stellar experts on sleep and sleep research, associate professor of medicine and psychiatry at Baylor College of Medicine in Houston, Texas, and secretary of the World Association of Sleep Medicine, along with Amir Sharafkhaneh, MD, PhD, associate professor of medicine at Baylor College of Medicine, medical director of the Sleep Laboratory at the Michael DeBakey Veterans Administration Hospital in Houston, and program director of the Sleep Medicine Fellowship program at Baylor College of Medicine. In this article, they provide an overview of sleep medicine for the non–sleep professional. The history of sleep medicine, the neuroanatomy of normal and abnormal sleep, sleep nomenclature, and the range of sleep disorders are discussed.

The next article is authored by Eric Larson, PhD, assistant professor of physical medicine and rehabilitation at Northwestern University's Feinberg School of Medicine in Chicago and clinical neuropsychologist at the Rehabilitation Institute of Chicago, Illinois. In this article, the topic of insomnia is discussed. Key points covered include the causes, manifestations, epidemiology, and treatment of insomnia in various neurorehabilitation populations.

The important relationship between stroke and sleep disorders is discussed by Bernardo Selim, MD, assistant professor of medicine at the Mayo Clinic in Rochester, Minnesota, and Francoise Roux, MD, PhD, associate professor of medicine at Yale University School of Medicine, director of Sleep Study Services at the Veterans Administration Medical Center in West Haven, Connecticut, and program director of the Sleep Medicine Fellowship at Yale University School of Medicine. These authors illustrate the high risk of patients with stroke for having sleep apnea and the importance of evaluating these patients for obstructive or central sleep apnea and treating them appropriately.

The relationship between TBI and multiple sleep disorders is well described by Christian Baumann, MD, professor of neurology at the University of Zurich, Zurich, Switzerland. Prof Baumann is a world-renowned sleep researcher and a leader in the field of TBI.

The next paper is a comprehensive review of sleep and epilepsy by Drs Sudha Tallavajula and Jeremy Slater. Dr Slater is Associate Professor of Neurology at the University of Texas Medical School at Houston and Director of the Texas Comprehensive Epilepsy Program. Dr Tallavajhula is Assistant Professor of Neurology at the University of Texas Medical School at Houston and Director of the Neurophysiology and Sleep Disorders Center at St. Joseph's Medical Center in Houston. This is an excellent treatment of seizure disorders and sleep from Aristotle to the most recent evidence based concepts.

The next paper is comprehensive review of sleep and movement disorders as they relate to neurorehabilitation. The authors of this paper are James Barker, MD, who is director of the division of Pulmonary, Critical Care and Sleep Medicine at Scott and White Healthcare as well as Professor of Medicine at Texas A&M College of Medicine

Sleep Med Clin 7 (2012) xi–xii
http://dx.doi.org/10.1016/j.jsmc.2012.08.006

and Shirley Jones, MD who is an assistant professor of Internal Medicine at Texas A&M College of Medicine and the Scott and White Sleep Disorders Center.

The next paper explains the important sleep related complications of spinal cord injury, which include circadian rhythm disturbances, insomnia, movement disorders and hypoventilation.

The next article, by Portaluppi et al, is an excellent review of chronobiology, endogenous biologic rhythms, and biologic clocks in the environment of neurorehabilitation. Francesco Portaluppi, MD, PhD, is associate professor of internal medicine at the University of Ferrara, Italy, and head of the Hypertension Center at the University Hospital S. Ana in Ferrara, where he works with Fabio Fabbian, MD. Michael Smolensky, PhD is a professor in the Department of Biomedical Engineering at the University of Texas at Austin, visiting professor at the University of Texas Health Science Center at Houston School of Public Health, and coeditor-in-chief of the journal *Chronobiology International*. Eric Haus, MD, is professor of pathology and laboratory medicine at the University of Minnesota. These 4 authors are experts in chronobiology and circadian rhythms with major research contributions to the field.

The following paper gives an illustrative review of what is currently known about the diagnosis and management of sleep related problems associated with neuromuscular diseases by Madeleine Grigg-Damberger, MD, Professor of Neurology, University of New Mexico School of Medicine, Lana K. Wagner, MD Sleep Medicine Fellow, University of New Mexico School of Medicine, and Lee K. Brown, MD, Professor of Internal Medicine and Pediatrics, University of New Mexico School of Medicine.

The next paper is an excellent review of sleep and congenital disorders seen in neuro-rehabilitation by Stamatia Alexiou, MD and Lee Brooks, MD, who is Professor of Pediatrics at the University of Pennsylvania and the Children's Hospital of Philadelphia.

The last article which covers sleep problems related to central nervous system infections, concentrating on the most recent fascinating discoveries, is by Gilbert Seda, MD, PhD. Sleep Medicine Fellow, Teofilo Lee-Chiong, MD, Professor

of Medicine, and John Harrington, MD Associate Professor of Medicine all at the University of Colorado National Jewish Health in Denver.

Richard J. Castriotta, MD
Professor and Director
Division of Pulmonary, Critical Care and
Sleep Medicine
University of Texas Health Science
Center at Houston
Houston, TX, USA

Sleep Disorders Center
Memorial Hermann Hospital–Texas Medical Center
Houston, TX, USA

Mark C. Wilde, Psy.D
Clinical Neuropsychologist
Department of Physical Medicine and
Rehabilitation
University of Texas Medical School at Houston
Houston, TX, USA

E-mail addresses:
Richard.J.Castriotta@uth.tmc.edu (R.J. Castriotta)
Mark.C.Wilde@uth.tmc.edu (M.C. Wilde)

## REFERENCES

1. Castriotta RJ, Murthy JN. Sleep disorders in patients with traumatic brain injury: a review. CNS Drugs 2011;25(3):175–85.
2. Roux F, D'Ambrosio C, Mohsenin V. Sleep related breathing disorders and cardiovascular disease. Am J Med 2000;108(5):396–402.
3. Tsai JC. Neurological and neurobehavioral sequelae of obstructive sleep apnea. NeuroRehabilitation 2010;26(1):85–94.
4. Reimer MA, Flemmons WW. Quality of life in sleep disorders. Sleep Med Rev 2003;7(4):335–49.
5. Wilde MC, Castriotta RJ, Lai JM, et al. Cognitive impairment in patients with traumatic brain injury and obstructive sleep apnea. Arch Phys Med Rehabil 2007;88(10):1284–8.
6. Makley MJ, English JB, Drubach DA, et al. Prevalence of sleep disturbance in closed head injury patients in a rehabilitation unit. Neurorehabil Neural Repair 2008;22(4):341–7.

# Introduction to Sleep Medicine

Max Hirshkowitz, PhD, DABSM[a,b,c,*],
Amir Sharafkhaneh, MD, PhD, DABSM[a,c]

## KEYWORDS

• Sleep medicine • Physiologic • Sleep regulation

## KEY POINTS

• The sleep disturbances provoked by frequent awakening adversely affect all aspects of health.
• Sleep can be a sensitive marker, and serves as a bellwether of overall health.

## HISTORY

### Sleep Physiology

Sleep medicine's roots date back to Henri Peiron who published *Le Probleme Physiologique du Sommeil* in 1913.[1] Peiron considered sleep from a physiologic perspective and performed research supporting the hypnotoxin theory of sleep regulation. He induced sleepiness by injecting alert dogs with serum from sleep-deprived dogs. Approximately a decade and a half later, in 1929 the "father of electroencephalography," Johannes Berger,[2] demonstrated the difference between brain activity during wakefulness and sleep. That same year, Constantin Von Economo[3] proposed a sleep-regulatory hypothalamic brain site based on his clinical experience with patients suffering from encephalitis. The first continuous all-night sleep studies were performed in 1936-1937 by Loomis and colleagues[4] as part of an intellectual exploration at the Loomis's Tuxedo Park laboratory. The first sleep stage classification arose from their work. Their classification did not include a description of the sleep stage later illustrated by Aserinsky and Kleitmann[5] (1953) that was ultimately named rapid eye movement (REM) sleep. REM sleep fascinated many researchers because of its association with dreams, what Freud had regarded as the "royal road to the unconscious."[6]

Long before sleep medicine developed, circadian rhythm had been described in plants and animals. Jean Jacques d'Ortous de Mairan[7] demonstrated heliotrope leaf opening and closing independent of sunlight in 1729. After more than 2 centuries of experimentation, the term "biological clock" was coined in 1935 by Bunning[8] and conceptually framed as a part of the sleep-wake cycle. In 1972, Robert Y. Moore's work[9] established the circadian pacemaker in the suprachiasmatic nuclei (SCN), and soon after mapped the retinohypothalamic projection as the pathway linking light and darkness to the sleep-wake circadian rhythm.

### Sleep Disorders

In 1945 Karl-Axel Ekbom coined the term "restless legs."[10] This sleep disorder had been initially described back in 1672 by Sir Thomas Willis, who noted that arm and leg movements were associated with sleep disturbances.[11] Although many descriptions of the restless legs syndrome (RLS) followed, it was Ekbom who provided a comprehensive report, clearly characterized the symptoms, differentiated it from other disorders, and estimated its prevalence. He also linked RLS to anemia. His work languished for many years but was revived in the past decade by Walters and Hening.[12]

Sleep apnea was described first by Gastaut and colleagues[13] (1965) in morbidly obese patients. The moniker "Pickwickian" was attached because

a Menninger Department of Psychiatry, Baylor College of Medicine, Houston, TX, USA; b Department of Medicine, Baylor College of Medicine, Houston, TX, USA; c Department of Medicine, Michael E. DeBakey Veterans Affairs Medical Center, Houston, TX, USA
* Corresponding author. MED VAMC Sleep Center 111i, 2002 Holcombe Boulevard, Houston, TX 77030.
*E-mail address:* maxh@bcm.tmc.edu

Sleep Med Clin 7 (2012) 577–585
http://dx.doi.org/10.1016/j.jsmc.2012.08.004
1556-407X/12/$ – see front matter © 2012 Published by Elsevier Inc

Charles Dickens had described such individuals, including their excessive sleepiness, in his fictional work *The Pickwick Papers*. Over time, it was realized that sleep apnea also occurs in patients who are not morbidly obese, and in 1978 the book *Sleep Apnea Syndromes* was published.[14] Positive airway pressure therapy was developed by Sullivan and colleagues[15] and was found to be an effective treatment; commercially available devices became available in 1982.

A quite different sleep disorder associated with excessive sleepiness (ie, narcolepsy) had been described in the medical literature back in 1880 by Gelineau.[16] However, this disorder was also associated with cataplexy that was triggerable by emotion. Sleep paralysis and hallucinations during transition between sleep and waking were also features. The link between narcolepsy and REM sleep emerged in the 1960s, and in 1962 Bedrich Roth[17] penned the book *Narkolepsie und Hypersomnie*. The discovery of hypocretin as the genetic underpinning for this disorder was a landmark discovery.[18]

## Nosology

1979 marked the birth of the first "official" diagnostic classification of sleep and arousal disorders, which was published in the fledgling journal *Sleep*.[19] This nosology represented the most complete cataloging of sleep disorders and rapidly became the standard. The nosology was reorganized and expanded in 1990 under Michael Thorpy's chairmanship, and the International Classification of Sleep Disorders (ICSD) resulted.[20] The year before marked the publication of the first edition of *Principles and Practice of Sleep Medicine* (edited by Meir Kryger, Thomas Roth, and William C. Dement), which became the de facto textbook of the field.[21] The second edition of ICSD was published in 2005 and **Table 1** shows is basic configuration.[22]

## CROSSROADS

Sleep medicine, nearly 100 years now from its original conception, finds itself at an important crossroads. Sleep medicine is now recognized by the American Board of Medical Specialties (ABMS). In addition, the Accreditation Council for Graduate Medical Education (ACGME) accredits sleep medicine fellowship training programs. Thus, sleep medicine has unquestionably entered the mainstream of professional medicine. With this entrance, the forces and currents of the mainstream now control its destiny more than the ideas, wishes, and principles of its founders and proponents. Sleep medicine arose largely from

a laboratory science and its traditional orientation focused on research, methodology, diagnostics, classification, and epidemiology. As the field has matured, more attention has been paid to therapeutics, disease management, and outcome assessment. Public health and economics, 2 major currents of the mainstream, now enter the picture. Sleep medicine must adapt to economic demands and prove its worth in terms of improving health if it is to survive. Much work is needed with respect to sleep disorders and functional disabilities, disease burden, and positive outcomes produced by therapeutic interventions.

Leading the way in this endeavor are research projects providing evidence that sleep disorders (and in particular sleep-related breathing disorders) are associated with major medical problems. The link between sleep apnea and hypertension, heart disease, and cerebrovascular disease raised awareness that sleep disorders are important.[23,24] The icing on the cake will be when successful treatment of sleep disorders is proven to reverse or reduce the burden of these illnesses. Another area of progress has been clear links between motor vehicle accidents and excessive sleepiness (and sleep disorders that produce excessive sleepiness). The relationship between sleep problems and workplace productivity (and on-the-job accidents) has grabbed the attention of regulators, safety officers, and corporate managers. We have begun to see regulations targeting hours of service, sleep disorder screening, and sleep disorder therapeutic compliance, especially in the transportation industry. Rules are likely to become stricter, more specific, and more strongly enforced in the future. Thus, sleep clinicians will be at another crossroads, the one intersecting patient advocacy and regulatory restrictions. This position may be an uncomfortable one for many of us. Clinicians intrinsically devote themselves to patient care and reflexively advocate for their patients. We now find ourselves in a regulatory role in order to promote public safety. Furthermore, motor vehicle regulations are determined on a state-by-state basis, and reporting laws may conflict with federal Health Insurance Portability and Accountability Act (HIPAA) Privacy Rules.

## UNDERLYING DYSFUNCTION OF SLEEP GENERATOR, WAKE GENERATOR, AND COORDINATION OF SLEEP AND WAKE GENERATORS

Basic mechanisms coordinating and governing sleep and wakefulness include (1) homeostatic sleep drive, (2) circadian rhythms, and (3) autonomic nervous system balance.[25] Homeostatic

**Table 1**
**Sleep diagnostic categories according to the international classification of sleep disorders, 2nd edition**

I. INSOMNIA
1. Adjustment Insomnia
2. Psychophysiological Insomnia
3. Paradoxical Insomnia
4. Idiopathic Insomnia
5. Insomnia due to Mental Disorder
6. Inadequate Sleep Hygiene
7. Behavioral Insomnia of Childhood
8. Insomnia due to Drug or Substance
9. Insomnia due to Medical Condition
10. Insomnia Not Due to Substance or Known Physiological Condition, Unspecified (*Nonorganic Insomnia, NOS*)
11. Physiological (*Organic*) Insomnia, Unspecified

II. SLEEP RELATED BREATHING DISORDERS
A. Central Sleep Apnea Syndromes
1. Primary Central Sleep Apnea
2. Central Sleep Apnea Due to Cheyne Stokes Breathing Pattern
3. Central Sleep Apnea Due to High-Altitude Periodic Breathing
4. Central Sleep Apnea Due to Medical Condition Not Cheyne Stokes
5. Central Sleep Apnea Due to Drug or Substance
6. Primary Sleep Apnea of Infancy
B. Obstructive Sleep Apnea Syndrome
7. Obstructive Sleep Apnea, Adult
8. Obstructive Sleep Apnea, Pediatric
C. Sleep Related Hypoventilation/Hypoxemic Syndrome
9. Sleep Related Nonobstructive Alveolar Hypoventilation, Idiopathic
10. Congenital Central Alveolar Hypoventilation Syndrome
D. Sleep Related Hypoventilation/Hypoxemia Due to Medical Condition
11. Sleep Related Hypoventilation/Hypoxemia Due to Pulmonary Parenchymal or Vascular Pathology
12. Sleep Related Hypoventilation/Hypoxemia Due to Lower Airway Obstruction
13. Sleep Related Hypoventilation/Hypoxemia Due to Neuromuscular & Chest Wall Disorders
E. Other Sleep Related Breathing Disorder
14. Sleep Apnea/Sleep Related Breathing Disorder, Unspecified.

III. HYPERSOMNIA OF CENTRAL ORIGIN NOT DUE TO A CIRCADIAN RHYTHM SLEEP DISORDER, SLEEP RELATED BREATHING DISORDER, OR OTHER CAUSE OF DISTURBED NOCTURNAL SLEEP.
1. Narcolepsy With Cataplexy
2. Narcolepsy Without Cataplexy
3. Narcolepsy Due to Medical Condition
4. Narcolepsy, Unspecified
5. Recurrent Hypersomnia
15. Kleine-Levin Syndrome
16. Menstrual-Related Hypersomnia
6. Idiopathic Hypersomnia With Long Sleep Time
7. Idiopathic Hypersomnia Without Long Sleep Time
8. Behaviorally Induced Insufficient Sleep Syndrome
9. Hypersomnia Due to Medical Condition
10. Hypersomnia due to Drug or Substance
11. Hypersomnia Not Due to Substance or Known Physiological Condition (*Nonorganic Hypersomnia, NOS*)
12. Physiological (Organic) Hypersomnia, Unspecified (*Organic Hypersomnia, NOS*)

IV. CIRCADIAN RHYTHM SLEEP DISORDERS
1. Circadian Rhythm Sleep Disorder, Delayed Sleep Phase Type
2. Circadian Rhythm Sleep Disorder, Advanced Sleep Phase Type
3. Circadian Rhythm Sleep Disorder, Irregular Sleep-Wake Type
4. Circadian Rhythm Sleep Disorder, Free Running Type
5. Circadian Rhythm Sleep Disorder, Jet Lag Type (*Jet Lag Disorder*)
6. Circadian Rhythm Sleep Disorder, Shift Work Type (*Shift Work Disorder*)
7. Circadian Rhythm Sleep Disorder Due to Medical Condition
8. Other Circadian Rhythm Sleep Disorder
9. Other Circadian Rhythm Sleep Disorder Due to Drug or Substance

V. PARASOMNIAS
A. Disorders of Arousal (From NREM Sleep)
1. Confusional Arousals
2. Sleepwalking
3. Sleep Terrors
B. Parasomnias Usually Associated with REM Sleep
4. REM sleep behavior disorder (including parasomnia overlap disorder and status disociatus)
5. Recurrent Isolated Sleep Paralysis
6. Nightmare Disorder
C. Other Parasomnias
7. Sleep Related Dissociative Disorder
8. Sleep Enuresis
9. Sleep Related Groaning (Catathrenia)
10. Exploding Head Syndrome
11. Sleep Related Hallucinations
12. Sleep Related Eating Disorder
13. Parasomnia, Unspecified
14. Parasomnia Due to Drug or Substance
15. Parasomnia due to Medical Condition

VI. SLEEP RELATED MOVEMENT DISORDERS
1. Restless Legs Syndrome
2. Periodic Limb Movement Disorder
3. Sleep Related Leg Cramps
4. Sleep Related Bruxism
5. Sleep Related Rhythmic Movement
6. Sleep Related Movement Disorder, Unspecified
7. Sleep Related Movement Disorder Due to Drug of Substance.
8. Sleep Related Movement Disorder Due to Medical Condition

VII. ISOLATED SYMPTOMS, APPARENTLY NORMAL VARIANTS, AND UNRESOLVED ISSUES.
1. Long Sleeper
2. Short Sleeper
3. Snoring
4. Sleep Talking
5. Sleep Starts (*Hypnic Jerk*)
6. Benign Sleep Myoclonus of Infancy
7. Hypnagogic Foot Tremor and Alternating Leg Muscle Activation during sleep.
8. Propriospinal Cyclones at Sleep Onset
9. Excessive Fragmentary Myoclonus

VIII. OTHER SLEEP DISORDERS
1. Other physiological (Organic) Sleep Disorders
2. Other Sleep disorder Not Due to Substance or Known Physiological Conditions.
3. Environmental Sleep Disorder

regulation of sleepiness parallels that for thirst, hunger, and sex. Sleepiness increases as a function of the duration of prior wakefulness. Homeostatic process is thought to be mediated hypothalamically. The hypnotoxin theory represents an early mechanistic approach to explaining sleep homeostasis. An alternative theory, one in which neurotransmitters are depleted during wakefulness and must be replenished by sleep, has also been proposed. Of course, both are correct at some level. However, homeostasis is inadequate to explain our sleep-wake behaviors. Most individuals reach peak alertness in the late evening, just before they become sleepy. Why someone would reach peak alertness at 8 PM after being awake all day contradicts the homeostatic prediction. Thus another factor must be involved to regulate the sleep-wake cycle, and this is the circadian rhythm. As previously mentioned, the sleep-wake circadian rhythm is regulated by the suprachiasmatic nucleus and it provides a wakefulness stimulus to offset accumulating homeostatic drive for sleep. When SCN activation declines, homeostatic drive asserts itself and the individual becomes very sleepy. Autonomic activation provides a mechanism to override the usual dynamics of the sleep-wake process. Increasing sympathetic activation can reduce sleepiness, at least temporarily. Thus, noradrenergic (and dopaminergic) responses to emergency situations protect the individual from being at the mercy of their sleep-wake cycle; it allows wakefulness to supersede sleep for a period of time so that life-threatening situations can sometimes be averted.

## NORMAL SLEEP

Because sleep is conceptualized as something done by the brain, the traditional measurement approach involves recording electroencephalographic (EEG) activity. An assortment of fairly unique EEG events occur during sleep (**Fig. 1**), and these can be used to classify sleep into stages. Electrooculographic (EOG) and electromyographic (EMG) activity were added to further differentiate specific sleep categories and characterize their features. Systems for sleep staging were developed to summarize sleep patterns in an attempt to find commonalities between individuals and to characterize a normal sleep pattern. An assortment of early sleep stage systems finally gave way to establishment of the standardized manual in 1968.[26] This scoring system remained the standard for 39 years, ultimately being updated by the American Academy of Sleep Medicine Manual for the Scoring of Sleep and Associated Events (2007).[27]

EEG activity recorded from central, occipital, and frontal derivations, EOG activity from the right and left eyes' outer canthi, and EMG recorded from the submentalis are summarized for each 30 seconds of recording (or epoch). Sleep stage scoring involves dividing the recording into epochs and classifying each as W (wake) or sleep stage N1, N2, N3, and R (REM). Stages 1, 2, or 3 are collectively referred to as non-REM (NREM) sleep.[28] EEG, EOG, and EMG characteristics vary for wakefulness and the different sleep stages. N1 is characterized by low-voltage mixed-frequency EEG without K-complexes, spindles, or rapid eye movements, and less than 15 seconds of alpha EEG activity. Vertex sharp waves may be present. N2 sleep is characterized by sleep spindles or K-complexes but less than 5 seconds of high-amplitude delta EEG activity (slow waves) per epoch. N3 sleep is scored if more than 5 seconds of slow-wave activity occurs. REM sleep is characterized by low-voltage mixed-frequency EEG activity (but devoid of spindles or K-complexes) accompanied by rapid eye movements and nearly absent submentalis EMG activity.

A healthy young adult will sleep 85% to 95% of their time in bed. Sleep onset should occur within 15 to 20 minutes after retiring, and nocturnal awakenings should be brief. N2 sleep typically occupies approximately half the night's sleep, with N3 accounting for 10% to 20%, N1 for 1% to 5%, and REM sleep for 20% to 25%. Inconsequential differences in stage distributions are found between young adult men and women, but these can increase with advancing age. NREM and REM repeat in 90- to 120-minute long cycles and **Fig. 2** shows a typical night for a healthy young adult. Sleep architecture can be generalized as beginning with NREM sleep, having slow-wave activity predominate in the first third of the night, having REM sleep predominate in the latter half of the night, and containing 4 to 6 individual REM sleep episodes that successively lengthen during the sleep period.[29]

## PRESENTATIONS: INSOMNIA, HYPERSOMNIA, AND PARASOMNIA

Patients with sleep disorders often present with multiple nighttime symptoms and related daytime consequences. The main categories of presenting complaints include insomnia, excessive sleepiness, and unusual or unwanted behaviors occurring during sleep or arising from sleep (parasomnias). Insomnia in adults may include: difficulty falling sleep, difficulty maintaining sleep, and/or early morning awakening. By contrast, in pediatrics the insomnia may present as bedtime

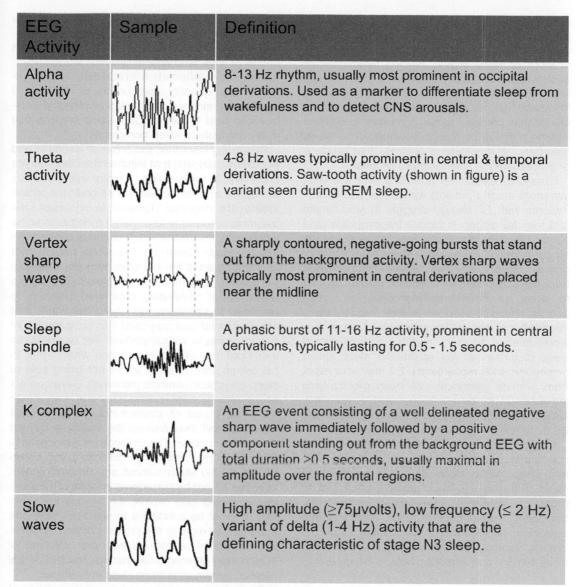

| EEG Activity | Sample | Definition |
|---|---|---|
| Alpha activity | | 8-13 Hz rhythm, usually most prominent in occipital derivations. Used as a marker to differentiate sleep from wakefulness and to detect CNS arousals. |
| Theta activity | | 4-8 Hz waves typically prominent in central & temporal derivations. Saw-tooth activity (shown in figure) is a variant seen during REM sleep. |
| Vertex sharp waves | | A sharply contoured, negative-going bursts that stand out from the background activity. Vertex sharp waves typically most prominent in central derivations placed near the midline |
| Sleep spindle | | A phasic burst of 11-16 Hz activity, prominent in central derivations, typically lasting for 0.5 - 1.5 seconds. |
| K complex | | An EEG event consisting of a well delineated negative sharp wave immediately followed by a positive component standing out from the background EEG with total duration >0.5 seconds, usually maximal in amplitude over the frontal regions. |
| Slow waves | | High amplitude (≥75µvolts), low frequency (≤ 2 Hz) variant of delta (1-4 Hz) activity that are the defining characteristic of stage N3 sleep. |

**Fig. 1.** EEG waveforms characterizing sleep and wakefulness.

resistance and/or inability to sleep independently. According to the latest classification of sleep disorders, diagnosis of insomnia should be considered if the aforementioned complaints are associated with daytime consequences, including: daytime sleepiness, fatigue, or malaise; impaired attention, concentration, or memory; social or vocational dysfunction or poor school

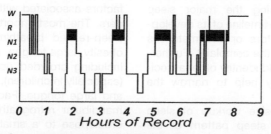

**Fig. 2.** Sleep Stage Histogram for a Normal, Young Adult Subject.

performance; mood disturbance or irritability; daytime sleepiness; motivation, energy, or initiative reduction; proneness for errors or accidents at work or while driving; tension headaches or gastrointestinal symptoms in response to sleep loss; and concerns or worries about sleep. Insomnia may be primary, but usually there are identifiable causes. Other comorbid conditions include medical or mental illnesses, other sleep disorders, or medications or drugs that produce or perpetuate the sleeplessness problem.

Excessive sleepiness (ES) is a very common symptom among patients with sleep disorders.[30] Patients with ES usually struggle to stay awake and may fall asleep in various inappropriate (and sometimes dangerous) situations (eg, while driving an automobile). ES naturally arises from acute or chronic sleep deprivation. Sleepiness can result from not scheduling an adequate amount of time for sleep, a mismatch between circadian rhythm and the timing of sleep (eg, jet lag), frequent sleep interruptions due to environmental factors (eg, environmental noise), and/or disease-related sleep disturbances (eg, obstructive sleep apnea or periodic limb movements). ES may also result from primary dysfunction of sleep mechanisms (eg, brain injury or neurodegenerative diseases). Finally, in some cases the specific cause of the ES is not clear (eg, idiopathic hypersomnia).

Parasomnias are undesirable behaviors, physical events, or experiences that occur during entry into sleep, within sleep, or during arousal from sleep. Parasomnias encompass a wide assortment of abnormal sleep-related movements, behaviors, emotions, perceptions, dreaming, and autonomic nervous system functioning. Examples include nightmares, sleep walking, sleep bruxism, sleep terrors, and exploding head syndrome.

## DIAGNOSTIC WORKUP

As with any illness, initial workup of sleep disorders relies heavily on eliciting a detailed history and performing a comprehensive physical examination (where indicated). One differentiating point in the workup of sleep disorders is the importance of interviewing the bed partner. A detailed history focuses on first identifying the major sleep complaint, establishing the timeline of its development, and identifying factors or circumstances that aggravate or improve the complaint. Furthermore, the interviewer should identify other associated symptoms that may help to narrow the differential diagnoses.

As part of comprehensive workup of sleep complaints, the detailed sleep pattern of the patient should be explored. The bedtime and wake time during weekdays and weekends, the subject's latency to fall asleep, number and duration of naps, effect of naps (refreshing or not), and details of work (and specifically shift work) constitute important information. In addition, use of stimulants (eg, quantity and timing of caffeinated beverages), alcohol, and timing of physical exercise can help to identify poor sleep hygiene that may contribute to sleep complaints.

Regarding insomnia, the onset of insomnia and the circumstance(s) that initiated the insomnia are important. In many cases, a major event such as the loss of a job or the death of a significant person initiates the insomnia. However, in most cases the insomnia resolves in less than 3 months. In some individuals, the insomnia will continue beyond this initial period. Identifying the sleep pattern, not only during adult life but also from the time that the patient may remember, will help to identify the tendency for developing prolonged insomnia in response to stressors. Identifying the habits that are developed and may feed into prolongation of this insomnia is very important. For example, an individual may start feeling tense when trying to fall asleep and ruminate about not being able to sleep (psychophysiologic insomnia). Development of psychophysiologic insomnia can perpetuate the initial phase of stressor-induced adjustment insomnia, and thus prolong the insomnia beyond the initial 3 months. The consequence of insomnia also should be explored, as difficulty falling asleep or maintaining sleep without any daytime consequences will not be considered insomnia. The interviewer should also explore the various behaviors that may not be conducive to sleep, as these are important as regards the proper initiation of sleep. Such behaviors can include reading or watching TV in bed or any other activities that may result in central nervous system stimulation close to bedtime.

Regarding parasomnias, detailed description of the events will be helpful in narrowing down the differential diagnosis. NREM parasomnias mostly happen at the earlier stages of sleep and closer to sleep onset. By contrast, REM-related parasomnias often occur late in the night when REM periods increase in duration and intensity.

Physical examination may help to identify factors associated with some of the sleep disorders. The most important findings are related to sleep-related breathing disorders, and include obesity, large tongue, upper airway abnormalities including crowded upper airways, large tonsils (especially in children), long uvula and soft palate, and large tongue. Facial abnormalities including mandibular retrognathia and micrognathia may predispose to a small airway and increase the risk of obstructive sleep apnea. Features of endocrine disorders such as hypothyroidism and acromegaly may be seen in some patients with obstructive sleep apnea. However, lack of the aforementioned findings does not rule out clinically significant obstructive sleep apnea.

## DIFFERENTIAL DIAGNOSIS

Differential diagnosis for insomnia includes disorders of circadian rhythm disturbances, conditions that cause sleep disruption such as restless leg syndrome, a variety of chronic medical conditions that may interrupt sleep (eg, chronic obstructive pulmonary disease and congestive heart failure), and environmental factors that may disturb sleep (eg, noise, high temperature, light, or even a bed partner that snores). Use of medications, stimulants (eg, caffeinated beverages), alcohol, and recreational drugs may also cause insomnia. Psychiatric conditions (eg, mood disorders and posttraumatic stress disorder) are commonly associated with insomnia. Many comorbid forms of insomnia may result in a maladaptive behavior presenting as psychophysiological insomnia. Unfortunately, insomnia sometimes has no identifiable causal or exacerbating factors (ie, idiopathic insomnia).

Differential diagnosis of excessive daytime sleepiness revolves around the adequacy and integrity of sleep. Disorders that result in sleep interruptions often present as ES. The interrupting factors can be environmental (eg, noise), respiratory events and snoring, leg movement, chest pain or dyspnea, waking up for frequent urination, or waking up because of reflux. The second category of causal factors for excessive daytime sleepiness is inadequate sleep time, which includes various forms of insomnia including circadian rhythm disorders and insufficient sleep because of lifestyle or work load. The third category of disorders presenting with ES includes disease patients who sleep for an adequate amount of time but remain sleepy. These conditions include disorders such as organic hypersomnia, including stroke. Use of recreational drugs also may also produce hypersomnia.

The differential diagnosis for parasomnias mainly includes NREM and REM parasomnias. Common parasomnias include nocturia, bruxism, and leg cramps. Some parasomnias are secondary to sleep-related breathing disorders while others can be drug induced. The major differential diagnosis for parasomnias involving prominent sleep-related behaviors (especially if injurious) is epilepsy. A detailed history and an extensive nocturnal EEG recording may help to differentiate seizure from other parasomnias.

## ASSESSMENT
### In the Office

Various diagnostic tests can help to narrow the differential diagnoses or confirm the diagnosis. Use of history and a focused physical examination should guide selection of subsequent diagnostic testing. Questionnaires and psychometric instruments can also provide valuable information. A good starting point is to determine the patient's sleep-wake schedule, especially if the chief complaint is insomnia or ES. Self-reported bedtimes and rising times (both on weekdays and weekends), possibly augmented by a sleep diary, can provide invaluable data. In a typical sleep diary, a patient not only tracks retiring and waking times, but also document how long it takes to fall asleep, how many hours thought to be slept, how many awakenings occurred, overall sleep quality (refreshingness), the use of stimulants (eg, caffeinated beverages), use and timing of medications (that may affect sleep), naps, and exercise times and frequency. The sleep diary will help obtain an overall picture of a patient's sleep-wake cycle and identify possible factors that may negatively affect sleep duration and quality. These self-reported data can be validated using objective measures obtained with actigraphy (see section on home testing). It is also standard procedure to administer a sleepiness questionnaire (eg, the Epworth Sleepiness Scale), a mood-screening instrument (eg, Zung Depression Scale or Beck Depression Inventory), possibly an anxiety scale, and some sort of generalized questionnaire on sleep problems. Because so many patients are referred for assessment of possible sleep-related breathing disorders, indexing the symptoms of sleep-disordered breathing and estimating severity with a validated instrument is strongly recommended (eg, the STOP-BANG questionnaire, Berlin Questionnaire, or Multivariable Apnea Prediction Scale).

Blood, urine, and other fluids drawn to further investigate possible sleep and fatigue issues also provide ancillary diagnostic information. Clinical laboratory testing for ferritin levels (for patients with possible RLS), thyroid function tests for patients with fatigue, urinalysis for drug screening, and HLA typing represent some of the analyses ordered at the sleep center.

### In the Laboratory

Attended laboratory sleep studies (also called polysomnography) are commonly used to diagnose sleep-related breathing disorders and to determine therapeutic positive airway pressure needed to eliminate breathing pathophysiologies.[31] Laboratory polysomnography, synchronized with video recording, is also indicated to diagnose other sleep disorders and to differentiate parasomnias from sleep-related seizure.[32,33] The Multiple Sleep Latency Test (MSLT) is a procedure primarily used to confirm narcolepsy. In addition, it provides objective documentation of sleepiness. MSLT provides 4 or 5 nap opportunities, scheduled at 2-hour intervals throughout the day, beginning approximately 2 hours after rising from a prior night's laboratory sleep study. During each test session, polysomnographic parameters are recorded while the patient attempts to relax and not resist falling asleep. Maintenance of Wakefulness Testing (MWT) also provides patients with test sessions scheduled at 2-hour intervals; however, the patient is instructed to resist falling asleep. The success, partial success, or failure at remaining awake provides objective measures of the patient's ability to overcome drowsiness in a nonstimulating environment. Four 40-minute test sessions are recorded while EEG, EOG, and submentalis EMG parameters are recorded. The Suggested Immobilization Test (SIT) is used for the diagnosis of RLS. During a SIT procedure, the patient semi-reclines in bed with legs outstretched and eyes open for 60 minutes before bedtime. The patient is instructed not to move but to remain awake. Polysomnographic recordings, including leg EMG derivations, are made concurrently to determine whether abnormal muscle activity and/or irresistible movements occur.

### Home Testing

As previously mentioned, actigraphy can be used to augment sleep diaries. A wristwatch-like device records movement using accelerometers.[31] Data are stored in memory for several days or weeks. Actigraphs commonly also monitor light levels using a photosensor. Information about a patient's sleep schedule, rest-activity cycle, and circadian patterns can be deduced from data collected.

Home sleep testing (HST) includes measures used principally to confirm sleep-disordered breathing in symptomatic patients.[34] Cardiopulmonary recorders with oximetry represent the most common configuration. HST is a confirmation technique only; it does not rule out sleep-related breathing disorders because it is prone to artifact and is less sensitive than laboratory polysomnography. Nonetheless, in patients with severe sleep apnea, HST clearly documents the pathophysiology, and treatment can thus proceed.

### SLEEP'S PRESUMED FUNCTIONS IN RELATION TO NEUROREHABILITATION AND RELEVANT SLEEP DISORDERS

In Macbeth, Shakespeare muses on "Sleep that knits up the ravelled sleeve of care, the death of each day's life, sore labor's bath, balm of hurt minds, great nature's second course, chief nourisher in life's feast."[35] Although scientific disagreements invariably arise when colleagues discuss the "function of sleep," all generally agree with Shakespeare that sleep is essentially a restorative process. The healing power of sleep and its necessity to rejuvenate or recharge us after a long day's activity seems incontrovertible. Research focused on the underlying biology finds sleep critical for both somatic and psychological restoration as well as being responsive to changing demands placed on the body and mind.

Sleep-related breathing disorders are especially relevant to rehabilitation. The sleep disturbances provoked by frequent awakening adversely affects all aspects of health.[23] Increased blood pressure, autonomic dysregulation, possible insulin resistance, neuroendocrine imbalances, cardiac afterload, and cerebrovascular insult can all result from sleep apnea. Some sleep disorders are also associated with alterations in cytokines and inflammatory markers. Furthermore, consequent hypoxemia (especially in patients with comorbid lung disease) compromises the individual further by precipitating cardiac arrhythmia and lowering seizure threshold. A wide assortment of conditions increases the risk for sleep-disordered breathing, especially spinal injury and neurodegenerative disorders. Neurodegenerative disorders also increase the risk for RLS and the parasomnia REM sleep behavior disorder (which can also be prodromal for Parkinson disease).[36]

Sleep can also provide prognostic indications. Patients with cerebrovascular infarcts in whom sleep spindles do not return after several days usually have a poor outcome. By contrast, overall improvement in sleep quality usually signals good recovery. Sudden adverse changes in sleep and sleep-related phenomena are seldom good omens. If a patient suddenly begins to have vivid dreams, this usually indicates that a sleep disturbance is awakening them from REM sleep (if one does not awaken, dreams are not remembered).[37] The disturbance can arise from a failure of the dream process to defuse dream anxieties (possibly from being overwhelmed) or simply from an awakening caused by a breathing disorder (that often adversely affects REM more than NREM sleep). Sleep can be a sensitive marker because it is fragile, but also because it is resilient. In a sense, sleep serves as a bellwether of overall health.

### REFERENCES

1. Pieron H. Le probleme physiologique du sommeil. Paris: Masson; 1913.
2. Berger H. Ueber das elektroenkephalogramm des menschen. J Psychol Neurol 1930;40:160–79.

3. Economo V. Encephalitis lethargica: its sequelae and treatment. London (England): Oxford University Press; 1931.

4. Loomis AL, Harvey N, Hobart GA. Cerebral states during sleep, as studied by human brain potentials. J Exp Psychol 1937;21:127–44.

5. Aserinsky E, Kleitman N. Regularly occurring periods of eye motility, and concomitant phenomena. Science 1953;118:273–4.

6. Freud S. The interpretation of dreams. New York: Avon; 1980.

7. de Mairan JJ. Observation botanique. Histoire de L'academie Royale des Sciences. 1729:35–6.

8. Biinning E. Die physiologische Uhr. Berlin-Göttingen-Heidelberg: Springer; 1963.

9. Moore RY, Eichler VB. Loss of a circadian adrenal corticosterone rhythm following suprachiasmatic lesions in the rat. Brain Res 1972;42:201–6.

10. Ekbom KA. Preface. Acta Med Scand 1945;121:7–8.

11. Coccagna G, Vetrugno R, Lombardi C, et al. Restless legs syndrome: an historical note. Sleep Med 2004;5:279–83.

12. Walters AS, Hickey K, Maltzman J, et al. A questionnaire study of 138 patients with restless legs syndrome: the 'Night-Walkers' survey. Neurology 1996;46(1):92–5.

13. Gastaut H, Tassinari CA, Duron B. Polygraphic study of the episodic diurnal and nocturnal (hypnic and respiratory) manifestations of the Pickwickian syndrome. Brain Res 1965;2:167–86.

14. Guilleminault C, Dement WC, editors. Sleep apnea syndromes. New York: Alan R Liss, Inc; 1978.

15. Sullivan CE, Issa FG, Berthon-Jones M, et al. Reversal of obstructive sleep apnoea by continuous positive airway pressure applied through the nares. Lancet 1981;1(8225):862–5.

16. Gelineau GB. De la narcolepsie. Lancette Fr 1880; 53:626–8.

17. Roth B. Narcolepsy and hypersomnia. Basel (Switzerland): Karger; 1980.

18. Nishino S, Ripley B, Overeem S, et al. Hypocretin (orexin) deficiency in human narcolepsy. Lancet 2000;355(9197):39–40.

19. Association of Sleep Disorders Centers. Diagnostic classification of sleep and arousal disorders, 1st edition. Prepared by the Sleep Disorders Classification Committee, H. P. Roffwarg, Chairman. Sleep 1979;2:1–137.

20. ICSD. The International Classification of Sleep Disorders: diagnostic and coding manual. Diagnostic Classification Steering Committee, Thorpy, M. J., chairman. Rochester (MN): American Sleep Disorders Association; 1990.

21. Kryger MH, Roth T, Dement WC, editors. Principles and practice of sleep medicine. Philadelphia: WB Saunders; 1989.

22. American Academy of Sleep Medicine. International Classification of Sleep Disorders: diagnostic and coding manual. 2nd edition. Westchester (IL): American Academy of Sleep Medicine; 2005.

23. Hirshkowitz M. The clinical consequences of obstructive sleep apnea and associated excessive sleepiness. J Fam Pract 2008;57(Suppl 8):S9–16.

24. Yaggi HK, Concato J, Kernan WN, et al. Obstructive sleep apnea as a risk factor for stroke and death. N Engl J Med 2005;353:2034–41.

25. Hirshkowitz M, Moore CA, Minhoto G. The basics of sleep. In: Pressman MR, Orr WC, editors. Understanding sleep: the evaluation and treatment of sleep disorders. Washington, DC: American Psychological Association; 1997. p. 11–34.

26. Rechtschaffen A, Kales A. A manual of standardized, techniques and scoring system for sleep stages in human subjects. NIH Publication No. 204. Washington DC: US Government Printing Office; 1968.

27. Iber C, Ancoli-Israel S, Chesson A, et al. The AASM manual for the scoring of sleep and associated events: rules, terminology and technical specifications. 1st edition. Westchester (IL): American Academy of Sleep Medicine; 2007.

28. Hirshkowitz M, Sharafkhaneh A. Clinical polysomnography and the evolution of recording and scoring technique. In: Chokroverty S, editor. Sleep disorders medicine. 3rd edition. Philadelphia: Saunders Elsevier; 2009. p. 229–52.

29. Hirshkowitz M. Normal human sleep: an overview. Med Clin N Am 2004;88:551–65.

30. Hirshkowitz M. Description of hypersomnias. In: Kushida C, (editor). Sleep disorders; 2012, (in press).

31. Hirshkowitz M. Introduction to sleep medicine diagnostics in adults. In: Barkoukis TJ, Matheson JK, Ferber R, et al, editors. Therapy in sleep medicine. Philadelphia: Elsevier; 2012. p. 28–40.

32. Mahowald MW, Cramer-Bornemann MA. NREM sleep parasomnias. In: Kryger MH, Roth T, Dement WC, editors. Principles and practice of sleep medicine. Philadelphia: Elsevier/Saunders; 2005. p. 889–96.

33. Standards of Practice Committee of the American Academy of Sleep Medicine. Practice parameters for the indications for polysomnography and related procedures: an update for 2005. Sleep 2005;28: 499–521.

34. Hirshkowitz M, Sharafkhaneh A. Comparison of portable monitoring with laboratory polysomnography for diagnosing sleep-related breathing disorders: scoring and interpretation. Sleep Med Clin 2011;6:283–92.

35. Shakespeare W. The tragedy of Macbeth. In: Eliot CW, editor. The Harvard classics. New York: PF Collier and Son; 1909-14.

36. Schenck CH, Bundlie SR, Mahowald MW. Delayed emergence of a parkinsonian disorder in 38% of 29 older men initially diagnosed with idiopathic rapid eye movement sleep behaviour disorder. Neurology 1996;46:388–93.

37. Hirshkowitz M, Gokcebay N. Theories concerning the function of REM sleep and the meaning of dreams. Dir Psychiatry 1992;6:1–7.

# Sleep Disorders in Neurorehabilitation: Insomnia

Eric B. Larson, PhD, ABPP

## KEYWORDS

- Sleep initiation and maintenance disorders • Neurologic disorder • Assessment • Treatment
- Rehabilitation

## KEY POINTS

- Insomnia is a disorder that is defined by subjective complaint concerning the duration and quality of sleep.
- Elevated prevalence of insomnia has been described in traumatic brain injury, stroke, Parkinson disease, spinal cord injury, and neuromuscular disease.
- Psychotherapy is an effective treatment of insomnia, although neurocognitive factors often interfere with participation.

## INTRODUCTION

Definitions of insomnia are provided in the International Classification of Sleep Disorders 2nd Edition (ICSD-2),[1] the Diagnostic and Statistical Manual of Psychiatric Disorders 4th Edition (DSM-IV),[2] and the International Classification of Diseases 10th Edition (ICD-10).[3] All definitions rely at least partly on self-report of subjective complaints of either unsatisfactory quantity or unsatisfactory quality of sleep. In the ICSD-2, diagnostic criteria are organized into 3 broad categories: (1) complaint of difficulty in initiating or maintaining sleep or waking up early morning or nonrestorative sleep; (2) these difficulties occur despite adequate opportunity for sleep; and (3) complaint of any 1 of 9 different forms of daytime impairment that are believed to be related to the sleep difficulty, ranging from somatic symptoms (eg, headaches and gastrointestinal distress) to functional impairment (eg, problems at school or work). Similarly, the DSM-IV specifies 2 criteria that also largely rely on self-report: (1) complaint of initiating or maintaining sleep or nonrestorative sleep and (2) consequent clinically significant distress or functional impairment

(**Box 1**). Last, the ICD-10 criteria specify (1) complaint of difficulty falling asleep or maintaining sleep or poor sleep quality, (2) occurrence at least 3 times a week for 1 month, (3) preoccupation or excessive concern about these problems and resulting impairment, and (4) sleep problems resulting in marked distress or interfering with activities of daily living. Unlike the above clinical definitions, research often specifies quantitative criteria including sleep onset latency of at least 30 minutes, wake time after sleep onset (WASO) of at least 30 minutes, or sleep efficiency of less than 85%.[4] As addressed later in the discussion of objective assessment technologies, such observable, quantitative criteria become particularly important in studies of neurologic populations who may not be able to communicate subjective complaints or who have limited awareness of their symptoms.

## EFFECT ON TREATMENT OUTCOME

In neurologically intact individuals, reduced sleep is associated with numerous health problems, including hypertension,[5] decreased ventilatory drive,[6] increased sympathetic cardiovascular activation,[7]

Supported by the US Department of Education, National Institute on Disability and Rehabilitation Research, Grant #HI33N060014 through the Midwest Regional Traumatic Brain Injury Model System: Innovative Approaches to Improve Cognition, Function, and Community Living.
Department of Physical Medicine and Rehabilitation, Rehabilitation Institute of Chicago, Feinberg School of Medicine, Northwestern University, 345 East Superior Street, Chicago, IL 60611, USA
E-mail address: elarson@ric.org

and possibly diabetes mellitus and obesity.[8] In patients with depression, insomnia contributes to lower self-ratings on health-related quality of life.[9] Studies of general medical populations have shown that insomnia increases the risk of psychiatric symptoms and delirium.[10] In a study of older patients at a skilled-care geriatric hospital in Japan, presence of insomnia was associated with increased risk of mortality at a 2-year follow-up.[11] Across many diagnostic groups, insomnia increases risk for injury (eg, sustained in falls) and increases burden on caregivers.

## ETIOLOGY

Insomnia can be a direct result of disturbances of neurochemical systems and cerebral structures that regulate wakefulness and sleep.[12,13] Although reduced wakefulness can result from dysregulation of acetylcholine, histamine, norepinephrine, serotonin, dopamine, and orexin, reduced sleep is associated with changes in GABA, adenosine, and melatonin. Sleep disturbance is also a direct consequence of injury or illness that results in lesions to the brain stem, thalamus, or anterior basal regions such as the suprachiasmatic nucleus.

Neurologic injury and illness also contributes to sleep disturbance through indirect mechanisms such as pain or emotional distress. Pain causes frequent periods of "alpha-delta sleep," which is the intrusion of "wake" alpha waves (8–13 Hz) into the electroencephalography (EEG) of nonrapid eye movement sleep, especially the deep sleep that is characterized by slow delta waves (0.5–2 Hz). This intrusion contributes to a subjective perception of poor sleep quality.[14] Prolonged hospitalization and adjustment to new disabilities can also contribute to insomnia, especially in the inpatient setting where, "patients may experience heightened emotional or cognitive activity at bedtime because they can be tense, may worry or ruminate: factors which are all linked to difficulty falling asleep."[4]

## NEUROLOGIC DISORDERS AND INSOMNIA

Insomnia is frequently observed in neurologic disorders including traumatic brain injury (TBI), stroke, Parkinson disease (PD), spinal cord injury (SCI), and neuromuscular disorders.[4,12,15]

### Traumatic Brain Injury

#### Epidemiology
After reviewing 21 studies of insomnia in TBI totaling 2816 subjects across all levels of severity, it was estimated that 40% of patients experience symptoms of insomnia.[16] This percentage is higher than the prevalence in the general population and in nonneurologic rehabilitation patients.[17] Those with less severe TBI appear to have a higher prevalence of insomnia.[18] It may be that those with severe TBI are unaware of their insomnia and therefore they may underreport it.

#### Associated factors/mechanism
Polysomnography showed that compared with neurologically intact controls, TBI patients experienced more awakenings, but the groups did not differ on sleep onset latency, sleep efficiency, or arousal index.[19] Although this study showed a strong concordance between self-report and objective awakenings, other researchers have demonstrated that self-report in this population may be inaccurate compared with objectively measured sleep latency, sleep efficiency, and WASO.[20]

Zeitzer and colleagues[16] proposed a model in which traumatic injury contributes first to a predisposition to insomnia through both structural changes and altered biochemistry in the brain. In their model, disruption of hypocretin-1, dopamine, and serotonin levels appear to elevate the predisposition to insomnia, especially in moderate to severe injuries. These investigators suggest that the insomnia symptoms may increase further in the presence of psychiatric comorbidities, the second trauma-related factor, including depression, pain, and anxiety, although they point out that there are no studies that specifically address the effect of psychiatric disorders on insomnia in TBI patients. However, indirect support is found for this hypothesis. TBI patients who sustained their injury in an assault have a higher prevalence of insomnia than those who sustained their injury in an accident, suggesting the additional emotional trauma resulting from assault contributes to sleep disturbance.[19]

Another 2-factor model of sleep dysregulation was proposed in which initially, direct physical damage and secondarily, neuropathologic events cause disruption of cerebral function, which contributes to sleep problems.[21] This model further proposes that later in recovery, behavioral and affective factors exert a stronger influence on sleep. Such multifactorial models provide a rationale for treatment that includes both pharmaceutical and behavioral interventions.

### Effect on outcome

Mahmood and colleagues[22] found that in TBI patients, poor performance on measures of cognitive functioning was associated with sleep disturbance, after controlling for sex and injury severity. It was also reported that sleep efficiency is correlated with orientation and predicted emergence from posttraumatic amnesia.[23] In a sample of TBI patients, a group with poor sleep had greater deficits on a sustained attention task than a group with good sleep.[24] In addition to cognitive impairment, behavior problems also have been associated with reduced sleep. When compared with other acute inpatient rehabilitation populations, TBI patients with sleep disturbance experienced an increased frequency of problems, including disruption of morning orientation, therapy sessions, meals, and community activities.[25] Insomnia was also associated with elevated depression and anxiety in TBI patients.[26]

## Stroke

### Epidemiology

Prevalence of insomnia symptoms in stroke patients has been estimated to be about 68%.[27] Using the DSM-IV definition, 37.5% of stroke patients meet diagnostic criteria for insomnia.[28]

### Associated factors/mechanism

The relationship between stroke and insomnia is complex in that sleep disturbance is both a risk factor and a consequence of cerebrovascular disease. Obstructive sleep apnea may precede stroke and place patients at elevated risk for stroke.[29] Although 56.7% of stroke patients complain of insomnia symptoms, 38.6% of patients report their insomnia predated their stroke, and 18.1% report that it was caused by their stroke.[28]

Examination of sleep EEG in stroke patients showed that compared with healthy controls, these patients had greater WASO and lower sleep efficiency.[30] Amount of slow wave sleep and stroke volume were correlated: size of stroke on digital imaging was associated with more time in slow wave sleep.

### Effect on outcome

The amount of slow wave sleep is associated with poorer outcome as measured by The Modified Rankin Scale score at discharge.[30] Amount of slow wave sleep is also associated with attention during the acute phase, but it is sleep efficiency that has the strongest association with attention later in recovery.[31] The investigators also reported that both slow wave and rapid eye movement (REM) sleep were associated with memory later in recovery.

However, others do not report a clear association between sleep and outcome in stroke. In a moderately large sample of patients with paramedian thalamic stroke, sleep architecture was not associated with cognitive function.[32] In a small, nonrandomized clinical trial of hypnotic medication, a group of stroke patients with insomnia did not exhibit greater functional impairment or depression than stroke patients without insomnia.[33] At baseline, the insomnia group also did not exhibit more impairment on the Mini-Mental State Examination or several other cognitive measures, although they did exhibit greater deficits on more demanding tasks such as an auditory continuous performance test and a backward digit span subtest. The investigators argued that after completing a course of treatment with sedative hypnotic medication, the stroke patients with insomnia achieved cognitive and functional outcomes that were equivalent to the stroke patients without insomnia.

## Parkinson Disease

### Epidemiology

About two-third of patients with PD have sleep initiation insomnia and as many as 90% of those patients also have sleep maintenance insomnia associated with frequent awakenings.[34,35] A large prospective population-based study showed that 54% to 60% of patients with PD had insomnia over a 3-year period.[36] About one-third of PD patients described their sleep disturbance as moderate to severe.[37]

### Associated factors/mechanism

Insomnia in PD has been associated with both the disease itself and side effects from medication. The cardinal motor symptoms of movement disorders such as tremors, dystonia, and rigidity appear during sleep, resulting in awakening.[38,39] Sleep disturbance results from pathology of the serotonergic neurons of the dorsal raphe nucleus, noradrenergic neurons of the locus coeruleus, and cholinergic neurons of the pedunculopontine nucleus.[40] High-dose dopaminergic agonists can result in hallucinations, nightmares, and increased arousal, whereas side effects of levodopa can include increased sleep latency.[41]

## Spinal Cord Injury and Neuromuscular Disorders

### Epidemiology

In a comparison with TBI patients, 72% of patients with SCI reported poor sleep quality and 56% indicated they suffered from insomnia on a self-report measure.[18] Sleep disturbance also has an elevated prevalence in amyotrophic lateral sclerosis and myotonic dystrophy.[42]

### Associated factors/mechanism

Cervical SCI has been reported to have poorer sleep efficiency than thoracic SCI, the latter of which was comparable to healthy controls.[43] It is suggested that insomnia in SCI patients can be at least partly explained by decreased secretion of melatonin during the night. Another factor that appears to contribute to insomnia in this population is sleep-disordered breathing, which is particularly prevalent in SCI patients with tetraplegia, increased neck circumference, and who are taking cardiac medications or who have lived with their injuries for longer duration.[44]

In amyotrophic lateral sclerosis also, insomnia can result from sleep-related respiratory disturbance[45]; this is particularly problematic when neuromuscular pathology results in disturbed diaphragmatic ventilation and increased reliance on intercostal muscles, the latter of which are affected by REM sleep atonia.[46] In this population, sleep maintenance insomnia and frequent nighttime awakenings secondary to sleep-disordered breathing may respond well to continuous positive airway pressure or bilevel positive airway pressure.[47]

## ASSESSMENT

Objective technology for assessment includes polysomnography and actigraphy. Paper and pencil measures include self-report instruments, clinical rating scales, sleep logs, and sleep diaries. Although objective measures allow accurate measurement of sleep duration, sleep efficiency, and other variables relevant to insomnia, paper and pencil measures are used for qualitative assessment. A debate continues about the accuracy of such measures in populations with cognitive impairment in which historian reliability is often compromised.

### Polysomnography

The polysomnography is considered the gold standard of sleep measurement. Based on electroencephalogram, electro-oculogram, electromyogram, airflow measurement, arterial saturation, and movement, duration of total sleep and of specific stages of sleep is calculated.

### Actigraphy

An actigraph is an electronic device that is used to measure periods of sleep and wakefulness through detecting movement while attached to the wrist, ankle, or waist. An actigraphy algorithm for sleep-wake assessment was found to have agreement rates with polysomnography scores that ranged between 91% and 93%.[48] This technology has allowed objective measurement of sleep efficiency in individuals with neurologic impairment who may have difficulty tolerating a polysomnogram because of agitation. Such objective measurement is particularly important when that impairment also interferes with accuracy of self-report. For this reason, actigraphy algorithm has been used for several studies of sleep disturbance in TBI.[23,49–53] However, it has been pointed out that the device is probably inaccurate in its description of sleep and wakefulness in low-functioning patients such as those in a minimally conscious state.[54] Investigators also raised concerns about validity in individuals with paresis, spasticity, or contractures because reduced movement for those patients is due to other factors than sleep.

### Sleep Logs

Routine monitoring of patients during inpatient treatment may include a sleep log in which staff (usually nurses) record hourly observations on sleep and wakefulness. Disagreement with objective measures has been attributed to common practice of basing a rating for a time period on a brief observation.[54] However, there is anecdotal evidence that staff observations are an essential complement to objective measures to ensure that devices are attached correctly.

### Sleep Diaries

Clinicians who treat sleep disorders often instruct their patients to record the duration of nighttime sleep and daytime naps in a diary. In a sample of patients with narcolepsy and in normal controls, sleep diaries were found to have acceptable agreement with sleep duration calculated with polysomnograph monitoring.[55] In a sample of TBI patients, objective data from polysomnography showed that subjective ratings had overestimated sleep disturbance, although the accuracy of self-report was no worse for the brain-injured group than it was for neurologically intact controls.[20]

### The Insomnia Severity Index

The Insomnia Severity Index (**Fig. 1**) is made up of 7 questions assessing symptoms of insomnia on a 5-point Likert scale.[56] The questions measure

## Insomnia Severity Index (ISI)

Subject ID: _____ Date: _____

For each question below, please circle the number corresponding most accurately to your sleep patterns in the **LAST MONTH.**

For the first three questions, please rate the **SEVERITY** of your sleep difficulties.

1. Difficulty falling asleep:

| None | Mild | Moderate | Severe | Very Severe |
|------|------|----------|--------|-------------|
| 0 | 1 | 2 | 3 | 4 |

2. Difficulty staying asleep:

| None | Mild | Moderate | Severe | Very Severe |
|------|------|----------|--------|-------------|
| 0 | 1 | 2 | 3 | 4 |

3. Problem waking up too early in the morning:

| None | Mild | Moderate | Severe | Very Severe |
|------|------|----------|--------|-------------|
| 0 | 1 | 2 | 3 | 4 |

4. How **SATISFIED**/dissatisfied are you with your current sleep pattern?

| Very Satisfied | Satisfied | Neutral | Dissatisfied | Very Dissatisfied |
|----------------|-----------|---------|--------------|-------------------|
| 0 | 1 | 2 | 3 | 4 |

5. To what extent do you consider your sleep problem to **INTERFERE** with your daily functioning (e.g., daytime fatigue, ability to function at work/daily chores, concentration, memory, mood).

| Not at all Interfering | A Little Interfering | Somewhat Interfering | Much Interfering | Very Much Interfering |
|------------------------|----------------------|----------------------|------------------|-----------------------|
| 0 | 1 | 2 | 3 | 4 |

6. How **NOTICEABLE** to others do you think your sleeping problem is in terms of impairing the quality of your life?

| Not at all Noticeable | A little Noticeable | Somewhat Noticeable | Much Noticeable | Very Much Noticeable |
|-----------------------|---------------------|---------------------|-----------------|----------------------|
| 0 | 1 | 2 | 3 | 4 |

7. How **WORRIED**/distressed are you about your current sleep problem?

| Not at all | A Little | Somewhat | Much | Very Much |
|------------|----------|----------|------|-----------|
| 0 | 1 | 2 | 3 | 4 |

### Guidelines for Scoring/Interpretation:

Add scores for all seven items = _____
Total score ranges from 0-28

| | |
|------|---|
| 0-7 | = No clinically significant insomnia |
| 8-14 | = Subthreshold insomnia |
| 15-21 | = Clinical insomnia (moderate severity) |
| 22-28 | = Clinical insomnia (severe) |

**Fig. 1.** Insomnia Severity Index. (*Courtesy of* Charles Morin, Quebec QC. © Morin, C.M. [1993, 1996, 2000, 2006.])

severity of sleep disturbance, satisfaction with sleep, disruption of daily functioning, prominence of resulting impairment, and resulting emotional distress. This measure includes forms for self-report, family report, and clinician rating. The self-report form has been demonstrated to have acceptable reliability and validity.[57]

### Other Self-Report Measures

The Pittsburgh Sleep Quality Index[58] and the Epworth Sleepiness Scale[59] are also self-report measures that have been validated and are frequently used in sleep research. However, although both of these measures assess aspects of sleep disturbance related to insomnia (subjective perception of quality of sleep and daytime sleepiness), neither was designed to measure the primary symptoms of insomnia itself.

### TREATMENT

Although medication is consistently found to be the most widely used treatment of insomnia in the general population, behavioral interventions have been found to be just as effective if not superior.[60] Medication use may be particularly problematic for neurologic patients who are undergoing rehabilitation because some sedative hypnotic medications have adverse effects on those populations. However, patients with neurologic disorders often have limited capacity to participate in psychotherapy because of cognitive impairment. Alternative treatments are currently under study as described in the later discussion.

## Psychotherapy

In cognitive psychotherapy for insomnia, the patient identifies and reconsiders dysfunctional beliefs that are associated with the emotional distress that can cause sleep disturbance. Cognitive behavioral psychotherapists combine this form of office-based therapy with several behavioral interventions (often implemented at home), including stimulus control therapy, sleep restriction, and relaxation. Stimulus control techniques teach the patient to associate stimuli such as a particular time of day (bedtime) and a particular place (the bedroom) with a response, which is rapid sleep onset. Sleep restriction exercises actually induce a mild state of sleep deprivation, which subsequently results in improved consolidation and efficiency of sleep. Relaxation training involves instruction in mental and physical exercises that reduce the autonomic arousal that interferes with sleep. A meta-analysis has shown strong effect sizes for cognitive behavioral treatment, comparable to outcome studies for hypnotic medications.[61]

## Medication

Sedative hypnotic medications include benzodiazepines and GABA agonists, both of which have been found to be safe and effective short-term treatments for insomnia in neurologically intact samples.[62] However, in patients with a neurologic diagnosis, many such agents have adverse cognitive effects when at peak plasma levels and some have residual effects after waking.[63] There is also evidence that certain sedative-hypnotics impede neuronal plasticity that underlies recovery from neurologic injury or illness.[64,65] A large percentage of individuals with orthopedic or neurologic disability take sleeping pills, but there is limited evidence of efficacy in this population, and their use is discouraged because of adverse effects on daytime alertness and gait stability.[66]

## Acupuncture

After an initial report that acupuncture is an effective treatment of insomnia in stroke,[67] this finding was replicated in a randomized double-blinded trial.[68] The latter study also found that compared with a sham acupuncture group, a group of stroke patients who underwent real acupuncture exhibited reduced heart-rate variability, which suggested that the intervention reduced hyperactivity of the sympathetic nervous system. A randomized controlled trial involving TBI patients also found an association between acupuncture and a reduced subjective complaint of insomnia, although objective measures of sleep duration did not differ between groups.[53]

## Management of Environmental Factors

There is sparse data regarding the management of environmental factors in neurorehabilitation units, but, like all hospital environments, these units exhibit conditions commonly found in other hospital units that have been studied. Environmental noise and patient care activities account for 30% of awakenings of patients in an intensive care unit.[69] An examination of a critical care setting showed that nursing routines included an average of almost 43 nighttime activities per patient, resulting in frequent sleep interruption.[70] Investigators observed that routine daily baths were given between 2 AM and 5 AM for 55 of 147 nights studied. A recent comprehensive algorithm to maximize healthy sleep in a hospital setting emphasized the importance of scheduling routine patient care activities so that they minimize interruption of sleep during the night.[71]

## Bright Light Therapy

Circadian rhythm disorders are frequently misdiagnosed as insomnia as seen in the article by Smolensky and Portaluppi in this issue. Many older adults fail to receive sufficient bright light to synchronize their circadian system and that this is particularly problematic in individuals who are receiving residential care (eg, skilled nursing facility or subacute rehabilitation).[72] A subsequent randomized controlled trial showed that placement in a residential setting with high levels of ambient light during the day was associated with improved sleep and lower ratings of physical and cognitive disability.[73] Further study of this intervention in specific neurologic populations is needed.

## Exercise

Physical exercise is one particularly powerful nonpharmacologic intervention that can have dramatic and far-reaching effects on sleep.[74] Sleep was examined in a sample of sedentary older adults who participated in a randomized controlled trial comparing a group that participated in a 16-week aerobic exercise program and a group that engaged in nonphysical activity.[75] The aerobic exercise group experienced superior improvement in subjective ratings of overall sleep quality and in objective measures of sleep latency, sleep duration, and sleep efficiency. Neurologic patients often have motor impairment that complicates exercise, which may explain the lack of studies of this intervention as a treatment of insomnia. However, because motor impairment may result in a sedentary lifestyle that exacerbates insomnia, the impact of physical therapy and home exercise programs on sleep among neurologic patients would appear to be a promising avenue for future research.

## REFERENCES

1. American Academy of Sleep Medicine. The international classification of sleep disorders: diagnostic and coding manual. 2nd edition. Westchester (IL): American Academy of Sleep Medicine; 2005.

2. American Psychiatric Association. Task Force on DSM-IV. Diagnostic and statistical manual of mental disorders: DSM-IV. 4th edition. Washington, DC: American Psychiatric Association; 1994.

3. World Health Organization. The ICD-10 classification of mental and behavioural disorders: clinical descriptions and diagnostic guidelines. Geneva (Switzerland): World Health Organization; 1992.

4. Ouellet MC, Beaulieu-Bonneau S. Sleep disorders in rehabiliation patients. In: Stone JH, Blouin M, editors. International encyclopedia of rehabilitation. 2012.http://cirrie.buffalo.edu/encyclopedia/en/article/43/

5. Gangwisch JE, Heymsfield SB, Boden-Albala B, et al. Short sleep duration as a risk factor for hypertension: analyses of the first National Health and Nutrition Examination Survey. Hypertension 2006; 47(5):833–9.

6. Schiffman PL, Trontell MC, Mazar MF, et al. Sleep deprivation decreases ventilatory response to $CO_2$ but not load compensation. Chest 1983;84(6):695–8.

7. Zhong X, Hilton HJ, Gates GJ, et al. Increased sympathetic and decreased parasympathetic cardiovascular modulation in normal humans with acute sleep deprivation. J Appl Physiol 2005;98(6):2024–32.

8. Knutson KL, Spiegel K, Penev P, et al. The metabolic consequences of sleep deprivation [literature review]. Sleep Med Rev 2007;11(3):163–78.

9. McCall WV, Blocker JN, D'Agostino R Jr, et al. Treatment of insomnia in depressed insomniacs: effects on health-related quality of life, objective and self-reported sleep, and depression. J Clin Sleep Med 2010;6(4):322–9.

10. Kahn-Greene ET, Killgore DB, Kamimori GH, et al. The effects of sleep deprivation on symptoms of psychopathology in healthy adults. Sleep Med 2007;8(3):215–21.

11. Manabe K, Matsui T, Yamaya M, et al. Sleep patterns and mortality among elderly patients in a geriatric hospital. Gerontology 2000;46(6):318–22.

12. Avidan AY. Clinical neurology of insomnia in neurodegenerative and other disorders of neurological function. Rev Neurol Dis 2007;4(1):21–34.

13. Young JS, Bourgeois JA, Hilty DM, et al. Sleep in hospitalized medical patients, part 1: factors affecting sleep. J Hosp Med 2008;3(6):473–82.

14. Moldofsky H. Sleep and fibrositis syndrome. Rheum Dis Clin North Am 1989;15(1):91–103.

15. Mayer G, Jennum P, Riemann D, et al. Insomnia in central neurologic diseases - Occurrence and management. Sleep Med Rev 2011;15(6):369–78.

16. Zeitzer JM, Friedman L, O'Hara R. Insomnia in the context of traumatic brain injury. J Rehabil Res Dev 2009;46(6):827–36.

17. Beetar JT, Guilmette TJ, Sparadeo FR. Sleep and pain complaints in symptomatic traumatic brain injury and neurologic populations. Arch Phys Med Rehabil 1996;77(12):1298–302.

18. Fichtenberg NL, Millis SR, Mann NR, et al. Factors associated with insomnia among post-acute traumatic brain injury survivors. Brain Inj 2000;14(7):659–67.

19. Parcell DL, Ponsford JL, Rodman JR, et al. Poor sleep quality and changes in objectively recorded sleep after traumatic brain injury: a preliminary study. Arch Phys Med Rehabil 2008;89(5):843–50.

20. Ouellet MC, Morin CM. Subjective and objective measures of insomnia in the context of traumatic brain injury: a preliminary study. Sleep Med 2006; 7(6):486–97.

21. Thaxton L, Myers MA. Sleep disturbances and their management in patients with brain injury [literature review]. J Head Trauma Rehabil 2002;17(4):335–48.

22. Mahmood O, Rapport LJ, Hanks RA, et al. Neuropsychological performance and sleep disturbance following traumatic brain injury. J Head Trauma Rehabil 2004;19(5):378–90.

23. Makley MJ, Johnson-Greene L, Tarwater PM, et al. Return of memory and sleep efficiency following moderate to severe closed head injury. Neurorehabil Neural Repair 2009;23(4):320–6.

24. Bloomfield IL, Espie CA, Evans JJ. Do sleep difficulties exacerbate deficits in sustained attention following traumatic brain injury? J Int Neuropsychol Soc 2010;16(1):17–25.

25. Worthington AD, Melia Y. Rehabilitation is compromised by arousal and sleep disorders: results of a survey of rehabilitation centres. Brain Inj 2006; 20(3):327–32.

26. Verma A, Anand V, Verma NP. Sleep disorders in chronic traumatic brain injury. J Clin Sleep Med 2007;3(4):357–62.

27. Palomaki H, Berg A, Meririnne E, et al. Complaints of poststroke insomnia and its treatment with mianserin. Cerebrovasc Dis 2003;15(1–2):56–62.

28. Leppavuori A, Pohjasvaara T, Vataja R, et al. Generalized anxiety disorders three to four months after ischemic stroke. Cerebrovasc Dis 2003;16(3):257–64.

29. Shamsuzzaman AS, Gersh BJ, Somers VK. Obstructive sleep apnea: implications for cardiac and vascular disease. JAMA 2003;290(14):1906–14.

30. Muller C, Achermann P, Bischof M, et al. Visual and spectral analysis of sleep EEG in acute hemispheric stroke. Eur Neurol 2002;48(3):164–71.

31. Siccoli MM, Rolli-Baumeler N, Achermann P, et al. Correlation between sleep and cognitive functions after hemispheric ischaemic stroke. Eur J Neurol 2008;15(6):565–72.

32. Hermann DM, Siccoli M, Brugger P, et al. Evolution of neurological, neuropsychological and sleep-wake disturbances after paramedian thalamic stroke. Stroke 2008;39(1):62–8.

33. Kim CR, Chun MH, Han EY. Effects of hypnotics on sleep patterns and functional recovery of patients with subacute stroke. Am J Phys Med Rehabil 2010;89(4):315–22.

34. Chokroverty S. Sleep and degenerative neurologic disorders. Neurol Clin 1996;14(4):807–26.

35. Frucht SJ, Greene PE, Fahn S. Sleep episodes in Parkinson's disease: a wake-up call. Mov Disord 2000;15(4):601–3.

36. Verbaan D, van Rooden SM, Visser M, et al. Nighttime sleep problems and daytime sleepiness in Parkinson's disease. Mov Disord 2008;23(1):35–41.

37. Tandberg E, Larsen JP, Karlsen K. A community-based study of sleep disorders in patients with Parkinson's disease. Mov Disord 1998;13(6):895–9.

38. Fish DR, Sawyers D, Allen PJ, et al. The effect of sleep on the dyskinetic movements of Parkinson's disease, Gilles de la Tourette syndrome, Huntington's disease, and torsion dystonia. Arch Neurol 1991;48(2):210–4.

39. Partinen M. Sleep disorder related to Parkinson's disease. J Neurol 1997;244(4 Suppl 1):S3–6.

40. Stocchi F, Barbato L, Nordera G, et al. Sleep disorders in Parkinson's disease. J Neurol 1998;245(Suppl 1): S15–8.

41. Pappert EJ, Goetz CG, Niederman FG, et al. Hallucinations, sleep fragmentation, and altered dream phenomena in Parkinson's disease. Mov Disord 1999;14(1):117–21.

42. Happe S. Excessive daytime sleepiness and sleep disturbances in patients with neurological diseases: epidemiology and management. Drugs 2003; 63(24):2725–37.

43. Scheer FA, Zeitzer JM, Ayas NT, et al. Reduced sleep efficiency in cervical spinal cord injury; association with abolished night time melatonin secretion. Spinal Cord 2006;44(2):78–81.

44. Stockhammer E, Tobon A, Michel F, et al. Characteristics of sleep apnea syndrome in tetraplegic patients. Spinal Cord 2002;40(6):286–94.

45. Arnulf I, Similowski T, Salachas F, et al. Sleep disorders and diaphragmatic function in patients with amyotrophic lateral sclerosis. Am J Respir Crit Care Med 2000;161(3 Pt 1):849–56.

46. Barthlen GM, Lange DJ. Unexpectedly severe sleep and respiratory pathology in patients with amyotrophic lateral sclerosis. Eur J Neurol 2000;7(3): 299–302.

47. Butz M, Wollinsky KH, Wiedemuth-Catrinescu U, et al. Longitudinal effects of noninvasive positive-pressure ventilation in patients with amyotrophic lateral sclerosis. Am J Phys Med Rehabil 2003; 82(8):597–604.

48. Sadeh A, Sharkey KM, Carskadon MA. Activity-based sleep-wake identification: an empirical test of methodological issues. Sleep 1994;17(3):201–7.

49. Ayalon L, Borodkin K, Dishon L, et al. Circadian rhythm sleep disorders following mild traumatic brain injury. Neurology 2007;68(14):1136–40.

50. Kaufman Y, Tzischinsky O, Epstein R, et al. Long-term sleep disturbances in adolescents after minor head injury. Pediatr Neurol 2001;24(2):129–34.

51. Masel BE, Scheibel RS, Kimbark T, et al. Excessive daytime sleepiness in adults with brain injuries. Arch Phys Med Rehabil 2001;82(11):1526–32.

52. Nagtegaal JE, Kerkhof GA, Smits MG, et al. Traumatic brain injury-associated delayed sleep phase syndrome. Funct Neurol 1997;12(6):345–8.

53. Zollman FS, Larson EB, Wasek-Throm LK, et al. Acupuncture for treatment of insomnia in patients with traumatic brain injury: a pilot intervention study. J Head Trauma Rehabil 2011;27(2):135–42.

54. Zollman FS, Cyborski C, Duraski SA. Actigraphy for assessment of sleep in traumatic brain injury: case series, review of the literature and proposed criteria for use. Brain Inj 2010;24(5):748–54.

55. Rogers AE, Caruso CC, Aldrich MS. Reliability of sleep diaries for assessment of sleep/wake patterns. Nurs Res 1993;42(6):368–72.

56. Morin CM. Insomnia: psychological assessment and management. New York: Guilford Press; 1993.

57. Bastien CH, Vallieres A, Morin CM. Validation of the Insomnia Severity Index as an outcome measure for insomnia research. Sleep Med 2001;2(4): 297–307.

58. Buysse DJ, Reynolds CF 3rd, Monk TH, et al. The Pittsburgh Sleep Quality Index: a new instrument for psychiatric practice and research. Psychiatry Res 1989;28(2):193–213.

59. Johns MW. A new method for measuring daytime sleepiness: the Epworth sleepiness scale. Sleep 1991;14(6):540–5.

60. NIH State of the Science Conference statement on Manifestations and Management of Chronic Insomnia in Adults statement. J Clin Sleep Med 2005;1(4): 412–21.

61. Murtagh DR, Greenwood KM. Identifying effective psychological treatments for insomnia: a meta-analysis. J Consult Clin Psychol 1995;63(1):79–89.

62. Mendelson WB, Roth T, Cassella J, et al. The treatment of chronic insomnia: drug indications, chronic use and abuse liability. Summary of a 2001 New Clinical Drug Evaluation Unit meeting symposium. Sleep Med Rev 2004;8(1):7–17.

63. Larson EB, Zollman FS. The effect of sleep medications on cognitive recovery from traumatic brain injury. J Head Trauma Rehabil 2010;25(1):61–7.

64. Goldstein LB. Neuropharmacology of TBI-induced plasticity. Brain Inj 2003;17(8):685–94.

65. Seibt J, Aton SJ, Jha SK, et al. The non-benzodiazepine hypnotic zolpidem impairs sleep-dependent cortical plasticity. Sleep 2008;31(10):1381–91.

66. Freter SH, Becker MR. Predictors of restful sleep in a rehabilitation hospital. Am J Phys Med Rehabil 1999;78(6):552–6.

67. Kim YS, Lee SH, Jung WS, et al. Intradermal acupuncture on shen-men and nei-kuan acupoints in patients with insomnia after stroke. Am J Chin Med 2004; 32(5):771–8.

68. Lee SY, Baek YH, Park SU, et al. Intradermal acupuncture on shen-men and nei-kuan acupoints improves insomnia in stroke patients by reducing the sympathetic nervous activity: a randomized clinical trial. Am J Chin Med 2009;37(6):1013–21.

69. Gabor JY, Cooper AB, Crombach SA, et al. Contribution of the intensive care unit environment to sleep disruption in mechanically ventilated patients and healthy subjects. Am J Respir Crit Care Med 2003; 167(5):708–15.

70. Tamburri LM, DiBrienza R, Zozula R, et al. Nocturnal care interactions with patients in critical care units. Am J Crit Care 2004;13(2):102–12 [quiz: 114–5].

71. Young JS, Bourgeois JA, Hilty DM, et al. Sleep in hospitalized medical patients, part 2: behavioral and pharmacological management of sleep disturbances. J Hosp Med 2009;4(1):50–9.

72. Ancoli-Israel S, Klauber MR, Jones DW, et al. Variations in circadian rhythms of activity, sleep, and light exposure related to dementia in nursing-home patients. Sleep 1997;20(1):18–23.

73. Riemersma-van der Lek RF, Swaab DF, Twisk J, et al. Effect of bright light and melatonin on cognitive and noncognitive function in elderly residents of group care facilities: a randomized controlled trial. JAMA 2008;299(22):2642–55.

74. Kubitz KA, Landers DM, Petruzzello SJ, et al. The effects of acute and chronic exercise on sleep. A meta-analytic review. Sports Med 1996;21(4):277–91.

75. Reid KJ, Baron KG, Lu B, et al. Aerobic exercise improves self-reported sleep and quality of life in older adults with insomnia. Sleep Med 2010;11(9): 934–40.

# Stroke and Sleep Disorders

Bernardo Selim, MD[a], Francoise J. Roux, MD, PhD[b],*

## KEYWORDS

- Sleep-disordered breathing • Obstructive sleep apnea • Central apnea • Cheyne-Stokes respiration
- Sleep-wake disorders • Stroke

## KEY POINTS

- Screening for obstructive sleep apnea (OSA) or central sleep apnea should be implemented in all stroke patients.
- Other sleep disorders such as insomnia and hypersomnia should be addressed because they can also adversely affect poststroke rehabilitation.
- Treating patients with OSA with continuous positive airway pressure improves vascular risk factors for stroke such as hypertension, atrial fibrillation, metabolic syndrome, and cognitive function.

## INTRODUCTION

Each year, about 795,000 people experience a new or recurrent stroke. Approximately 610,000 are first attacks and 185,000 are recurrent attacks. Despite the recent steady decline of stroke deaths, stroke continues to be the third leading cause of death in the United States and the second in the world.[1] It also accounts for the leading cause of long-term disability, institutionalization, and increase in health care costs.[2,3] The identification and management of modifiable risk factors are crucial for the development of primary and secondary preventive strategies.[4] There is accumulating literature that indicates that sleep-disordered breathing (SDB) is a prevalent and treatable risk factor for the development of cerebrovascular events.[5] SDB has also been independently associated to specific cardiovascular risk factors, such as hypertension; myocardial ischemia; fatal and nonfatal cardiovascular events; and arrhythmias such as atrial fibrillation, diabetes, and stroke.[6-8] Therefore, the diagnosis and optimal treatment of SDB is critical among patients with stroke during the acute and chronic phase of neurorehabilitation.

## NORMAL CEREBRAL HEMODYNAMIC CHANGES DURING SLEEP

At night, cerebral hemodynamics is influenced by the various stages of sleep. During nonrapid eye movement sleep, sympathetic activity decreases and parasympathetic tone predominates with concomitant reduction of heart rate, blood pressure (blood pressure dip of 10%–15% from awake baseline), cardiac output, systemic vascular resistance, and respiratory frequency. Rapid eye movement (REM) sleep, more frequent in the second half of the night, is characterized by phasic oscillations of sympathetic and parasympathetic activity translating into increased cerebral and spinal flow as well as elevation of systemic blood pressure and heart rate. As a consequence, blood pressure falls to its lowest level in the first part of the night, followed by a marked surge in the morning hours. These sleep-related fluctuations in systemic hemodynamics are compensated by the local cerebrovascular autoregulation system of blood flow, ensuring a constant range of perfusion pressure to the central nervous system.[9,10]

a Section of Pulmonary, Critical Care and Sleep Medicine, Mayo Clinic Sleep Center, Mayo Clinic, 200 First Street SW, Rochester, Minnesota 55905, USA; b Section of Pulmonary and Critical Care and Sleep Medicine, Yale Sleep Center, Yale University School of Medicine, 333 Cedar Street, Post Office Box 208057, New Haven, CT 06520-8057, USA
* Corresponding author.
E-mail address: francoise.roux@yale.edu

Sleep Med Clin 7 (2012) 597–607
http://dx.doi.org/10.1016/j.jsmc.2012.08.007

## DEFINITION, CLASSIFICATION, AND PATHOPHYSIOLOGY OF SDB

SDB is characterized either by cyclical nocturnal flow limitation secondary to upper airways collapse (obstructive sleep apnea [OSA]) or by cyclical nocturnal cessation of respiratory efforts (central sleep apnea [CSA]). An apnea is defined as cessation of airflow for at least 10 seconds in the presence of thoracoabdominal ventilatory efforts. The Sleep Heart Health Study, a large, multicenter trial designed to relate cardiovascular disease with polysomnographic findings, defined hypopnea as a 30% reduction in airflow or chest wall movement from baseline movement for at least 10 seconds and accompanied by oxygen desaturation of 4% or greater.[11] The apnea-hypopnea index (AHI) is the sum of apneas and hypopneas per hour of sleep. An AHI of greater than equal to 5 per hour established the diagnosis of OSA according to the criteria of the American Academy of Sleep Medicine.[12] It is estimated that in Western countries, 24% of men and 15% of women have OSA and 4% of men and 2% of women have OSA with symptoms of daytime sleepiness. Unfortunately, up to 80% of cases remain undiagnosed.[13,14] As a result of cyclical airflow limitation events related to OSA, several nocturnal physiologic stressors arise: (1) cyclical hypoxemic events of varying frequency, duration, and severity; (2) cyclical swings of negative intra-thoracic pressures while attempting to breath against an occluded upper airway (Muller maneuver); and (3) cyclical sympathetic nerve surges at the end of each respiratory event.[15] These intermittent, OSA-associated physiologic stressors provide a perfect milieu for development of cerebrovascular events.

## ASSOCIATION OF OSA AND STROKE

Early case series and case-control studies, some using snoring as a surrogate of objective diagnosis of OSA, have suggested an association between OSA and stroke.[16–18] However, a direct causal relationship has been difficult to establish for several reasons: (1) studies about prevalence of OSA in patients with stroke are affected by selection bias of stroke survivors transferred to rehabilitation units; (2) multiple cardiovascular comorbidities identified as risk factors for stroke (hypertension, diabetes, etc.) are commonly associated with patients with sleep apnea; and (3) cerebrovascular events themselves might also compromise the respiratory centers precipitating or exacerbating CSA and OSA, making the temporal cause-effect relationship more difficult to establish.

### Epidemiology of OSA in the Stroke Population

Several observational studies have noted a high prevalence of sleep apnea in subjects studied shortly after an acute stroke.[19–21] In a recent published meta-analysis of 2343 patients with ischemic or hemorrhagic stroke and transient ischemic attack (TIA), the frequency of SDB with AHI greater than 5 was 72% (95% confidence interval [CI], 60–81) and with AHI greater than 20 was 38% (95% CI, 31–46).[22] Neither stroke severity nor anatomic location or type of stroke (ischemic vs hemorrhagic) has been shown to predict the presence or severity of OSA,[23] implying that OSA is a risk factor rather than a consequence of stroke. There was no difference in the prevalence of OSA in TIA patients in comparison to stroke patients,[24] also suggesting that OSA preceded the development of stroke. Immediately after an acute stroke, CSA may be more common than OSA and may influence stroke outcome. In the postacute recovery phase and during rehabilitation, OSA is more common than CSA.[20,23] Three months after an acute stroke, approximately 50% of patients still exhibit a residual obstructive AHI of greater than or equal to 10 per hour.[23]

### Risk of Stroke in the OSA Population

To establish the causal nature of an association requires an analysis of incident events in prospective cohort studies. Since 2005, well-designed prospective studies have shown that sleep apnea is a predisposing risk factor for stroke. In men, untreated severe OSA (AHI >30) was found to significantly increase the risk of fatal and nonfatal cardiovascular events, including stroke in comparison to healthy population. Even after adjusting for demographic and traditional cardiovascular confounders, untreated severe OSA significantly increased the risk of fatal (odds ratio 2.87, 95% CI 1.17–7.51) and non-fatal (3.17, 1.12–7.51) cardiovascular events compared with healthy participants.[6] A cross-sectional analysis of a population-based study (Wisconsin Sleep Cohort Study) showed that moderate to severe OSA (AHI ≥20) was associated with approximately 4-fold increased risk of having had a stroke (OR, 4.33; 95% CI, 1.32–14.24; P = .02) in comparison to those without OSA.[25] Also in 2005, a referral-based observational cohort study showed that OSA is associated with an almost 2-fold increased incidence of a composite outcome of stroke mortality in a 6-year follow-up period. This association remained statistically significant even after adjusting for confounding factors such as age, race, gender, hyperlipidemia, atrial fibrillation, and even hypertension (hazard ratio [HR], 1.97; 95% CI,

1.12–3.48; $P$ = .01).[8] Furthermore, this study showed a dose effect between increased severity of SDB and increased risk of stroke, another postulate of causal relationship. A population-based longitudinal study of elderly adults showed that severe OSA (AHI $\geq$30) increased the incidence of first-time ischemic stroke in a 6-year follow-up, after adjusting for confounding factors.[26] Finally, the Sleep Heart Health Study, a multicenter prospective cohort study of a large community-based sample, showed that men with moderate to severe OSA have three times higher risk for new onset ischemic stroke than those without OSA after adjusting for traditional cardiovascular confounders.[27] Overall, these various studies strongly support the concept that SDB precedes stroke and may contribute to the development of stroke.

## Significance of OSA in Stroke Population

The relationship between OSA and stroke patients is relevant not only because of the high prevalence of OSA in the stroke population but also because of the poorer outcomes after stroke, including prolong hospitalization, increased functional disability, and higher mortality in comparison to those patients without OSA.[28,29] Ten-year follow-up data of patients with stroke have shown an increased risk of death in those patients with OSA (adjusted OR, 1.76; 95% CI, 1.05–2.95; $P$ = .03) that is independent of age, sex, BMI, smoking, hypertension, diabetes, atrial fibrillation, Mini-Mental State Examination Score, and Barthel index of activities of daily living.[30] Long-term stroke-related mortality in OSA patients was associated with an initial high AHI; older age; and presence of hypertension, diabetes, and coronary heart disease.[31,32]

## Potential Physiopathology Linking OSA and Stroke

There are multiple mechanisms by which OSA may lead to the development of stroke. In OSA patients, cyclical physiologic stressors such as recurrent hypoxemia, intrathoracic pressure swings, and sympathetic tone surge are the result of recurrent nocturnal respiratory events (apneas and hypopneas).[15] These physiologic stressors may contribute to potential mechanistic pathways of transient cerebral ischemia or stroke, such as:

### Chronic hypertension and nocturnal blood pressure swings

Chronic hypertension is a well-established risk factor for developing stroke. The Wisconsin Sleep Cohort Study demonstrated almost a 3-fold increased risk of incident hypertension in OSA patients (AHI >15/h) over a period of 4-year follow-up (OR 2.89, 95% CI, 1.46–5.64), independent of other known cardiovascular risk factors (baseline hypertension, age, sex, BMI, alcohol, and cigarette smoking).[7] However, a similar observational longitudinal study (Sleep Heart Health Study) found this relationship to be attenuated (OR, 1.51; 95% CI, 0.93–2.47) and not statistically significant after adjustment for baseline BMI.[33] Despite this discrepancy, probably based on diverse populations, sample sizes, varying diagnostic techniques, and different definitions of apneas and hypopneas, there is still a modest association between severe OSA (AHI >30) and future hypertension. Even in the absence of hypertension during the daytime, SDB is associated with cyclical surges of blood pressure during the night and lack of the physiologic drop of nocturnal blood pressure (dipping), increasing their risk for cardiovascular damage.[34] Pronounced spikes of systemic blood pressure at the end of each respiratory event are followed by abrupt drops in systemic blood pressure driven by withdrawal of the sympathetic tone and recovery of the dominant nocturnal parasympathetic (vagal) tone.[35]

### Reduction of cerebral blood flow and cyclical hypoxemia

Multiple cerebral blood flow studies by transcranial Doppler techniques have shown that blood velocity increases in the middle cerebral artery at the end of apnea, followed by an abrupt drop of blood velocity at apnea termination (onset of respiration), below resting values.[36,37] This change in blood flow velocity correlates temporally with surges in systemic blood pressure and intracranial pressure during the end of apnea, pointing to endothelial dysfunction and reduced compensatory cerebrovascular flow response as possible causes.[38] This loss of vascular autoregulation is considered to be secondary to wide blood pressure swings concomitant with oxidative stress from cyclical hypoxemia.[39] Cerebral perfusion, defined as the difference between arterial pressure and intracranial pressure, will be the lowest shortly after the end of apnea, when respiration restarts. These hemodynamic changes may predispose to ischemia in watershed areas of the brain.[40]

Endothelial cells produce several vasoactive and physiologically essential substances such as endothelin (ET-1), which induces vasoconstriction, and nitric oxide (NO), which results in vasodilation. The cyclical hypoxemia related to OSA events results in significant increase of ET-1 with consequent increase of blood pressure. NO is also diminished in OSA patients, contributing to impaired vasodilation and increased vascular tone. Even patients with mild OSA have been shown to have altered endothelium-dependent vasomotor relaxation.[38,41]

### Accelerated atherosclerosis and inflammation

The role of atherosclerosis as the cause of stroke in patients with SDB is supported by data reporting a higher prevalence of internal carotid artery atherosclerotic lesions in stroke patients with OSA than in those without OSA, even after adjusting for traditional cardiovascular risk factors.[42] Carotid intima-media thickness, a marker of preclinical atherosclerosis, has been shown to be increased among patients with OSA.[43] Cyclical hypoxemia and reoxygenation during nocturnal respirator events activates the transcription of hypoxia-inducible factor 1 and nuclear factor-kB, which in turn induce the expression of proinflammatory cytokines and adhesion molecules implicated in atherogenesis.[41,44] Furthermore, elevated markers of inflammation such as interleukin 6, tumor necrosis factor α, homocysteine, and C-reactive protein are elevated in patients with OSA and in patients with atherosclerosis without SDB.[45]

### Prothrombotic and hypercoagulable state

There is well-documented evidence regarding the prothrombotic state in patients with OSA. Compared with patients without OSA, those with OSA have increased platelet aggregation, higher levels of plasminogen activator inhibitor 1 (PAI-1) and fibrinogen.[46,47] PAI-1 is a major inhibitor of the fibrinolytic system by inhibiting tissue-type plasminogen activator. PAI-1 levels have been shown to be elevated in patients with stroke and also in OSA patients, suggesting an important role in the thrombosis-prone state.[48]

### Nocturnal arrhythmias, atrial fibrillation

In the general population, the presence of persistent and paroxysmal atrial fibrillation is potent predictor of first as well as recurrent stroke.[49] In SDB patients, the prevalence of nocturnal arrhythmias, especially atrial fibrillation, is higher among subjects with OSA than in those without OSA.[50] Compared with those without SDB and adjusting for age, sex, BMI, and cardiovascular risks, individuals with OSA had 4 times the odds of developing atrial fibrillation (OR, 4.02; 95% CI, 1.03–15.74).[51] Obesity and the magnitude of nocturnal oxygen desaturations, which results from cyclical respiratory events, are independent risk factors for atrial fibrillation in individuals younger than 65 years of age.[50] This interaction between OSA and atrial fibrillation has also been

shown having favorable response to continuous positive airway pressure (CPAP) treatment.[52]

### Diagnosis and Treatment of OSA in Stroke Patients

Based on the Adult Obstructive Sleep Apnea Task Force of the American Academy of Sleep Medicine, patients with history of stroke are considered at high risk for OSA, and a comprehensive sleep history should be obtained (Consensus) and polysomnographic study may be pursued (Option).[53] However, identification of OSA in stroke patients during rehabilitation may represent a clinical challenge. Based on current publications, screening questionnaires for OSA are not sensitive to identifying patients with high risk for OSA.[54] It is estimated that up to 36% of stroke patients with proven OSA by polysomnogram have normal sleep apnea questionnaires. Snoring history, hypersomnia, age, and stroke severity are not proved to directly predict presence of OSA in stroke patients in the first 24 hours after stroke.[24] Because 2 key clinical diagnostic criteria, excessive daytime sleepiness and obesity, do not appear to be prevalent in patients poststroke, the clinical suspicion and screening for OSA may be compromised.[55] Therefore, indications for polysomnography to diagnose OSA in the stroke population may differ from those in the nonstroke population, but future studies are needed to further characterize them.[56]

In general, management of patients with OSA, independent of presence of stroke, should target life style modifications such as cautious use of alcohol and sedative hypnotic drugs (Consensus).[53] Also, supine position in the acute recovery phase may influence OSA severity manifested by increased frequency and severity of oxygen desaturations. Therefore, positional therapy for acute stroke patients with OSA should be reinforced in rehabilitation units.[57]

In the general OSA population, CPAP is a well-established cost-effective treatment of moderate to severe OSA (Standard) and mild OSA (Option).[53,58] CPAP has been shown to improve cardiovascular prognosis in OSA patients, likely by reduction of (1) high levels of inflammatory cytokines and adhesion molecules, (2) excessive sympathetic tone, (3) vascular oxidative stress, and (4) reversal of coagulation abnormalities.[6,41,59,60] Regarding traditional cardiovascular risk factors associated with OSA and stroke, CPAP treatment of OSA patients without stroke has shown a modest reduction of SBP by 1.38 mm Hg (95% CI, 3.6 to −0.88; P = .23) and diastolic blood pressure (DBP) by 1.52 mm Hg (95% CI, 3.1

to −0.07; $P = .06$). In more severe OSA (mean AHI >30/h), CPAP reduced SBP by 3.03 mm Hg (95% CI, −6.7 to 0.61; $P = .10$) and DBP by 2.03 mm Hg (95% CI, 4.1 to −0.002; $P = .05$).[61] Although these reductions are small, they are clinically relevant. Studies have shown that a reduction of blood pressure of 1 to 5 mm Hg results in a risk reduction of stroke, major cardiovascular events, and death by more than 20%.[62] CPAP therapy was also found to reduce atrial fibrillation recurrence and to improve glycemic control.[52,63] There are no published guidelines by the American Academy of Sleep Medicine or the American Heart Association regarding CPAP treatment in the acute and subacute poststroke population with OSA.[53,64] There are limited data regarding the impact of noninvasive ventilation on morbidity and mortality in this population. In the first month of stroke, small observational studies of OSA patients in CPAP treatment have shown to improve depression, quality of life, and cognitive function.[65,66] In TIA patients, the use of autoset CPAP (APAP) was feasible acutely and associated with a statistical trend toward lowering recurrent vascular event rate and improved neurologic recovery.[67,68] In a prospective observational study at 5 years, CPAP treatment provided protection from the excessive cardiovascular mortality in patients with moderate to severe OSA who have suffered from a stroke when compared with those who have no tolerance for this treatment.[5] There is, however, a wide range of variability in CPAP compliance (25%–50%) in this population, which is in part explained by the spontaneous improvement of SDB severity concomitant with motor and cognitive residual sequelaes.[21,65,69] Accordingly, APAP may be considered as a valid alternative treatment option to the traditional fixed positive airway pressure (CPAP) in this patient population.[67,68]

## Impact of OSA in Rehabilitation of Stroke Patients

The presence of OSA is independently associated not only with increased hospitalization length but also with poorer functional abilities both on admission to and at discharge from rehabilitation services.[28,70] Even after adjusting for functional level on admission to inpatient rehabilitation, the severity of OSA is associated with a poorer gain in functional ability. Specifically in the poststroke population, the presence of OSA not only may increase the risk of recurrent stroke and death, but may also reduce motivation, decrease cognitive capacity, and prolong hospital rehabilitation. In a study of 61 patients admitted to a stroke rehabilitation unit, after matching for severity of stroke, patients with OSA had lower functional capacity (Functional Independence Measure Score, mean ± SEM 80.2 ± 3.6 vs 94.7 ± 4.3; $P<.05$) and spent significantly more days in rehabilitation (45.5 ± 2.3 vs 32.1 ± 2.7 d, $P<.005$).[28] In another small observational study, the presence of SDB and recurrent hypoxemia was associated with worse functional status measured by Barthel index on discharge, at 3 months and at 1-year poststroke follow-up. In this study, nocturnal hypoxemia was associated not only with worse functional outcome but also with higher mortality rate.[71] The pathophysiology by which OSA may lead to poor recovery is not well known. It is possible that cyclical hypoxemia may impair neuronal plasticity involved in functional recovery.[72] Little is known regarding the impact of CPAP treatment in the rehabilitation process of stroke patients with OSA. A randomized, open-label, parallel-group trial with blind assessment of functional outcomes was recently completed in Canada. Patients were assigned to standard rehabilitation alone (control group) or to CPAP (CPAP group). Compared with the control group, patients assigned to the CPAP group experienced improvement in the overall severity of stroke-related impairment based on improvement of the Canadian Neurologic Scale Score and also improvement of the motor component of the Functional Independence Measure, Chedoke-McMaster Stroke Assessment leg score, Stanford Sleepiness Scale, Epworth Sleepiness Scale, and the affective component of Beck Depression Inventory.[73] Still, larger longer-term trials are needed to determine whether such improvements in the functional, motor, and mood dimension could perpetuate over time.

## ASSOCIATION OF CSA AND STROKE

Various forms of SDB can be found in stroke patients, not only OSA but also central apneas or Cheyne-Stokes respiration. Cheyne-Stokes respiration is a form of central apnea characterized by cyclical breathing alternating between fluctuations of hyperpneas and hypopneas/apneas in a crescendo-decrescendo pattern.

### Epidemiology of CSA in the Stroke Population

Cheyne was the first to describe Cheyne-Stokes breathing in a patient with concomitant stroke and heart failure.[74] Parra and colleagues[23] examined prospectively the prevalence of SDB in patients presenting with a first-ever stroke or TIA in the acute phase and 3 months later when patients were considered in the stable phase of their cerebrovascular events using a portable respiratory recording. They found that 26% of these patients had evidence for Cheyne-Stokes breathing, which was not related to any specific neuroanatomic or vascular distribution. The reduction in the severity of the central apneas 3 months after the stroke suggests that central apneas might be a consequence of the neurologic insult. Earlier reports found that Cheyne-Stokes breathing was present in patients with extensive stroke and altered level of consciousness.[75] In contrast, a more recent prospective study in 93 noncomatose stroke patients using polysomnography confirmed that Cheyne-Stokes breathing was frequent but did not correlate to any particular neurologic topography or size of infarct.[76,77]

## Mechanisms of Disease and Prognosis

Cheyne-Stokes respiration occurs in many patients with congestive heart failure (CHF), and these patients have a worse prognosis than those without Cheyne-Stokes respiration.[78,79] In patients with CHF, Cheyne-Stokes respiration appears to be the result of instability of the central control of respiration. The hyperventilation and periodic breathing may be the result of stimulation of pulmonary vagal-irritant receptors by pulmonary congestion.[80] However, in stroke patients, the physiopathology of Cheyne-Stokes breathing has not been well defined. A prospective study involving 93 patients examined the physiopathologic correlates between Cheyne-Stokes breathing and stroke. The investigators found that Cheyne-Stokes breathing in stroke patients was associated with nocturnal hypocapnia and strongly correlated with the degree of left ventricular systolic dysfunction, especially if the ejection fraction was lower than 40%. There was no correlation between the central apneas and the type or location of the stroke.[81] In contrast, other investigators have found the presence of Cheyne-Stokes breathing in stroke patients who had no evidence for CHF.[20] Another study found a lack of correlation between central apneas and stroke localization and severity, suggesting that other mechanisms than brain damage could account for the respiratory abnormalities.[76]

A large cohort of conscious acute stroke patients showed that the presence of Cheyne-Stokes breathing was common and associated with a worse outcome such as disability or death at 3 months compared with stroke patients without Cheyne-Stokes breathing.[82] Similar results were found in a large cohort of stroke and transient ischemic attack patients observed for more than 2 years. The central apnea patients, especially with a Cheyne-Stokes breathing pattern, were more likely to die during this follow-up period.[32]

## Treatment Options in CSA

The treatment of SDB can be a challenge in stroke patients, especially in the acute phase. Hypoxemia should be corrected because it has been shown to worsen stroke outcome with an increased risk of death.[82] Oxygen therapy has been tried because it is easier to use than airway pressurization and should be better tolerated. A prospective study on the effect of oxygen therapy was conducted among stroke and heart failure patients with Cheyne-Stokes respiration. Oxygen therapy could reduce the frequency of the central apneas by more than 50% in most patients irrespective of the presence or absence of heart failure.[83] In respect to positional therapy, sleep in the supine position has been found to worsen Cheyne-Stokes breathing among heart failure and stroke patients.[84] Lateral positioning was beneficial to reduce the severity of central apneas but was only studied in heart failure patients with central apneas and not in a stroke population.[85] CPAP therapy has also been used for the treatment of central apneas but could only reduce the number of apneas and hypopneas per hour by about 50% in heart failure patients, without any qualitative improvement in sleep architecture.[86] Johnson and Johnson[87] showed that bilevel positive airway pressure worsened central apneas in 48% of patients with primary or stroke-related Cheyne-Stokes respiration and in 33% of patients with central apneas. A new mode of noninvasive ventilation called adaptive servo-ventilation was recently developed as a better physiologic approach to treat central apneas and Cheyne-Stokes respiration by applying variable pressure support, thereby preventing ventilatory overshoot and instability. This novel mode of therapy has been shown to be successful in patients with primary or cardiac failure–related Cheyne-Stokes respiration and superior to CPAP and oxygen therapy.[86,88] Finally, because the severity of central apneas might lessen with time after the acute phase of a stroke, an observational approach might be justified in patients who are reluctant to use noninvasive positive pressure ventilation.

## ASSOCIATION OF SLEEP-WAKE DISORDERS AND STROKE

Sleep and wake states encompass a complex interaction of neuronal networks with a delicate balance governing the transition from one state to the other. Stroke can create brain damage that can affect this fragile sleep-wake regulation.

Hypersomnia is a common complaint after stroke, present in about 20% to 40% of stroke patients. Significant hypersomnia in the acute phase of a stroke is frequently found in patients with large, deep hemispheric stroke.[89] The degree of hypersomnia can range from minimal to severe (>20 h/d) in unilateral or bilateral paramedian thalamic stroke patients. Hypersomnia can resolve after a few months in mild cases, whereas it can persist for more than 1 year in severe thalamic strokes.[24] A case of secondary narcolepsy with hypersomnia and low cerebrospinal fluid hypocretin level has also been described after hypothalamic stroke, most likely due to damage of the hypocretin neurons.[90] The Kleine-Levin syndrome, which consists of hypersomnia and hyperphagia, has been reported after multiple cerebral strokes.[91] The treatment of poststroke hypersomnia can be challenging but can improve with methylphenidate or modafinil.[92]

Conversely, some stroke patients might present with insomnia, and a large cohort study suggested that insomnia itself might be a risk factor for developing stroke.[93] Insomnia seems to be a frequent complaint after stroke. The prevalence of insomnia 3 months after ischemic stroke was examined in a large retrospective finish cohort study. The prevalence of insomnia was 37.5% in stroke patients when stringent criteria such as the Diagnostic and Statistical Manual of Mental Disorders IV criteria A-C were applied for insomnia. Among the insomnia patients, 38.6% had insomnia before stroke, whereas 18% developed insomnia after stroke. The new insomniacs had more often a major dominant stroke with more severe disability compared with the noninsomniacs.[94] Stroke-related brain damage in the frontal lobe area seems to predict insomnia symptoms after stroke as well as lesions in the brainstem.[95–97] Treatment of poststroke insomnia should obviously include good sleep hygiene. Mianserin was found to decrease insomnia symptoms better than placebo in stroke patients even in absence of concomitant depression.[98] Benzodiazepines should be used with caution in poststroke insomniacs, because use of benzodiazepine can promote the reemergence of neurologic symptoms in these patients and have numerous side effects.[99] Benzodiazepines can also worsen SDB, which is frequently found in these stroke patients. Sedative antidepressants might be a more favorable option, especially in patients with associated depression.

## MOVEMENT DISORDERS, PARASOMNIAS, AND STROKE

Restless leg syndrome (RLS) is characterized by an urge to move the legs, worse in the evening and relieved by movements. Periodic leg movement during sleep (PLMS) is defined by periodic episodes of stereotyped movements at night, most commonly involving the legs, which can be present in about 80% to 90% of RLS patients. Various case reports have described the occurrence of RLS and PLMS after stroke.[100] A large recent study has reported that 12% of stroke patients developed RLS within 1 week after an ischemic stroke. The investigators found that the anatomic substrates for the RLS symptoms were most frequently the basal ganglia/corona radiata and the pons.[101] It has been suggested that pyramidal tract and basal ganglia–brainstem axis lesions involved in motor functions could lead to RLS symptoms after an ischemic stroke.[102] Dopaminergic agents have been successfully used to treat poststroke PLMS/RLS.

REM sleep behavior disorder (RBD) is a parasomnia characterized by intermittent loss of muscle atonia during REM sleep, such that the patient presents with a violent behavior, acting out his dreams. RBD is usually more common in the setting of neurodegenerative disorders but has been described after the onset of a lacunar ischemic infarct in the pons.[103]

## CIRCADIAN RHYTHM VARIATIONS AND STROKE

Various cardiovascular events, including myocardial infarction and sudden death, display a circadian rhythmicity (6 AM and noon). A recent meta-analysis was conducted to determine when was the most vulnerable period to develop a stroke in a 24 hour period. Elliott[104] found that, irrespective of the type of the stroke, the increased risk for a stroke was also between 6 AM and noon time. It has been suggested that the circadian variability of the blood pressure could play a role in the circadian pattern of acute stroke.[105]

## SUMMARY

Sleep might represent a vulnerable period, especially in stroke patients. Patients with stroke have a high rate of undiagnosed OSA. Screening for OSA or CSA should be implemented in all stroke patients. Other sleep disorders such as insomnia, hypersomnia should be addressed because they can also adversely affect poststroke rehabilitation. Treating OSA patients with CPAP improves vascular risk factors for stroke such as hypertension, atrial fibrillation, metabolic syndrome, and cognitive function. However, the optimal time for screening and starting therapy is unknown, although early use of CPAP has been feasible and might be beneficial to prevent further vascular damage. Further studies are needed to determine whether CPAP treatment reduces stroke-related cardiovascular outcomes and improves prognosis.

## REFERENCES

1. Roger VL, Go AS, Lloyd-Jones DM, et al. Heart disease and stroke statistics–2011 update: a report from the American Heart Association. Circulation 2011;123(4):e18–209.

2. Brown DL, Boden-Albala B, Langa KM, et al. Projected costs of ischemic stroke in the United States. Neurology 2006;67(8):1390–5.

3. Centers for Disease Control and Prevention (CDC). Prevalence and most common causes of disability among adults–United States, 2005. MMWR Morb Mortal Wkly Rep 2009;58(16):421–6.

4. Wu CM, McLaughlin K, Lorenzetti DL, et al. Early risk of stroke after transient ischemic attack: a systematic review and meta-analysis. Arch Intern Med 2007;167(22):2417–22.

5. Martinez-Garcia MA, Soler-Cataluna JJ, Ejarque-Martinez L, et al. Continuous positive airway pressure treatment reduces mortality in patients with ischemic stroke and obstructive sleep apnea: a 5-year follow-up study. Am J Respir Crit Care Med 2009;180(1):36–41.

6. Marin JM, Carrizo SJ, Vicente E, et al. Long-term cardiovascular outcomes in men with obstructive sleep apnoea-hypopnoea with or without treatment with continuous positive airway pressure: an observational study. Lancet 2005;365(9464):1046–53.

7. Peppard PE, Young T, Palta M, et al. Prospective study of the association between sleep-disordered breathing and hypertension. N Engl J Med 2000; 342(19):1378–84.

8. Yaggi HK, Concato J, Kernan WN, et al. Obstructive sleep apnea as a risk factor for stroke and death. N Engl J Med 2005;353(19):2034–41.

9. Ainslie PN, Duffin J. Integration of cerebrovascular CO2 reactivity and chemoreflex control of breathing: mechanisms of regulation, measurement, and interpretation. Am J Physiol Regul Integr Comp Physiol 2009;296(5):R1473–95.

10. Vavilala MS, Lee LA, Lam AM. Cerebral blood flow and vascular physiology. Anesthesiol Clin North America 2002;20(2):247–64, v.

11. Punjabi NM, Newman AB, Young TB, et al. Sleep-disordered breathing and cardiovascular disease: an outcome-based definition of hypopneas. Am J Respir Crit Care Med 2008;177(10):1150–5.

12. Silber MH, Ancoli-Israel S, Bonnet MH, et al. The visual scoring of sleep in adults. J Clin Sleep Med 2007;3(2):121–31.

13. Young T, Evans L, Finn L, et al. Estimation of the clinically diagnosed proportion of sleep apnea syndrome in middle-aged men and women. Sleep 1997;20(9):705–6.

14. Young T, Palta M, Dempsey J, et al. The occurrence of sleep-disordered breathing among middle-aged adults. N Engl J Med 1993;328(17): 1230–5.

15. Dempsey JA, Veasey SC, Morgan BJ, et al. Pathophysiology of sleep apnea. Physiol Rev 2010;90(1): 47–112.

16. Dyken ME, Somers VK, Yamada T, et al. Investigating the relationship between stroke and obstructive sleep apnea. Stroke 1996;27(3):401–7.

17. Partinen M, Palomaki H. Snoring and cerebral infarction. Lancet 1985;2(8468):1325–6.

18. Tikare SK, Chaudhary BA, Bandisode MS. Hypertension and stroke in a young man with obstructive sleep apnea syndrome. Postgrad Med 1985;78(7): 59–60, 64–56.

19. Bassetti C, Aldrich MS. Sleep apnea in acute cerebrovascular diseases: final report on 128 patients. Sleep 1999;22(2):217–23.

20. Hermann DM, Siccoli M, Kirov P, et al. Central periodic breathing during sleep in acute ischemic stroke. Stroke 2007;38(3):1082–4.

21. Hui DS, Choy DK, Wong LK, et al. Prevalence of sleep-disordered breathing and continuous positive airway pressure compliance: results in chinese patients with first-ever ischemic stroke. Chest 2002;122(3):852–60.

22. Johnson KG, Johnson DC. Frequency of sleep apnea in stroke and TIA patients: a meta-analysis. J Clin Sleep Med 2010;6(2):131–7.

23. Parra O, Arboix A, Bechich S, et al. Time course of sleep-related breathing disorders in first-ever stroke or transient ischemic attack. Am J Respir Crit Care Med 2000;161(2 Pt 1):375–80.

24. Bassetti C, Aldrich MS, Chervin RD, et al. Sleep apnea in patients with transient ischemic attack and stroke: a prospective study of 59 patients. Neurology 1996;47(5):1167–73.

25. Arzt M, Young T, Finn L, et al. Association of sleep-disordered breathing and the occurrence of stroke. Am J Respir Crit Care Med 2005;172(11):1447–51.

26. Munoz R, Duran-Cantolla J, Martinez-Vila E, et al. Severe sleep apnea and risk of ischemic stroke in the elderly. Stroke 2006;37(9):2317–21.

27. Redline S, Yenokyan G, Gottlieb DJ, et al. Obstructive sleep apnea-hypopnea and incident stroke: the sleep heart health study. Am J Respir Crit Care Med 2010;182(2):269–77.

28. Kaneko Y, Hajek VE, Zivanovic V, et al. Relationship of sleep apnea to functional capacity and length of hospitalization following stroke. Sleep 2003;26(3): 293–7.

29. Yan-fang S, Yu-ping W. Sleep-disordered breathing: impact on functional outcome of ischemic stroke patients. Sleep Med 2009;10(7):717–9.

30. Sahlin C, Sandberg O, Gustafson Y, et al. Obstructive sleep apnea is a risk factor for death in patients with stroke: a 10-year follow-up. Arch Intern Med 2008;168(3):297–301.

31. Bassetti CL, Milanova M, Gugger M. Sleep-disordered breathing and acute ischemic stroke: diagnosis, risk factors, treatment, evolution, and long-term clinical outcome. Stroke 2006;37(4):967–72.

32. Parra O, Arboix A, Montserrat JM, et al. Sleep-related breathing disorders: impact on mortality of cerebrovascular disease. Eur Respir J 2004; 24(2):267–72.

33. O'Connor GT, Caffo B, Newman AB, et al. Prospective study of sleep-disordered breathing and hypertension: the Sleep Heart Health Study. Am J Respir Crit Care Med 2009;179(12):1159–64.

34. Kario K, Pickering TG, Matsuo T, et al. Stroke prognosis and abnormal nocturnal blood pressure falls in older hypertensives. Hypertension 2001;38(4): 852–7.

35. Phillips SA, Olson EB, Lombard JH, et al. Chronic intermittent hypoxia alters NE reactivity and mechanics of skeletal muscle resistance arteries. J Appl Physiol 2006;100(4):1117–23.

36. Balfors EM, Franklin KA. Impairment of cerebral perfusion during obstructive sleep apneas. Am J Respir Crit Care Med 1994;150(6 Pt 1):1587–91.

37. Hajak G, Klingelhofer J, Schulz-Varszegi M, et al. Sleep apnea syndrome and cerebral hemodynamics. Chest 1996;110(3):670–9.

38. Kato M, Roberts-Thomson P, Phillips BG, et al. Impairment of endothelium-dependent vasodilation of resistance vessels in patients with obstructive sleep apnea. Circulation 2000;102(21):2607–10.

39. Furtner M, Staudacher M, Frauscher B, et al. Cerebral vasoreactivity decreases overnight in severe obstructive sleep apnea syndrome: a study of cerebral hemodynamics. Sleep Med 2009;10(8):875–81.

40. Franklin KA. Cerebral haemodynamics in obstructive sleep apnoea and Cheyne-Stokes respiration. Sleep Med Rev 2002;6(6):429–41.

41. Jelic S, Lederer DJ, Adams T, et al. Vascular inflammation in obesity and sleep apnea. Circulation 2010;121(8):1014–21.

42. Dziewas R, Ritter M, Usta N, et al. Atherosclerosis and obstructive sleep apnea in patients with ischemic stroke. Cerebrovasc Dis 2007;24(1):122–6.

43. Szaboova E, Tomori Z, Donic V, et al. Sleep apnoea inducing hypoxemia is associated with early signs of carotid atherosclerosis in males. Respir Physiol Neurobiol 2007;155(2):121–7.

44. Drager LF, Bortolotto LA, Krieger EM, et al. Additive effects of obstructive sleep apnea and hypertension on early markers of carotid atherosclerosis. Hypertension 2009;53(1):64–9.

45. Saletu M, Nosiska D, Kapfhammer G, et al. Structural and serum surrogate markers of cerebrovascular disease in obstructive sleep apnea (OSA): association of mild OSA with early atherosclerosis. J Neurol 2006;253(6):746–52.

46. Bokinsky G, Miller M, Ault K, et al. Spontaneous platelet activation and aggregation during obstructive sleep apnea and its response to therapy with nasal continuous positive airway pressure. A preliminary investigation. Chest 1995;108(3): 625–30.

47. Mehra R, Xu F, Babineau DC, et al. Sleep-disordered breathing and prothrombotic biomarkers: cross-sectional results of the Cleveland Family Study. Am J Respir Crit Care Med 2010;182(6):826–33.

48. von Kanel R, Natarajan L, Ancoli-Israel S, et al. Day/Night rhythm of hemostatic factors in obstructive sleep apnea. Sleep 2010;33(3):371–7.

49. Sacco RL, Boden-Albala B, Abel G, et al. Race-ethnic disparities in the impact of stroke risk factors: the northern Manhattan stroke study. Stroke 2001;32(8):1725–31.

50. Gami AS, Pressman G, Caples SM, et al. Association of atrial fibrillation and obstructive sleep apnea. Circulation 2004;110(4):364–7.

51. Mehra R, Benjamin EJ, Shahar E, et al. Association of nocturnal arrhythmias with sleep-disordered breathing: the Sleep Heart Health Study. Am J Respir Crit Care Med 2006;173(8):910–6.

52. Kanagala R, Murali NS, Friedman PA, et al. Obstructive sleep apnea and the recurrence of atrial fibrillation. Circulation 2003;107(20):2589–94.

53. Epstein LJ, Kristo D, Strollo PJ Jr, et al. Clinical guideline for the evaluation, management and long-term care of obstructive sleep apnea in adults. J Clin Sleep Med 2009;5(3):263–76.

54. Srijithesh PR, Shukla G, Srivastav A, et al. Validity of the Berlin Questionnaire in identifying obstructive sleep apnea syndrome when administered to the informants of stroke patients. J Clin Neurosci 2011;18(3):340–3.

55. Arzt M, Young T, Peppard PE, et al. Dissociation of obstructive sleep apnea from hypersomnolence and obesity in patients with stroke. Stroke 2010; 41(3):e129–34.

56. Broadley SA, Jorgensen L, Cheek A, et al. Early investigation and treatment of obstructive sleep apnoea after acute stroke. J Clin Neurosci 2007; 14(4):328–33.

57. Brown DL, Lisabeth LD, Zupancic MJ, et al. High prevalence of supine sleep in ischemic stroke patients. Stroke 2008;39(9):2511–4.

58. Guest JF, Helter MT, Morga A, et al. Cost-effectiveness of using continuous positive airway pressure in the treatment of severe obstructive sleep apnoea/hypopnoea syndrome in the UK. Thorax 2008;63(10):860–5.

59. Chin K, Ohi M, Kita H, et al. Effects of NCPAP therapy on fibrinogen levels in obstructive sleep

apnea syndrome. Am J Respir Crit Care Med 1996; 153(6 Pt 1):1972–6.

60. Phillips CL, Yang Q, Williams A, et al. The effect of short-term withdrawal from continuous positive airway pressure therapy on sympathetic activity and markers of vascular inflammation in subjects with obstructive sleep apnoea. J Sleep Res 2007; 16(2):217–25.

61. Alajmi M, Mulgrew AT, Fox J, et al. Impact of continuous positive airway pressure therapy on blood pressure in patients with obstructive sleep apnea hypopnea: a meta-analysis of randomized controlled trials. Lung 2007;185(2):67–72.

62. Turnbull F, Blood Pressure Lowering Treatment Trialists' Collaboration. Effects of different blood-pressure-lowering regimens on major cardiovascular events: results of prospectively-designed overviews of randomised trials. Lancet 2003; 362(9395):1527–35.

63. Dawson A, Abel SL, Loving RT, et al. CPAP therapy of obstructive sleep apnea in type 2 diabetics improves glycemic control during sleep. J Clin Sleep Med 2008;4(6):538–42.

64. Summers D, Leonard A, Wentworth D, et al. Comprehensive overview of nursing and interdisciplinary care of the acute ischemic stroke patient: a scientific statement from the American Heart Association. Stroke 2009;40(8):2911–44.

65. Sandberg O, Franklin KA, Bucht G, et al. Nasal continuous positive airway pressure in stroke patients with sleep apnoea: a randomized treatment study. Eur Respir J 2001;18(4):630–4.

66. Wessendorf TE, Wang YM, Thilmann AF, et al. Treatment of obstructive sleep apnoea with nasal continuous positive airway pressure in stroke. Eur Respir J 2001;18(4):623–9.

67. Bravata DM, Concato J, Fried T, et al. Auto-titrating continuous positive airway pressure for patients with acute transient ischemic attack: a randomized feasibility trial. Stroke 2010;41(7):1464–70.

68. Bravata DM, Concato J, Fried T, et al. Continuous positive airway pressure: evaluation of a novel therapy for patients with acute ischemic stroke. Sleep 2011;34(9):1271–7.

69. Palombini L, Guilleminault C. Stroke and treatment with nasal CPAP. Eur J Neurol 2006;13(2):198–200.

70. Cherkassky T, Oksenberg A, Froom P, et al. Sleep-related breathing disorders and rehabilitation outcome of stroke patients: a prospective study. Am J Phys Med Rehabil 2003;82(6):452–5.

71. Good DC, Henkle JQ, Gelber D, et al. Sleep-disordered breathing and poor functional outcome after stroke. Stroke 1996;27(2):252–9.

72. Thomas RJ, Rosen BR, Stern CE, et al. Functional imaging of working memory in obstructive sleep-disordered breathing. J Appl Physiol 2005;98(6): 2226–34.

73. Ryan CM, Bayley M, Green R, et al. Influence of continuous positive airway pressure on outcomes of rehabilitation in stroke patients with obstructive sleep apnea. Stroke 2011;42(4):1062–7.

74. Cheyne JA. Case of apoplexy in which the fleshy part of the heart was converted into fat. Dublin Hosp Rep 1818;2:216–23.

75. Brown HW, Plum F. The neurologic basis of Cheyne-Stokes respiration. Am J Med 1961;30(6): 849–60.

76. Bassetti C, Aldrich MS, Quint D. Sleep-disordered breathing in patients with acute supra- and infra-tentorial strokes. A prospective study of 39 patients. Stroke 1997;28(9):1765–72.

77. Bonnin-Vilaplana M, Arboix A, Parra O, et al. Sleep-related breathing disorders in acute lacunar stroke. J Neurol 2009;256(12):2036–42.

78. Hanly PJ, Zuberi-Khokhar NS. Increased mortality associated with Cheyne-Stokes respiration in patients with congestive heart failure. Am J Respir Crit Care Med 1996;153(1):272–6.

79. Javaheri S, Parker TJ, Liming JD, et al. Sleep apnea in 81 ambulatory male patients with stable heart failure. Types and their prevalences, consequences, and presentations. Circulation 1998; 97(21):2154–9.

80. Churchill ED, Cope O. The rapid shallow breathing resulting from pulmonary congestion and edema. J Exp Med 1929;49(4):531–7.

81. Nopmaneejumruslers C, Kaneko Y, Hajek V, et al. Cheyne-Stokes respiration in stroke: relationship to hypocapnia and occult cardiac dysfunction. Am J Respir Crit Care Med 2005;171(9):1048–52.

82. Rowat AM, Dennis MS, Wardlaw JM. Hypoxaemia in acute stroke is frequent and worsens outcome. Cerebrovasc Dis 2006;21(3):166–72.

83. Franklin KA, Eriksson P, Sahlin C, et al. Reversal of central sleep apnea with oxygen. Chest 1997; 111(1):163–9.

84. Sahlin C, Svanborg E, Stenlund H, et al. Cheyne-Stokes respiration and supine dependency. Eur Respir J 2005;25(5):829–33.

85. Szollosi I, Roebuck T, Thompson B, et al. Lateral sleeping position reduces severity of central sleep apnea / Cheyne-Stokes respiration. Sleep 2006; 29(8):1045–51.

86. Teschler H, Dohring J, Wang YM, et al. Adaptive pressure support servo-ventilation: a novel treatment for Cheyne-Stokes respiration in heart failure. Am J Respir Crit Care Med 2001;164(4):614–9.

87. Johnson KG, Johnson DC. Bilevel positive airway pressure worsens central apneas during sleep. Chest 2005;128(4):2141–50.

88. Banno K, Okamura K, Kryger MH. Adaptive servo-ventilation in patients with idiopathic Cheyne-Stokes breathing. J Clin Sleep Med 2006;2(2): 181–6.

89. Vock J, Achermann P, Bischof M, et al. Evolution of sleep and sleep EEG after hemispheric stroke. J Sleep Res 2002;11(4):331–8.

90. Scammell TE, Nishino S, Mignot E, et al. Narcolepsy and low CSF orexin (hypocretin) concentration after a diencephalic stroke. Neurology 2001; 56(12):1751–3.

91. Drake ME Jr. Kleine-Levin syndrome after multiple cerebral infarctions. Psychosomatics 1987;28(6): 329–30.

92. Bassetti CL, Valko P. Poststroke hypersomnia. Sleep Med Clin 2006;1(1):139–55.

93. Elwood P, Hack M, Pickering J, et al. Sleep disturbance, stroke, and heart disease events: evidence from the Caerphilly cohort. J Epidemiol Community Health 2006;60(1):69–73.

94. Leppavuori A, Pohjasvaara T, Vataja R, et al. Insomnia in ischemic stroke patients. Cerebrovasc Dis 2002;14(2):90–7.

95. Chen YK, Lu JY, Mok VC, et al. Clinical and radiologic correlates of insomnia symptoms in ischemic stroke patients. Int J Geriatr Psychiatry 2011;26(5): 451–7.

96. Freemon FR, Salinas-Garcia RF, Ward JW. Sleep patterns in a patient with a brain stem infarction involving the raphe nucleus. Electroencephalogr Clin Neurophysiol 1974;36(6):657–60.

97. Furie KL, Kasner SE, Adams RJ, et al. Guidelines for the prevention of stroke in patients with stroke or transient ischemic attack: a guideline for healthcare professionals from the American heart association/American stroke association. Stroke 2011;42(1):227–76.

98. Palomaki H, Berg A, Meririnne E, et al. Complaints of poststroke insomnia and its treatment with mianserin. Cerebrovasc Dis 2003;15(1–2):56–62.

99. Lazar RM, Fitzsimmons BF, Marshall RS, et al. Reemergence of stroke deficits with midazolam challenge. Stroke 2002;33(1):283–5.

100. Sechi G, Agnetti V, Galistu P, et al. Restless legs syndrome and periodic limb movements after ischemic stroke in the right lenticulostriate region. Parkinsonism Relat Disord 2008;14(2):157–60.

101. Lee SJ, Kim JS, Song IU, et al. Poststroke restless legs syndrome and lesion location: anatomical considerations. Mov Disord 2009;24(1):77–84.

102. Kang SY, Sohn YH, Lee IK, et al. Unilateral periodic limb movement in sleep after supratentorial cerebral infarction. Parkinsonism Relat Disord 2004; 10(7):429–31.

103. Xi Z, Luning W. REM sleep behavior disorder in a patient with pontine stroke. Sleep Med 2009; 10(1):143–6.

104. Elliott WJ. Circadian variation in the timing of stroke onset: a meta-analysis. Stroke 1998;29(5): 992–6.

105. Casetta I, Granieri E, Fallica E, et al. Patient demographic and clinical features and circadian variation in onset of ischemic stroke. Arch Neurol 2002;59(1):48–53.

# Traumatic Brain Injury and Sleep-Wake Disorders

Christian R. Baumann, MD

## KEYWORDS

- TBI • Sleep-wake disorders • Rehabilitation

## KEY POINTS

- Traumatic brain injury (TBI) is defined as an alteration in brain function or other evidence of brain pathology caused by an external force.
- One of the most recent estimates of the prevalence of US civilian residents living with disability following a TBI is 3.2 million.
- Sleep-wake disturbances, such as impaired vigilance or insomnia, and sleep medication, such as benzodiazepines, negatively affect these sequelae in patients with TBIs.

## INTRODUCTION

Traumatic brain injury (TBI) is a prevalent worldwide problem. In the following article, the literature on sleep-wake disorders (SWD) and TBI are reviewed with the objective of providing the reader with a solid understanding of the relationship between TBI and SWD. One of the most recent estimates of the prevalence of US civilian residents living with a disability following a TBI is 3.2 million.[1]

These numbers reveal that TBI belongs among the most prevalent problems encountered in hospitals and outpatient clinical practice. They also reveal that many patients have chronic neurologic impairment following TBI, including neuropsychological and psychiatric symptoms, as well as SWD.[2] In the following, it is shown that these reported proportions of 1:20 (80 000 patients with irreversible neurologic impairment in a total of 1 600 000 patients with TBI) might be a significant underestimation of longstanding neurologic problems after TBI because SWD seem to be much more prevalent after TBI.

## NEUROLOGIC SEQUELAE AFTER TBI

The most common sequela of mild to moderate TBI is postconcussive syndrome, which includes headaches, irritability, dizziness, tinnitus, lethargy, and SWD.[3] These symptoms may persist for weeks, months, and even years. Along with these, multiple neuropsychiatric consequences may complicate the course after TBI, including depression; anxiety; aggressiveness; and cognitive deficits, primarily in the domains of attention, executive functioning, and memory.[4] These deficits may not improve with time.

SWD, such as impaired vigilance or insomnia, and also sleep medication, such as benzodiazepines, negatively affect these sequelae in patients with TBI.[5,6] For instance, it has been shown that sustained attention is impaired in patients with TBI with SWD.[7] In TBI with underlying obstructive sleep apnea, sustained attention and memory are both worse than in patients with TBI without sleep-disordered breathing.[8] In the same line, a study of 443 patients with mild TBI revealed that patients with SWD are more likely to suffer from concomitant headaches, depressive symptoms, and irritability.[9]

Patients with severe TBI or with proven traumatic damage to brain tissue often have additional deficits, such as motor or sensory deficits, tendon reflex asymmetries, and cerebellar or cranial nerve symptoms.

Department of Neurology, University Hospital Zurich, Frauenklinikstrasse 26, Zurich 8091, Switzerland
E-mail address: christian.baumann@usz.ch

Sleep Med Clin 7 (2012) 609–617
http://dx.doi.org/10.1016/j.jsmc.2012.08.002
1556-407X/12/$ – see front matter © 2012 Elsevier Inc. All rights reserved.

## EPIDEMIOLOGY AND CHARACTERISTICS OF POSTTRAUMATIC SWD

Traumatic injuries to the brain are very heterogeneous about the kind, localization, and severity of trauma, which sets strict boundaries to systematic epidemiologic and clinical studies. Furthermore, most of the few studies on posttraumatic SWD have been performed in retrospective settings, which does not allow drawing conclusions regarding the epidemiology of posttraumatic SWD.

Cohen and coworkers[10] published one of the first systematic studies on SWD following TBI. The investigators obtained SWD in 22 hospitalized patients with recent TBI and in 77 discharged patients with TBI who experienced their trauma about 2 to 3 years ago. They applied questionnaires and found SWD in 73% of patients with recent TBI and in 52% of discharged patients with previous TBI. The most common complaint in patients with recent TBI was insomnia (81%), whereas excessive daytime sleepiness was more prevalent in patients with TBI 2 to 3 years ago (73%) (**Fig. 1** is the original illustration from this article). Furthermore, the investigators found that SWD in discharged patients with TBI were associated with neuropsychological impairment and poor occupational outcome.

The first systematic and prospective studies on posttraumatic SWD have been published recently. Six months after TBI, the author's group systematically recorded SWD in 65 consecutive patients.[11] For this purpose, they applied structured interviews; questionnaires with validated scales, such as the Epworth sleepiness scale (ESS); and electrophysiological sleep laboratory examinations, including actigraphy, nocturnal polysomnography, and multiple sleep latency tests.[11] Furthermore,

they assessed levels of the wake-promoting hypothalamic neuropeptide hypocretin (orexin) in the cerebrospinal fluid and HLA alleles that are associated with narcolepsy. In 47 patients (72% of the population), trauma-related SWD have been identified, which were not present before the trauma (**Fig. 2**). SWD occurred regardless of the localization or the severity of the trauma and was not associated with gender, clinical outcome, or HLA typing but with significant impairment of quality of life. The most prevalent sleep-wake disturbance following TBI was impaired daytime vigilance (excessive daytime sleepiness with mean sleep latencies <8 minutes on multiple sleep latency test or with pathologic scores on the ESS in 38% and fatigue in 17%). Posttraumatic hypersomnia (increased sleep need per 24 hours: ≥2 hours more than before TBI) was observed in 22%. On the other hand, insomnia was found only in 5% of the patients with TBI. The author's group identified 2 patients who fulfilled the criteria of the current *International Classification of Sleep Disorders, Second Edition* (ICSD-2) for narcolepsy without cataplexy,[12] but patients with posttraumatic narcolepsy with cataplexy were not present in their population. Hypocretin levels were significantly lower in patients with posttraumatic excessive daytime sleepiness (EDS).

In a follow-up study 3 years after TBI in 51 of the same patients, the author's group applied structured interviews and validated questionnaires to assess the long-term outcome of posttraumatic SWD.[13] In this study, they found that most SWD persisted; posttraumatic SWD were still found in 67%, with posttraumatic hypersomnia being the most common (27%). Excessive daytime sleepiness was less prevalent (12%) than 6 months after

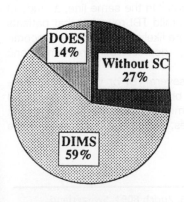

**Hospitalised Patients**

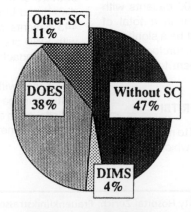

**Discharged Patients**

**Fig. 1.** Distribution of sleep complaints (SC) in early and late groups of patients with TBI. DIMS, disorders in initiating and maintaining sleep; DOES, disorders of excessive daytime somnolence. (*From* Cohen M, Oksenberg A, Snir D, et al. Temporally related changes of sleep complaints in traumatic brain injured patients. J Neurol Neurosurg Psychiatry 1992;55:313–5.)

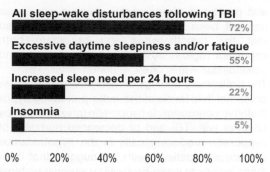

**Fig. 2.** Frequency of trauma-related SWD in the first prospective study in 65 consecutive patients with TBI. SWD have been assessed and characterized by interviews, questionnaires, and sleep laboratory examinations, including polysomnography, multiple sleep latency tests, and actigraphy.

TBI, but fatigue was more common (35%). Insomnia was found in 10%. Again, SWD were not associated with severity or localization of, or time interval since, the TBI. Insomnia, however, was linked to depressive symptoms. The results of the long-term outcome study highlight the chronic aspect of impairments caused by post-traumatic SWD and possibly reflect the lack of effective treatment.[14]

Regarding the high prevalence of sleepiness as opposed to much less common insomnia in patients with TBI, a Canadian group made observations that corroborate this finding. The member of this group recorded daytime electroencephalography and nocturnal polysomnography and assessed validated questionnaires in 21 athletes with and without multiple sport-related concussions.[15] Concussed athletes reported impaired quality of night sleep, but polysomnographic recordings did not reveal any differences between concussed and nonconcussed athletes. However, waking electroencephalogram (EEG) during daytime showed enhanced delta activity, suggesting that wakefulness rather than sleep might be impaired after TBI.

Almost at the same time as the study conducted by the author's group, another prospective clinical and sleep laboratory study of 87 patients at least 3 months (64 ± 118 months) after TBI applied nocturnal polysomnography; the multiple sleep latency test (MSLT); the psychomotor vigilance test; and validated scales, such as the ESS. The investigators found abnormal sleep studies in 46% of the examined population, with excessive daytime sleepiness as the most common finding (25%).[16] The latter was defined as mean sleep latencies on MSLT less than 10 minutes. In addition, psychomotor vigilance test results were worse in patients with low mean sleep latencies. In detail, 23% of patients had obstructive sleep apnea, 6% had narcolepsy (typical cataplexy was not reported), and 7% had periodic limb movements in sleep. Characteristics of TBI were not linked to excessive daytime sleepiness, but higher body mass indices and obstructive sleep apnea were more common in sleepy patients. Interestingly, sleepy patients reported better self-rated quality of life than nonsleepy patients, but cognitive outcomes as assessed with questionnaires were not influenced by the presence or absence of sleepiness.

A longitudinal observational study in 54 patients with closed TBI used interviews and applied scales to evaluate sleep problems within 3 months after trauma.[17] As compared with before TBI, patients reported more prevalent sleep disturbances, including shortness of breath and headache, and, more commonly, excessive daytime sleepiness. Anxiety as assessed with the Structured Clinical Interview for *DSM-IV* Axis 1 Disorders (SCID-IV) was the most consistent risk factor for the development of posttraumatic SWD.

Schreiber and colleagues[18] evaluated the sleep-wake pattern with polysomnography and MSLTs in 26 patients with prior minor TBI and with normal cranial computerized tomography. Minor TBI was defined as a brain concussion that can cause a short (up to 30 minutes) transient loss or impairment of consciousness, accompanied by vomiting or some degree of amnesia. They found significant alterations in nocturnal sleep architecture, with higher non–rapid eye movement (NREM) stage 2 amounts compared with controls (55% vs 47%) and lower amounts of REM sleep (21 vs 25%). The MSLTs revealed signs of excessive daytime sleepiness, with mean sleep latencies being much shorter in injured patients than in controls (6 vs 17 minutes).

In 2007, Verma and colleagues[19] conducted a retrospective study of 60 patients with TBI. Nothing was known about their sleep and wakefulness before the trauma. Three months up to 2 years following TBI, the following examinations were performed in different subsets of patients: nocturnal polysomnography (n = 54), MSLTs (n = 28), and a variety of different questionnaires. Subjective excessive daytime sleepiness, as assessed with the ESS, was present in 52%; 53% of patients who underwent MSLTs had mean sleep latencies less than 5 minutes. Nine of these patients had additional multiple sleep onset REM periods, which is a biomarker either of narcolepsy without cataplexy or of chronic sleep deprivation.[12,20] Insomnia as reported by patients was present in 25%.

## POSTTRAUMATIC EXCESSIVE DAYTIME SLEEPINESS

Excessive daytime sleepiness is characterized by a difficulty to prevent oneself from falling asleep during daytime. Already in 1983, Guilleminault and colleagues[21] noted the importance of recognizing excessive daytime sleepiness as a residual symptom after TBI. In their study, they found sleep apnea in a significant portion of their sleepy patients with TBI. Similarly, 18 years later, Masel and coworkers[22] investigated a case series of 71 patients with TBI enrolled consecutively into a residential rehabilitation program, and they performed nocturnal polysomnography MSLTs, and applied structured questionnaires. Mean sleep latencies less than 10 minutes were found in 47% and less than 5 minutes in 18% of their population. Among these sleepy patients, a relatively high prevalence of sleep apnea–hypopnea syndrome and periodic limb movement disorder was found, suggesting that these specific sleep disorders might account for excessive daytime sleepiness following TBI. In the same line, Castriotta and colleagues[23] provided a prospective cohort study including polysomnography and MSLTs in 10 patients with TBI with subjective excessive daytime sleepiness. They found that treatable SWD are common in patients with TBI with excessive daytime sleepiness, for they found a specific sleep disorder in every single patient, particularly sleep-disordered breathing but also narcolepsy.

More recent and prospective data, however, showed that in most patients with TBI, posttraumatic excessive daytime sleepiness cannot be explained by underlying SWD, neurologic, or other disorders.[11,16] Contrariwise, these data suggest that posttraumatic excessive daytime sleepiness is directly related to the neuronal injury itself. The underlying pathophysiology, however, is not known. A clear association between TBI characteristics, such as severity or localization of the trauma,

and posttraumatic excessive daytime sleepiness has not been found.[11,16] Early studies revealed that the hypothalamus and brainstem—both important regions in the regulation of sleep and wakefulness—are often lesioned after TBI.[24,25] The preliminary findings of mildly decreased cerebrospinal fluid levels of the wake-promoting hypothalamic neuropeptide hypocretin (orexin) in sleepy patients with TBI and of decreased numbers of hypocretin-producing cells in the hypothalamus of deceased patients with TBI suggest that traumatic lesions to wake-promoting neuronal systems might contribute to posttraumatic excessive sleepiness (**Fig. 3**).[11,26]

In narcolepsy, another disorder with severe excessive daytime sleepiness, hypocretin levels are markedly decreased and hypocretin-producing neurons are almost completely lost.[27] The existence of posttraumatic narcolepsy, however, is still a matter of debate. Previous studies suggested that narcolepsy might be common after TBI.[22,23] However, narcolepsy with cataplexy, which is characterized by loss of muscle tone with strong emotions, is exceedingly rare after TBI. Furthermore, there is evidence that the present diagnostic criteria for narcolepsy without cataplexy might be unspecific and lead to a large number of false-positive diagnoses of narcolepsy.[20,28]

### Diagnosis and Management

In patients with TBI, excessive daytime sleepiness can be assessed by interviews; questionnaires, such as the ESS or the Karolinska Sleepiness Scale; and more objectively by sleep laboratory examinations, such as the MSLT. During this test, patients are asked to go to bed for 20 minutes every 2 hours at daytime, and the latencies to falling asleep are measured. In patients with excessive daytime sleepiness, mean sleep latencies for all 4 to 5 tests are typically less than 5 to 8 minutes. Furthermore, to rule out other causes of excessive

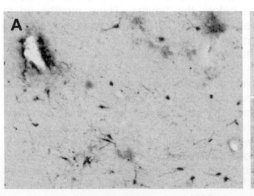
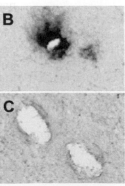

**Fig. 3.** Besides numerical loss of hypocretin cells, patients with TBI have dense perivascular hypocretin immunoreactivity within the hypothalamic hypocretin field (*A, B*) but not in adjacent areas (*C*).

daytime sleepiness, such as a specific SWD (eg, sleep apnea, periodic limb movements during sleep) or other disorders (eg, hypothyroidism), appropriate tests, including laboratory and polysomnography studies, should be performed.

Excessive daytime sleepiness impairs daytime functioning and the quality of life of patients with TBI[11,16]; therefore, treatment is warranted. But until now, no specific therapy for posttraumatic excessive daytime sleepiness has been tested or approved. If an underlying disorder can be identified, it should be treated[29]; obstructive sleep apnea should be treated with continuous positive airway pressure (CPAP), and periodic limb movements may be treated with dopaminergic drugs, if necessary. Castriotta and colleagues[29] found that the treatment of sleep disorders after TBI, such as sleep apnea, may result in polysomnographic resolution, but excessive daytime sleepiness or neuropsychological dysfunction may persist.

The stimulant modafinil is used to treat excessive daytime sleepiness in a variety of disorders. In contrast to the first encouraging case reports and small series, a recent study could not confirm a beneficial effect from modafinil, which is used for the treatment of excessive daytime sleepiness in different disorders, on posttraumatic excessive daytime sleepiness.[30] The author's prospective placebo-controlled and double-blind trial in 20 patients with TBI with excessive daytime sleepiness or fatigue, however, provides class I evidence that modafinil (100–200 mg daily) improves posttraumatic EDS but not fatigue compared with placebo (**Fig. 4**).[31] Nevertheless, facing the fact that treatment even with potent stimulants remains unsuccessful in many sleepy and fatigued patients with TBI, further studies to delineate treatment strategies for sleepy patients with TBI are urgently needed.

# POSTTRAUMATIC FATIGUE

Fatigue can be defined as a subjective experience and includes such symptoms as rapid inanition, persisting lack of energy, exhaustion, physical and mental tiredness, and apathy.[32] Definite conclusions regarding fatigue after TBI cannot be drawn because of the inconsistent definition of fatigue, the fact that the few present studies on posttraumatic fatigue used a multitude of different assessment scales that have not been validated properly, and the difficulty that fatigue cannot be measured by objective tests.

Fatigue as assessed by the Fatigue Impact Scale and the Fatigue Severity Scale was found to be common in patients with TBI.[33] In the study conducted by the author's group 3 years after TBI, the validated Fatigue Severity Scale was applied and identified fatigue in 35%.[13,34] Similarly, another study used the global fatigue index and observed that fatigue is more common and pronounced in patients with TBI compared with healthy controls.[35] The investigators found associations with other symptoms, such as pain, depression, and SWD, but not with specific TBI characteristics. This finding is in line with another recent study that found that fatigue is robustly correlated with gender, depression, pain, and memory and motor dysfunction; but there was no correlation between pituitary dysfunction and fatigue.[36]

## Diagnosis and Management

The pathophysiology of fatigue in general and also of posttraumatic fatigue is not known. Therefore, there are no laboratory tests to diagnose fatigue. Similarly, fatigue cannot be diagnosed based on specific electrophysiological sleep laboratory tests. Besides the possibility of structured interviews, there is a multitude of different fatigue assessment scales to diagnose and quantify fatigue. However, only a few of them have been validated, mostly in small studies and for specific disorders. The Fatigue Severity Scale is one of the most commonly used self-report questionnaires to measure fatigue and has recently been validated in a large sample.[34] A specific therapy for posttraumatic fatigue is not available. Treatment of concomitant depression, pain, or SWD might help alleviate fatigue in patients with TBI. In recent studies, modafinil failed to show beneficial effects on fatigue following TBI.[30,31]

# POSTTRAUMATIC HYPERSOMNIA

Hypersomnia is defined by increased sleep need per 24 hours and must be distinguished from excessive daytime sleepiness (increased daytime

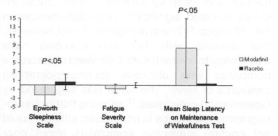

**Fig. 4.** In patients with TBI, modafinil (100–200 mg) improves subjective excessive daytime sleepiness, as assessed with the ESS, and enhances the ability to stay awake during nonstimulating conditions, as measured with the maintenance of wakefulness test. Fatigue, as assessed with the fatigue severity scale, is not improved by modafinil.

sleep propensity [ie, difficulty fighting sleep during the daytime]). In the literature, the 2 entities are mostly confounded. In fact, if somebody searches for specific information on posttraumatic hypersomnia, he or she is most likely to end up with studies on posttraumatic excessive daytime sleepiness, whereas specific studies on hypersomnia are exceedingly sparse.

In the context of TBI, a reasonable definition of posttraumatic hypersomnia could be increased sleep need of 2 hours or more compared with pre-TBI conditions. In the prospective study of 65 patients with TBI conducted by the author's group, this definition was applied and found that most patients with posttraumatic SWD had either hypersomnia or excessive daytime sleepiness/fatigue.[11] Furthermore, an association between severity of TBI and the presence of hypersomnia was found. In light of these findings, it could be hypothesized whether the primary SWD after TBI may be hypersomnia. Thus, patients whose psychosocial environment allows extended sleeping times per 24 hours may avoid increased sleep propensity at daytime, whereas in patients who cannot compensate the increased sleep need, excessive daytime sleepiness may occur. This hypothesis is supported by the finding of increased excessive daytime sleepiness/fatigue in patients between 30 and 50 years of age, whose social environment normally does not allow longer sleeping times (tight work schedules, families with young children) and of hypersomnia in younger or older patients.[11]

### Diagnosis and Management

Posttraumatic hypersomnia can be diagnosed by interviews, sleep logs that are filled in by patients, and by wrist actigraphy that measures motor activity and light and calculates time asleep and time awake during a defined period of usually 1 to 2 weeks. Regarding actigraphy, a recent article proposed criteria for its use in patients with TBI.[37] According to the proposed guidelines, patients should be cognitively fit and the device should be placed on the least affected limb in patients with paresis, significant spasticity, or contractures of one or more limbs. Furthermore, for patients with tetraparesis, the investigators stated that a wrist actigraphy device may not be an appropriate instrument for measurement of rest and activity; instead, placing it on the head rather than limbs or torso should be considered.

The cause of posttraumatic hypersomnia is not known, and a specific treatment is not available because there have been no systematic studies on this topic so far. Clinical practice tells us that treatment of posttraumatic hypersomnia is frustrating.

## POSTTRAUMATIC INSOMNIA

Insomnia is defined as a chronic inability to fall asleep or remain asleep for an adequate length of time at night. Previous studies yielded contradictory results on the prevalence of insomnia in patients with TBI. A prospective study based on sleep questionnaires observed a high prevalence (30%) of insomnia symptoms in 50 patients after TBI.[38] In a retrospective study comprising a population of 184 somnolent patients who suffered a TBI or a head-neck trauma (whiplash injury), almost half of the patients reported disturbed nocturnal sleep, which was mostly caused by nocturnal pain.[39]

Another study examined sleep-wake diaries of 63 patients with TBI and 63 healthy controls. The major finding was an increased number of nighttime awakenings and higher latencies from wakefulness to sleep in patients with TBI, particularly in those with mild injuries, anxiety, and depression.[40] Two years later, the same group published a report on polysomnographic findings in 10 patients with TBI and in 10 controls.[41] The investigators found that patients with TBI reported poorer sleep quality and higher levels of psychiatric symptoms, such as anxiety and depression. Polysomnographic recordings, on the other hand, revealed an increase in deep sleep (NREM 3), a reduction in REM sleep, and higher arousal indices. These changes in sleep covaried with anxiety and depression.

In a questionnaire study, more than 50% of 452 patients with TBI reported insomnia symptoms.[42] Risk factors associated with insomnia were milder injuries, higher levels of fatigue, depression, and pain. In the same direction, the same group compared 14 patients with TBI with 14 healthy good sleepers, and all subjective measures of sleep as assessed by the questionnaires revealed significant sleep disturbances in the TBI group.[43] The investigators found, however, that patients with TBI with insomnia have a tendency to overestimate their sleep disturbance compared with objective (polysomnographic) measures of sleep. The same was suggested by Gosselin and colleagues,[15] showing that polysomnographic recordings in concussed athletes could not confirm subjective complaints about poor nocturnal sleep quality.

Similarly, the prospective study by the author's group including objective sleep laboratory tests has found insomnia in only 5% of patients.[11] Together, these studies suggest that insomnia may be common but overestimated after TBI.

## Diagnosis and Management

Posttraumatic insomnia seems to be related to depression and anxiety.[38,42] Thus, the screening for and treatment of psychiatric comorbidities should be performed in patients that complain of posttraumatic insomnia. Hypnotic medications still remain the most frequent treatment of insomnia in clinical practice. Hypnotics are effective for the short-term relief of insomnia but exhibit side and tolerance effects. Newer treatment strategies, such as hypocretin antagonists, are currently being evaluated, but recent evolutions suggest that these compounds may not reach approval swiftly, if ever. A recent study suggested that psychologic interventions, including cognitive-behavioral therapies for insomnia, are a promising therapeutic strategy for patients with TBI.[44]

## POSTTRAUMATIC CIRCADIAN SWD

The findings pertaining to circadian SWD following TBI are sparse and rather inconclusive. Anecdotal reports on a posttraumatic delayed sleep phase syndrome have been published, but a study of 10 patients using questionnaires, sleep diaries, polysomnography, and saliva melatonin measurements failed to provide evidence of any shift in circadian timing of sleep after TBI.[45,46] Contrariwise, a recent study of 42 patients with minor TBI with complaints of insomnia have been examined by actigraphy, saliva melatonin, and oral temperature measurements.[47] The investigators found circadian SWD in 36% of these patients. Two types of circadian SWD were observed: delayed sleep

phase syndrome and irregular sleep-wake pattern (see **Fig. 2**). The observation of frequent circadian SWD following TBI further supports the assumption that posttraumatic insomnia might be overestimated (see paragraph on insomnia).

The exact pathophysiology of posttraumatic circadian SWD remains elusive. However, a recent observational study in observational study comparing 23 patients with TBI to 2 matched healthy subjects assessed polysomnographic sleep measures, salivary dim light melatonin onset (DLMO) time, and self-reported sleep quality, anxiety, and depression.[48] In this study, patients with TBI showed significantly lower levels of evening melatonin production, together with more frequent complaints of sleep problems and symptoms of depression or anxiety. The investigators concluded that reduced evening melatonin production caused by traumatic brain damage may indicate a disruption to circadian regulation of sleep and wakefulness.

## Diagnosis and Management

The clinical diagnosis of circadian SWD is based on a detailed interview, sleep diaries, and actigraphy studies with or without additional saliva melatonin measurement (**Fig. 5**). Treatments with melatonin or bright light, which aim to synchronize the sleep-wake cycle with the environmental dark-light cycle, are appropriate therapeutic strategies for these patients.[47]

In conclusion, present evidence suggests that excessive daytime sleepiness and hypersomnia (ie, enhanced sleep need per 24 hours) might be

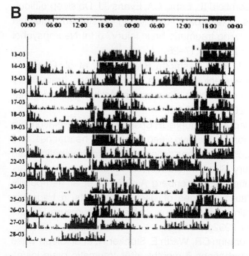

**Fig. 5.** Actigraphy findings of patients with delayed sleep phase syndrome (A) and irregular sleep-wake pattern (B). The horizontal lines show the times of the day and the vertical lines distinguish between different days of a 2-week observation period. Sleep episodes are represented by very low/nonexistent lines (*white areas*) and wake episodes by greater activity (*black areas*). (*From* Guilleminault C, Faull KF, Miles L, et al. Posttraumatic excessive daytime sleepiness: a review of 20 patients. Neurology 1983;33:1584–9; with permission.)

the most prevalent SWD following TBI. These SWD can be caused by underlying problems, such as sleep apnea or periodic limb movements during sleep, but they seem to be caused by the trauma itself in many patients. On the other hand, there are indications that posttraumatic insomnia might be overestimated. All studies, either retrospective or prospective, based on questionnaires or on sleep laboratory studies, suggest that posttraumatic SWD are frequent, impair quality of life and general outcome after TBI, and can persist for many years.

## REFERENCES

1. Maegele M, Engel D, Bouillon B, et al. Incidence and outcome of traumatic brain injury in an urban area in Western Europe over 10 years. Eur Surg Res 2007; 39:372–9.

2. Corrigan JD, Selassie AW, Orman JA. The epidemiology of traumatic brain injury. J Head Trauma Rehabil 2010;25:72–80.

3. Ingebrigtsen T, Waterloo K, Marup-Jensen S, et al. Quantification of post-concussion symptoms 3 months after minor head injury in 100 consecutive patients. J Neurol 1998;245:609–12.

4. Starkstein SE, Jorge R. Dementia after traumatic brain injury. Int Psychogeriatr 2005;17(Suppl 1):S93–107.

5. Mahmood O, Rapport LJ, Hanks RA, et al. Neuropsychological performance and sleep disturbance following traumatic brain injury. J Head Trauma Rehabil 2004;19:378–90.

6. Larson EB, Zollman FS. The effect of sleep medications on cognitive recovery from traumatic brain injury. J Head Trauma Rehabil 2010;25:61–7.

7. Bloomfield IL, Espie CA, Evans JJ. Do sleep difficulties exacerbate deficits in sustained attention following traumatic brain injury? J Int Neuropsychol Soc 2010;16:17–25.

8. Wilde MC, Castriotta RJ, Lai JM, et al. Cognitive impairment in patients with traumatic brain injury and obstructive sleep apnea. Arch Phys Med Rehabil 2007;88:1284–8.

9. Chaput G, Giguère JF, Chauny JM, et al. Relationship among subjective sleep complaints, headaches, and mood alterations following a mild traumatic brain injury. Sleep Med 2009;10:713–6.

10. Cohen M, Oksenberg A, Snir D, et al. Temporally related changes of sleep complaints in traumatic brain injured patients. J Neurol Neurosurg Psychiatry 1992;55:313–5.

11. Baumann CR, Werth E, Stocker R, et al. Sleep-wake disturbances 6 months after traumatic brain injury: a prospective study. Brain 2007;130:1873–83.

12. AASM (American Academy of Sleep Medicine). International classification of sleep disorders (ICSD-2), diagnostic and coding manual. 2nd edition. Westchester (IL): American Academy of Sleep Disorders Association; 2005.

13. Kempf J, Werth E, Kaiser PR, et al. Sleep-wake disturbances 3 years after traumatic brain injury. J Neurol Neurosurg Psychiatry 2010;81:1402–5.

14. Gosselin N, Tellier M. Patients with traumatic brain injury are at high risk of developing chronic sleep-wake disturbances. J Neurol Neurosurg Psychiatry 2010;81:1297.

15. Gosselin N, Lassonde M, Petit D, et al. Sleep following sport-related concussions. Sleep Med 2009;10:35–46.

16. Castriotta RJ, Wilde MC, Lai JM, et al. Prevalence and consequences of sleep disorders in traumatic brain injury. J Clin Sleep Med 2007;3:349–56.

17. Rao V, Spiro J, Vaishnavi S, et al. Prevalence and types of sleep disturbances acutely after traumatic brain injury. Brain Inj 2008;22:381–6.

18. Schreiber S, Barkai G, Gur-Hartman T, et al. Long-lasting sleep patterns of adult patients with minor traumatic brain injury (mTBI) and non-mTBI subjects. Sleep Med 2008;9:481–7.

19. Verma A, Anand V, Verma NP. Sleep disorders in chronic traumatic brain injury. J Clin Sleep Med 2007;3:357–62.

20. Marti I, Valko PO, Khatami R, et al. Multiple sleep latency measures in narcolepsy and behaviourally induced insufficient sleep syndrome. Sleep Med 2009;10:1146–50.

21. Guilleminault C, Faull KF, Miles L, et al. Posttraumatic excessive daytime sleepiness: a review of 20 patients. Neurology 1983;33:1584–9.

22. Masel BE, Scheibel RS, Kimbark T, et al. Excessive daytime sleepiness in adults with brain injuries. Arch Phys Med Rehabil 2001;82:1526–32.

23. Castriotta RJ, Lai JM. Sleep disorders associated with traumatic brain injury. Arch Phys Med Rehabil 2001;82:1403–6.

24. Crompton MR. Hypothalamic lesions following closed head injury. Brain 1971;94:165–72.

25. Crompton MR. Brainstem lesions due to closed head injury. Lancet 1971;1:669–73.

26. Baumann CR, Bassetti CL, Valko PO, et al. Loss of hypocretin (orexin) neurons with traumatic brain injury. Ann Neurol 2009;66:555–9.

27. Baumann CR, Bassetti CL. Hypocretins (orexins) and sleep-wake disorders. Lancet Neurol 2005;4: 673–82.

28. Mignot E, Lin L, Finn L, et al. Correlates of sleep-onset REM periods during the multiple sleep latency test in community adults. Brain 2006;129:1609–23.

29. Castriotta RJ, Atanasov S, Wilde MC, et al. Treatment of sleep disorders after traumatic brain injury. J Clin Sleep Med 2009;5:137–44.

30. Jha A, Weintraub A, Allshouse A, et al. A randomized trial of modafinil for the treatment of fatigue and excessive daytime sleepiness in individuals with

chronic traumatic brain injury. J Head Trauma Rehabil 2008;23:52–63.

31. Kaiser PR, Valko PO, Werth E, et al. Modafinil ameliorates excessive daytime sleepiness after traumatic brain injury. Neurology 2010;75:1780–5.

32. Chaudhuri A, Behan PO. Fatigue in neurological disorders. Lancet 2004;363:978–88.

33. LaChapelle DL, Finlayson MA. An evaluation of subjective and objective measures of fatigue in patients with brain injury and healthy controls. Brain Inj 1998;12:649–59.

34. Valko PO, Bassetti CL, Bloch KE, et al. Validation of the fatigue severity scale in a Swiss cohort. Sleep 2008;31:1601–7.

35. Cantor JB, Ashman T, Gordon W, et al. Fatigue after traumatic brain injury and its impact on participation and quality of life. J Head Trauma Rehabil 2008;23: 41–51.

36. Englander J, Bushnik T, Oggins J, et al. Fatigue after traumatic brain injury: association with neuroendocrine, sleep, depression and other factors. Brain Inj 2010;24:1379–88.

37. Zollman FS, Cyborski C, Duraski SA. Actigraphy for assessment of sleep in traumatic brain injury: case series, review of the literature and proposed criteria for use. Brain Inj 2010;24:748–54.

38. Fichtenberg NL, Zafonte RD, Putnam S, et al. Insomnia in a post-acute brain injury sample. Brain Inj 2002;16:197–206.

39. Guilleminault C, Yuen KM, Gulevich MG, et al. Hypersomnia after head-neck trauma: a medicolegal dilemma. Neurology 2000;54.653–9.

40. Parcell DL, Ponsford JL, Rajaratnam SM, et al. Self-reported changes to nighttime sleep after traumatic brain injury. Arch Phys Med Rehabil 2006;87: 278–85.

41. Parcell DL, Ponsford JL, Redman JR, et al. Poor sleep quality and changes in objectively recorded sleep after traumatic brain injury: a preliminary study. Arch Phys Med Rehabil 2008;89:843–50.

42. Ouellet MC, Beaulieu-Bonneau S, Morin CM. Insomnia in patients with traumatic brain injury: frequency, characteristics, and risk factors. J Head Trauma Rehabil 2006;21:199–212.

43. Ouellet MC, Morin CM. Subjective and objective measures of insomnia in the context of traumatic brain injury: a preliminary study. Sleep Med 2006; 7:486–97.

44. Ouellet MC, Morin CM. Efficacy of cognitive-behavioral therapy for insomnia associated with traumatic brain injury: a single-case experimental design. Arch Phys Med Rehabil 2007;88:1581–92.

45. Quinto C, Gellido C, Chokroverty S, et al. Posttraumatic delayed sleep phase syndrome. Neurology 2000;54:250–2.

46. Steele DL, Rajaratnam SM, Redman JR, et al. The effect of traumatic brain injury on the timing of sleep. Chronobiol Int 2005;22:89–105.

47. Ayalon L, Borodkin K, Dishon L, et al. Circadian rhythm sleep disorders following mild traumatic brain injury. Neurology 2007;68:1136–40.

48. Shekleton JA, Parcell DL, Redman JR, et al. Sleep disturbance and melatonin levels following traumatic brain injury. Neurology 2010;74:1732–8.

# Sleep and Epilepsy

Sudha S. Tallavajhula, MD*, Jeremy D. Slater, MD

## KEYWORDS

- Epilepsy • Sleep disturbances • Seizures • Sleep-Wake cycle • Sleep deprivation

## KEY POINTS

- Epilepsy and sleep have a well-studied, intricately woven relationship. Understanding this relationship and addressing sleep problems in epilepsy patients improves quality of life in this population.
- Certain seizure types and epilepsy syndromes have patterns of temporal synchrony with the sleep-wake cycle.
- Seizures, epilepsy and treatments used for epilepsy are all capable of affecting sleep patterns and subjective sleep quality. Conversely, treatment of sleep-disordered breathing has been shown to improve seizure control.

## INTRODUCTION

For more than 2000 years, scientists have recognized the bidirectional connection between sleep and epilepsy based on timing of seizures with respect to the sleep-wake cycle. In 350 BC, Aristotle noted "for sleep is like epilepsy, and, in a sense, actually is a seizure of this sort. Accordingly, the beginning of this malady takes place with many during sleep, and their subsequent habitual seizures occur in sleep, not in waking hours".[1] In the second century AD, Soranus of Ephesus wrote, among his recommendations for the treatment of epilepsy, "sleep must be undisturbed."[2] At the same time, Galen, in a commentary on Hippocrates Aphorisms, noted that "to sleep on the earth might induce the disease in adolescents."[2] Not long after the time of Hippocrates, Diocles of Carystus further observed that "to go to sleep on ones back might provoke an attack...."[2]

In the classic treatise, *Epilepsy and Other Chronic Convulsive Diseases*, William Gowers[3] documented one of the earliest formal studies of the timing of seizure occurrence in relationship to the sleep-wake cycle. He evaluated the timing of seizures in 840 institutionalized patients and found

that 21% occurred in a given patient only at night, 43% of the seizures occurred only during the day, and the remainder of the seizures occurred in patients by day and night. Seizures occurring just with waking or just with sleep onset occurred in 0.5% and 1% of patients, respectively. Two peaks were reported for the time of occurrence of nocturnal seizures. The first occurred roughly 2 hours past bedtime, and the second occurred between 4 and 5 AM. On longitudinal follow-up, he was able to conclude that the patients whose seizures only occur at night may eventually have them occur by day, but the nocturnal events will continue. But if a patient had only daytime seizures then went on to develop nocturnal seizures, the daytime seizures would disappear.[3] Although this study was limited because it only consisted of clinical reports, such early observations are still of interest, because patients who present with only nocturnal seizures feel they are at little risk for daytime events.

The same peak times noted by Gowers were observed by Langdon-Down and Brain,[4] who additionally identified a diurnal epilepsy with the first peak occurring shortly after waking between

Sudha Tallavajhula has no disclosures to report.
Jeremy Slater is on the speaker's bureau for UCB, Lundbeck and Cyberonics. He serves as a consultant for Lundbeck and Cyberonics.
Department of Neurology, University of Texas Health Sciences Center, 6431 Fannin, MSB 7.044, Houston, TX 77030, USA
* Corresponding author.
E-mail address: Sudha.S.Tallavajhula@uth.tmc.edu

Sleep Med Clin 7 (2012) 619–630
http://dx.doi.org/10.1016/j.jsmc.2012.10.001
1556-407X/12/$ – see front matter © 2012 Elsevier Inc. All rights reserved.

sleep.theclinics.com

7 and 8 AM. These findings were again limited to clinical observations, given that Berger's first report of the human electroencephalogram only appeared the same year.[5] The first report of the relationship of interictal epileptiform activity and sleep came from Gibbs and Gibbs in 1947,[6] and noted an increase in interictal epileptiform activity during sleep compared with the waking state. In 1953, Janz[7] described an epilepsy syndrome with seizures occurring within the first 2 hours after waking (awakening epilepsy). He was the first to note this type of epilepsy as having an identifiable organic cause only 10% of the time. Patients suffering from the "myoclonic epilepsy of Janz" seemed to have inherited their disease 12.5% of the time, and the onset of the seizures most often occurred between ages 10 and 25 years.[8]

The topic of epilepsy and sleep can be roughly divided into 2 parts. First, what is the effect of sleep on epilepsy? Second, what is the effect of epilepsy on sleep? Epilepsy and its treatment influence sleep. Sleep, arousal, and sleep deprivation influence epilepsy. Sleep state modulates both the occurrence of seizures and of interictal epileptiform discharges. Sleepiness and sleep disorders may coexist with epilepsy. Treatment of coexisting sleep disorders may improve seizure control in patients with epilepsy. Lennox and Lennox[9] summarized the complexity of this relationship: "Sleep itself is a mystery, and the problem of epilepsy is not simplified by having to consider the reciprocal relationship of sleep and seizures. Possibly investigators will need to unravel the mysteries of both to fully understand either."

## SLEEP AND SLEEP DEPRIVATION EFFECTS ON EPILEPSY

Patterns begin to emerge when examining the timing of seizures during sleep. Seizures predominate during non–rapid eye movement (NREM) sleep compared with REM[10–12] and are more likely to occur during the lighter stages of NREM sleep.[12,13] Partial seizures are more frequent during sleep than during wake, and when they occur during sleep are more likely to secondarily generalize.[10,12] When the anatomic origin is examined, seizures of frontal lobe origin are more likely to occur during normal sleep hours than during wake, but those of temporal, parietal, or occipital lobe origins show the opposite pattern.[12,14,15] The link between seizure recurrence, site of seizure origin, and circadian rhythm has been supported further by studies of the timing of seizures with respect to dim light melatonin onset.[16]

Subsequent research supported initial clinical impressions that seizures of frontal lobe origin

have their onset out of sleep, but those of temporal lobe origin are preceded by an arousal, and the onset occurs during the waking state.[10,17] Recordings from intracranial electrodes have found the actual onsets for all of these events tend to occur out of sleep; state transitions rather than arousals may facilitate some types of seizure recurrence.[11]

NREM sleep has been described as a physiologic state of relative neuronal synchronization, which facilitates the recruitment of the critical mass of neurons needed to initiate and sustain a seizure.[18] Generalized spike wave discharges preferentially occur during NREM sleep, particularly during the lighter stages when sleep spindles are present, supporting this idea of neuronal synchronization.[19,20] This finding, combined with animal model evidence of the transformation of sleep spindles into spike-wave discharges, led to the hypothesis that spike-wave discharges have their origin in the pathologically altered generation of sleep spindles.[21] More recent review of these clinical studies and animal data has raised questions about this proposition.[22] Interictal discharges are more frequent during sleep than wake.[23,24] This alone does not explain why seizures occur more frequently out of lighter stages of sleep or why certain seizures are triggered by arousals or awakenings.

Neuronal synchronization during NREM sleep results at least in part from underlying neurotransmitter changes. Pharmacologic agents, which synchronize electroencephalogram (EEG) (cholinergic and noradrenergic antagonists), tend to have proconvulsant effects, whereas agonists desynchronize EEG and have anticonvulsant effects.[25–27] Histaminergic neurons in the posterior hypothalamus are one of the major excitatory sources of cortical activation during arousal. In several animal models, increased brain histamine levels elevate seizure threshold and reduce the severity and duration of seizures[28] and delay the development of seizure onset in genetically susceptible mice.[29] First-generation antihistamines (H1 receptor antagonists) act as m-current potassium channel antagonists,[30] and the m-current potassium channel agonist, retigabine, has anticonvulsant properties.[31,32] Taken together, these findings explain the proconvulsant impact of commonly used antihistamines.

Patients frequently cite sleep deprivation as a trigger for seizure recurrence. This concept is supported by animal work, including the demonstration that cats are more susceptible to kindled and penicillin-induced seizures after sleep deprivation.[33,34] Either REM or total sleep deprivation accelerates the rate of kindling in the amygdala.[35] Transcranial magnetic stimulation found reduced short intracortical inhibition and increased intra-cortical facilitation in healthy volunteers after 24 hours of sleep deprivation; both are metrics suggesting increased cortical excitability.[36] An earlier study using only partial sleep deprivation failed to show the change in cortical excitability in normal controls but did show this increase in susceptible patients with juvenile myoclonic epilepsy.[37] Military studies reviewing the effects of sleep deprivation show that pilots are more likely to have their first generalized convulsion in the setting of sleep deprivation, and soldiers are more likely to have had prolonged sleep depriva-tion the night before seizure occurrence.[38,39] Anal-ysis of patient surveys and diaries found that sleep deprivation exacerbated seizures in patients with either temporal lobe or idiopathic generalized epilepsies.[40,41] However, acute sleep deprivation of hospitalized patients with medically refractory partial epilepsy failed to affect daily seizure frequency.[42] This finding may, in part, be caused by greater susceptibility to the effects of sleep deprivation in patients with idiopathic generalized epilepsies compared with those with epilepsies of focal onset.[43]

# THE EFFECTS OF EPILEPSY ON SLEEP

Comorbidities in patients with epilepsy and the secondary effects of these on sleep confound the environment for study of the effects of epilepsy on sleep in human subjects. Anxiety about the seizure disorder, coexistent depression and other psychiatric ailments, frequent arousals leading to sleep disruption, and effects of antiepileptic medi-cations among other variables cloud the picture in understanding exclusively the effect of epilepsy on sleep in human subjects. Animal studies have helped overcome some of these confounders. A sampling of some of these studies has been provided in **Table 1**.

A seizure acutely disrupts sleep quality, and epilepsy chronically produces alterations in sleep organization and architecture. Broadly speaking, sleep architecture in patients with epilepsy is char-acterized by a decrease in total sleep time, frequent awakenings, frequent stage shifts, and a decrease in deep sleep, particularly in REM sleep.

Touchon and colleagues[44] reported a reduction in total sleep time and decreased REM percentage resulting from nocturnal generalized and repetitive partial seizures. This significant decrease in REM

| Table 1<br>Some animal data on sleep architecture in models of epilepsy | |
|---|---|
| Cohen and Dement,[98] 1966,<br>Rondouin et al,[99] 1980 | Suppression of REM sleep after electroconvulsive shock and kindling in cats |
| Raol and Meti,[100] 1998 | Seizures induced by amygdala kindling led to short-term alterations in sleep phases, with an initial increase in deep SWS and REM sleep. Consecutive seizures resulted in increases in deep NREM and decreased light NREM and REM sleep |
| Ayala-Guerrero et al,[101] 2002 | NREM and REM sleep reduced in first 24 hours after kainic acid–induced SE, returning to baseline 4 days later |
| Yi et al,[102] 2004 | Time of seizure occurrence influences the effects of seizures on sleep in adult rats |
| Bastlund et al,[103] 2005 | Reduction in REM sleep and prolonged wakefulness after 15 weeks of status epilepticus (complex partial seizures induced by hippocampal electrical stimulation) |
| van Luijtelaar and Bikabaev,[104] 2007 | Drug-free naïve WAG/Rij rats had a longer lasting sleep cycle with reduced REM sleep time. Older animals showed a reduction in NREM sleep |
| Alfaro-Rodríguez et al,[105] 2009 | Carbamazepine protected against the damaging effects of kainic acid–induced seizures on sleep phases in rats |
| Matos G et al,[106] 2010 | After 60 days of status epilepticus in male adult rats after pilocarpine-induced temporal lobe epilepsy, reduction of REM sleep during the afternoon, increase in NREM Sleep and relaxed wakefulness early in the night, increase in NREM Sleep in the morning as well as decrease of sleep cycles throughout the light-dark cycle |

*Abbreviations:* SE, Status Epilepticus; SWS, slow wave sleep.

sleep was seen in patients of temporal lobe epilepsy only when multiple seizures occurred but not with a single seizure. In patients with temporal lobe seizures, polysomnographic recordings showed a significant decrease in REM sleep percentage even when seizures occurred on the previous day.[45]

When patients with primary generalized epilepsy and patients with focal epilepsy were evaluated, an increase in WASO and awakenings less than 2 minutes and greater than 2 minutes were found.[44] Total sleep time and proportion of NREM and REM sleep were unchanged. A possible mechanism proposed for sleep stage instability was an increase in norepinephrine and acetylcholine, with a corresponding decrease in gamma-amino-butyric acid (GABA). Patients with temporal lobe epilepsy were found to have significant sleep fragmentation with a decrease in efficiency index compared with frontal lobe epilepsy (FLE) and controls. However, no difference of sleep organization was seen in patients with FLE compared with controls.[17] Janz[8] reported a decrease in deep sleep in patients with generalized epilepsy. Barreto and colleagues[46] replicated these results and also described a decrease in sleep efficiency and stage 4 NREM sleep in patients with idiopathic generalized epilepsy. A more recent study of chronotype distribution reported that those with epilepsy were more morning oriented and had longer sleep duration on seizure-free days. The investigators suggest that epilepsy itself rather than seizure timing, which is often a feature of specified epilepsy syndromes, influences chronotype behavior and subjective sleep parameters.[47] In a study comparing medically refractory epilepsy patients with those with controlled epilepsy, patients in the former group were found to have significantly less total sleep time with delayed sleep latency and REM latency, poor sleep efficiency, frequent arousals, and WASO compared with the latter group. Notably, medically refractory epilepsy patients seem to think that they spent more time sleeping than their actual demonstrated sleep time by polysomnography.[48]

Fewer studies have investigated polysomnographic abnormalities specifically in children. Children with medically refractory epilepsy were found to have significantly lower sleep efficiency, higher arousal index, and a higher REM sleep percentage when compared with children with controlled epilepsy.[49] A more recent study[50] found a significant reduction of total sleep time, REM sleep, stage 3 NREM sleep, and sleep efficiency as well as an increase in WASO in children with drug-resistant epilepsy. Larson and colleagues[51] investigated sleep behaviors in children with epilepsy. In these families, there were increased rates of both parent-child room sharing ($P<.001$) and cosleeping ($P = .005$) compared with controls. Also, children with epilepsy were found to have greater sleep disturbances, particularly parasomnias, night awakenings, sleep duration, daytime sleepiness, sleep onset delay, and bedtime resistance. Parents of children with epilepsy also reported increased sleep dysfunction and were more fatigued than parents of children without epilepsy.

## HYPERSOMNOLENCE AND OTHER SLEEP COMPLAINTS IN EPILEPSY

Although sedation from antiepileptic drugs is usually the most commonly perceived reason for sleepiness in patients with epilepsy, other causes of hypersomnolence in the general population should be considered in the differential diagnosis. Particular attention should be paid to other possibilities like nocturnal seizure activity and psychiatric comorbidities. Treatment of sleep disorders and improved sleep hygiene often leads to improved seizure control and quality of life. **Box 1** contains a summary of some of the causes of sleepiness in epilepsy patients.

Many studies report the presence of daytime sleepiness (EDS) in the population of patients with epilepsy. The methods of assessing sleepiness vary. The Epworth Sleepiness Scale (ESS) is the most commonly administered tool. Given the subjectivity of this measure, percentages of those with EDS also are reported variably. Hence, it is controversial if hypersomnolence in these patients is in reality significantly higher than in the general population.[52] In earlier studies, EDS measured by the ESS was found in 28% of patients with epilepsy and 18% of control subjects with other neurologic disorders.[53] Further, in terms of predictors of sleepiness among the epilepsy patients, the

---

**Box 1**
**Causes of sleepiness in epilepsy patients**

1. Anti-epileptic medications

2. Nocturnal seizure activity leading to sleep disruption

3. Psychiatric comorbidities: anxiety and depression

4. Primary sleep disorders: sleep-disordered breathing, periodic limb movements in sleep (PLMS), restless legs syndrome, narcolepsy, and other hypersomnia syndromes, insufficient sleep syndrome, circadian rhythm disorders, poor sleep hygiene

5. Underlying cause of epilepsy itself

number or type of antiepileptic medication, seizure frequency, epilepsy syndrome (partial vs generalized), or the presence of sleep-related seizures were not found to be significant. Chen and colleagues[54] estimate the prevalence of EDS among patients with epilepsy at 20%, significantly increased compared with controls (7%). A Brazilian study with 99 unselected patients from an outpatient epilepsy clinic found EDS complaints in 47.5% of their population. EDS was most closely associated with anxiety and neck circumference.[55] In 50 patients with juvenile myoclonic epilepsy, EDS (ESS scores of more than 11) was documented in 17% and disturbed sleep was reported despite adequate seizure control. However, because these patients were on valproate monotherapy, the investigators concede that the role of this medication could be contributory.[56]

A study of sleep disorder symptoms in patients with simple partial, complex partial, and generalized seizures compared with normal control subjects reported significantly more sleep disorder symptoms in patients with simple partial and complex partial seizures, especially frequent night awakenings. Independent of seizure type, patients with more frequent seizures also had the most sleep disturbances.[57] In a study of 33 patients with nocturnal frontal lobe epilepsy (NFLE) and 27 controls, "tiredness after awakening" and "spontaneous mid-sleep awakenings" were found to be more frequent in NFLE patients than in controls (36.4% vs 11.1%, $P = .04$, and 50.0% vs 22.2%, $P = .03$).[58] An investigation of sleep hygiene based on a questionnaire compared 244 patients who had focal or generalized epilepsy with 205 healthy subjects and reported higher scores on ESS in those with snoring, apneas, or recurrent seizures in the last year, in the epilepsy patients.[52] Another questionnaire-based study from the Netherlands reported a 2-fold higher prevalence of sleep disturbance in patients with partial epilepsy when compared with controls. de Weerd and colleagues[59] reported an association between the presence of a sleep disturbance and impairment in quality of life. In a small case-control retrospective study with neuropsychological testing, 31 elderly patients with epilepsy were compared with 31 age-matched healthy controls. Although none of the controls had depression, 18% of the patients were depressed.[60]

## EFFECTS OF ANTIEPILEPTIC MEDICATIONS ON SLEEP

It is difficult to draw conclusions about the effects of antiepileptic medications (AEDs) given the complications from the effects of epilepsy itself on the patient's sleep. Hence, some of these data are also gathered from investigations on normal volunteers. A summary of the effects of some of the commonly used AEDs on sleep is provided in **Table 2**.

**Table 2**
**Antiepileptic drugs and effects on sleep**

| Medication | Effects on Sleep |
|---|---|
| Carbamazepine | Variable reports:<br>No significant effect (Legros and Bazil,[107] 2003)<br>Increased TST and SWS, decreased REM density with unchanged REM latency and percentage (Sammaritano and Sherwin,[108] 2000)<br>Acute decrease in REM, not seen chronically (Gigli et al,[109] 1997) |
| Phenytoin | Decrease in sleep efficiency, decrease in sleep latency, decrease in stages 1 and 2, decrease in REM, variable reports on effects on slow wave sleep |
| Valproate | Many studies report little or no effect. Some report increase in stage 1 sleep |
| Gabapentin | Increases SWS and REM sleep, reduces stage 1 sleep, reduces number of awakenings, improves sleep stability (Placidi et al,[110] 2000; Foldvary-Schaefer,[111] 2002) |
| Lamotrigine | Increases REM sleep, reduces SWS, reduces stage shifts, improves sleep stability (Placidi et al,[112] 2000) |
| Oxcarbazepine | Increases SWS and REM in rats (Ayala-Guerrero et al,[113] 2009) |
| Topiramate | No significant increase in daytime sleepiness measured by MSLT (Bonanni et al,[114] 2004) |
| Levetiracetam | Increase in TST, sleep efficiency and stages 2 and 4 (Bell et al,[115] 2002; Cicolin et al,[116] 2006; Cho et al,[117] 2011). Decrease in REM sleep time and percentage in patients (Zhou et al,[118] 2011) |
| Felbamate | Higher incidence of insomnia, alerting effect |

Abbreviations: SWS, slow wave sleep; TST, total sleep time.

Although AEDs are often thought to be paramount in causing sleepiness in the epilepsy population, a definite cause-and-effect relationship between these 2 factors is not proven.[61] When daytime sleep tendency was measured with mean sleep latency tests (MSLTs) in Swedish children with epilepsy, patients continued to have significantly higher sleep tendency even after discontinuation of their AEDs. This sleep tendency could be not be attributed to medications, recent seizures, or their disease.[62] Hence, it is important to examine other causes of hypersomnolence in this population. Primary sleep disorders should be suspected, especially in those on low doses of AEDs, on AED monotherapy, and with well-controlled seizures.

When medications are thought to be the primary cause of hypersomnolence, certain simple strategies may be used to alleviate symptoms:

1. Simplify drug regimen, if possible to monotherapy.
2. Switch to less sedating medications. In general, most of the more recently released antiepileptic medications are less sedating than the older drugs. If sedating medications cannot be avoided, they may be moved to the night, or their largest dose can be administered at night.
3. Switch to extended-release formulations.

When selecting AEDs for patients with epilepsy and sleep disorders, as in other patients with epilepsy, one should also bear in mind the effects of AEDs on the underlying sleep problem. For instance, barbiturates and benzodiazepines may worsen comorbid obstructive sleep apnea (OSA) by influencing upper airway muscle tone. AEDs that are known to be associated with weight gain (eg, valproate) may also worsen OSA. Patients with insomnia may benefit from the more sedative drugs, preferably taken at bedtime.

## PRIMARY SLEEP DISORDERS IN EPILEPSY

Identifying sleep disorders complicating epilepsy requires careful history taking. The time required is certainly worth the effort in comprehensively treating these patients with the goal of improving their quality of life. Initial studies focused on the co-occurrence of OSA with epilepsy[63–65] as well the potential of improved seizure control with treatment of OSA. Malow and colleagues[66] have worked extensively on this interface. In a large study, 63 epilepsy patients referred for either a combination of or isolated EDS, suspected OSA, or nocturnal spells were evaluated by polysomnography (PSG). MSLTs were also performed in 33 patients. OSA was diagnosed in 44 patients

(71%). Narcolepsy and insufficient sleep syndrome were diagnosed in one patient each. Although 11 patients had greater than 20 PLMs per hour, these were not associated with arousal. Thereafter, many studies have examined the relationship between OSA and epilepsy. A total of 10.2% of 283 adult patients with epilepsy studied by PSG were found to have coexistent OSA.[67] Kaleyias and colleagues[49] report a 20% prevalence of coexistent OSA and epilepsy in children.

In children with epilepsy and sleep disruption evaluated by polysomnography, uncontrolled epilepsy was found to be a risk factor for OSA.[68] A Brazilian study prospectively screening 98 adult patients with epilepsy for risk of OSA using the Berlin questionnaire placed the prevalence of this risk at 55.1%.[55] The risk was related primarily to large neck circumference, high body mass index and anxiety. More recently, in medically refractory epilepsy patients, diabetes and snoring were found to be predictive of a diagnosis of OSA.[69] Conversely, OSA was found to be a contributing risk factor for worsening seizure frequency in older adults with epilepsy.[70]

Less is known about the incidence of other sleep disorders in this population. Restless legs syndrome was described in 2 subjects taking methosuximide and phenytoin.[71] Two patients were found to have PLMs in a case series of 6 patients not on anticonvulsant therapy.[72] A case report of zonisamide-induced restless legs syndrome is also described.[73] Only isolated case reports of narcolepsy concurrent with epilepsy are found in the literature. In one case, a previously healthy 40-year-old man had hypersomnolence and narcolepsy before the subsequent appearance of complex partial seizures 18 months later; magnetic resonance imaging found a progressively enlarging lesion in the left frontotemporal region. His seizures were medically refractory and culminated in an episode of complex partial status epilepticus. He underwent a partial resection, and the pathology was found to be consistent with Rasmussen's syndrome. The authors raise the possibility of a common autoimmune etiology for the 2 disorders.[74] A second report described a 5-year-old boy who had a valproate-responsive myoclonic epilepsy at age 4 years and narcolepsy with cataplexy 6 months later.[75] Although the former case does suggest the possibility of a common underlying etiology, the latter could simply the coincidental occurrence of both conditions in a single patient (a statistical inevitability). Coexisting REM behavior disorder with epilepsy has been reported in 2 case series by the same group.[76,77] There are diagnostic dilemmas given the nature of involuntary nocturnal movements.

Parasomnias in epilepsy patients also present this diagnostic difficulty, because, in most cases, the diagnosis is based only on a history of involuntary nocturnal movements. An increased frequency of parasomnias has been reported not only in patients with NFLE, but also in their relatives when compared with controls.[78] The association was strongest with the NREM arousal disorders (such as sleep walking, sleep terrors, and confusional arousals). A questionnaire-based study described a higher occurrence of parasomnias ($P<.01$) among children with idiopathic generalized epilepsy when compared with siblings and healthy controls. They also found a higher density of paroxysmal EEG activity was related to parasomnias, suggesting that sleep fragmentation from epilepsy contributes to altered arousal mechanisms in these children.[79] In adults, an association between parasomnias and epilepsy was not found.[80]

Oliveira and colleagues[81] describe a decrease in EEG interictal epileptiform activity after continuous positive airway pressure (CPAP) therapy. In a pilot study, 3 adult patients and one child, all with coexistent epilepsy and OSA, had at least a 45% reduction in seizure frequency during CPAP treatment.[82] Several other studies have reported significant improvement in seizure frequency after the use of CPAP in CPAP-compliant patients with epilepsy and OSA.[83,84]

Melatonin has been studied to treat sleep disorders in children, and note should be made to its anticonvulsant effect seen in animal models.[85–89] Some studies in children with epilepsy have been reviewed in **Table 3**.

## VAGAL NERVE STIMULATION AND SLEEP

In treating patients with epilepsy who are treated with vagal nerve stimulation (VNS), it is worthwhile to keep in mind the association with sleep-disordered breathing described in literature. In 4 epilepsy patients who were evaluated with PSG before and after 3 months of treatment with VNS, consistent sleep-related decreases in airflow and effort synchronized to VNS activation were identified.[90] Although these events did not meet clinical criteria for apneas and hypopneas, it was noticed that they occurred more frequently during VNS activation. In one of the patients who had a pretreatment apnea-hypopnea index of 4, the post-treatment apnea-hypopnea index increased to 11.3. Stimulus frequency, when reduced, helped ameliorate VNS-related apneas and hypopneas. No such significant effect was seen with altering stimulus intensity, pulse width, or signal on time. VNS-induced airway changes or alterations in sleep architecture were suggested as possible causes of these respiratory events. In a subsequent communication, Murray and colleagues[91] suggested that tachypnea accompanying VNS stimulation was somehow related to sleep-disordered breathing. Increases in esophageal pressure were also seen with respiratory events, which, in one patient, responded to CPAP therapy.[92] Malow and colleagues[93] also describe increase in daytime alertness with VNS treatment at low stimulus intensities, likely caused by enhanced cholinergic activation. A case report of a medication-resistant epilepsy patient with VNS, for whom adequate CPAP titration could be achieved only with the VNS device turned off, raises the question of whether these patients should undergo polysomnographic studies (both diagnostic and therapeutic) with the device turned off.[94] Papacostas and colleagues[95] report a case of a woman with medication-resistant epilepsy in whom VNS induced central sleep apnea, which resolved on adjustment of VNS parameters. In children on VNS therapy, changes in respiratory patterns are

| Table 3 Melatonin in epilepsy | |
|---|---|
| **Authors** | **Results of Study** |
| Coppola et al,[119] 2004 | In 25 patients (children, adolescents, and young adults) with mental disabilities, melatonin in nightly doses of 3 mg escalated up to 9 mg if necessary improved sleep latency and other subjective parameters of sleep |
| Gupta et al,[120] 2005 | In 31 children with epilepsy, oral melatonin reduced parasomnias and improved sleep latency and quality |
| Elkhayat et al,[121] 2010 | Oral melatonin in children with intractable epilepsy resulted in significant improvement in bedtime resistance, sleep latency and duration, frequent awakenings, sleep-walking, EDS, nocturnal enuresis, bruxism, sleep apnea, and ESS scores as well as reduction in seizure severity |
| Uberos et al,[122] 2011 | Nightly oral 3-mg dose of melatonin improved sleep efficiency and seizure frequency |

also described, although no significant hypoxia or hypercapnia have been reported.[96]

When evaluating patients on VNS therapy, the possibility of either inducing or worsening pre-existing sleep-disordered breathing should be kept in mind. Reducing the stimulus frequencies or the signal off time when feasible are strategies to minimize this effect. If necessary, PSG studies before and after VNS device implantation and after VNS parameter adjustment in symptomatic patients should be considered.

## SUMMARY

The bidirectional nature of the interaction between epilepsy and sleep is revealed in multiple observations. Interictal epileptiform discharges and the timing of seizures in some epilepsy syndromes show patterns of temporal synchrony with the sleep-wake cycle. Sleep deprivation is associated with an increase in cortical excitability. Both seizures and epilepsy are capable of altering sleep microarchitechture and macroarchitecture, sleep-related behaviors, and subjective sleep quality. Patients with epilepsy have a variety of sleep-related symptoms, which may be caused by AEDs or primary sleep disorders. Recognition of sleep deprivation as a cause of lowering of seizure threshold is a frequently addressed topic in the seizure clinic now and in the past. However, discussion of the patient's sleep patterns, with particular attention to possible sleep disorders that are coexistent with epilepsy, is often overlooked. Because sleep disturbances have been found to be one of the main predictors in quality of life in epilepsy,[97] and because there are effective treatments available, addressing these efficiently is integral to the overall management strategy for these patients.

## REFERENCES

1. Aristotle. On sleep and sleeplessness. [Beare JI, Trans.; 350 BCE]. Available at: http://classics.mit.edu/Aristotle/sleep.html. Accessed October 1, 2012.
2. Temkin O. The falling sickness. Baltimore (MD): The Johns Hopkins University Press; 1994. p. 48.
3. Gowers WR. Epilepsy and other chronic convulsive diseases. New York: William Wood & Company; 1885. p. 162–4.
4. Langdon-Down M, Brain WR. Time of day in relation to convulsion in epilepsy. Lancet 1929;1: 1029–32.
5. Berger H. Über das Elektrenkephalogramm des Menchen. European Archives of Psychiatry and Clinical Neuroscience 1929;87(1):527–70.
6. Gibbs EL, Gibbs FA. Diagnostic and localizing value of electroencephalographic studies in sleep. Res Publ Assoc Res Nerv Ment Dis 1947;26:366–76.
7. Janz D. Matutinal epilepsies; comparison with nocturnal and sleep epilepsies. Arch Psychiatr Nervenkr Z Gesamte Neurol Psychiatr 1953; 191(1):73–96.
8. Janz D. The grand mal epilepsies and the sleeping-waking cycle. Epilepsia 1962;3:69–109.
9. Lennox WG, Lennox MS, editors. Epilepsy and related disorders, vol. 2. Boston: Little, Brown; 1960. p. 773.
10. Bazil CW, Walczak TS. Effects of sleep and sleep stage on epileptic and nonepileptic seizures. Epilepsia 1997;38(1):56–62.
11. Malow A, Bowes RJ, Ross D. Relationship of temporal lobe seizures to sleep and arousal: a combined scalp-intracranial electrode study. Sleep 2000;23(2):231–4.
12. Herman ST, Walczak TS, Bazil CW. Distribution of partial seizures during the sleep-wake cycle. Neurology 2001;56:1453–9.
13. Minecan D, Natarajan A, Marzec M, et al. Relationship of epileptic seizures to sleep stage and sleep depth. Sleep 2002;25(8):899–904.
14. Karafin M, St Louis EK, Zimmerman MB, et al. Bimodal ultradian seizure periodicity in human mesial temporal lobe epilepsy. Seizure 2010; 19(6):347–51.
15. Pavlova MK, Woo Lee J, Yilmaz F, et al. Diurnal pattern of seizures outside the hospital. Neurology 2012;78:1488–92.
16. Hofstra WA, Gordijn MC, van der Palen J, et al. Timing of temporal and frontal seizures in relation to the circadian phase: a prospective pilot study. Epilepsy Res 2011;94:158–62.
17. Crespel A, Coubes P, Baldy-Moulinier M. Sleep influence on seizures and epilepsy effects on sleep in partial frontal and temporal lobe epilepsies. Clin Neurophysiol 2000;111(Suppl 2):S54–9.
18. Steriade M, Contreras D, Amzica F. Synchronized sleep oscillations and their paroxysmal developments. Trends Neurosci 1994;17(5):201–7.
19. Kellaway P, Frost JD Jr, Crawley JW. Time modulation of ictal and interictal spike-and-wave activity in generalized epilepsy. Trans Am Neurol Assoc 1979;104:92–3.
20. Kellaway P. Time modulation of spike-and-wave activity in generalized epilepsy. Ann Neurol 1980; 8(5):491–500.
21. Gloor P, Fariello RG. Generalized epilepsy: some of its cellular mechanisms differ from those of focal epilepsy. Trends Neurosci 1988;11(2):63–8.
22. Leresche N, et al. From sleep spindles of natural sleep to spike and wave discharges of typical absence seizures: is the hypothesis still valid? Pflugers Arch 2012;463:201–12.

23. Mayanagi Y. The influence of natural sleep on focal spiking in experimental temporal lobe epilepsy in the monkey. Electroencephalogr Clin Neurophysiol 1977;43(6):813–24.

24. Asano E, et al. Effect of sleep on interictal spikes and distribution of sleep spindles on electrocorticography in children with focal epilepsy. Clin Neurophysiol 2007;118(6):1360–8.

25. Pelletier MR, Corcoran ME. Infusions of alpha-2 noradrenergic agonists and antagonists into the amygdala: effects on kindling. Brain Res 1993; 632(1–2):29–35.

26. Shouse MN, et al. The alpha 2-adrenoreceptor agonist clonidine suppresses seizures, whereas the alpha 2-adrenoreceptor antagonist idazoxan promotes seizures in amygdala-kindled kittens: a comparison of amygdala and pontine microinfusion effects. Epilepsia 1996;37(8):709–17.

27. Foldvary-Schaefer N, Grigg-Damberger M. Sleep and epilepsy: what we know, don't know, and need to know. J Clin Neurophysiol 2006;23(1):4–20.

28. Scherkl R, Hashem A, Frey HH. Histamine in brain-its role in regulation of seizure susceptibility. Epilepsy Res 1991;10:111–8.

29. Yawata I, et al. Role of histaminergic neurons in development of epileptic seizures in EL mice. Brain Res Mol Brain Res 2004;132:13–7.

30. Sato I, Munakata M, Iinuma K. Histamine H1 antagonists block M-currents in dissociated rat cortical neurons. Brain Res 2005;1057:81–7.

31. Rundfeldt C, Netzer R. The novel anticonvulsant re tigabine activates M-currents In Chinese hamster ovary-cells tranfected with human KCNQ2/3 subunits. Neurosci Lett 2000;282(1–2):73–6.

32. Tatulian L, et al. Activation of expressed KCNQ potassium currents and native neuronal M-type potassium currents by the anti-convulsant drug retigabine. J Neurosci 2001;21:5535–45.

33. Shouse MN, Sterman MB. Acute sleep deprivation reduces amygdala-kindled seizure thresholds in cats. Exp Neurol 1982;78(3):716–27.

34. Shouse MN. Sleep deprivation increases susceptibility to kindled and penicillin seizure events during all waking and sleep states in cats. Sleep 1988; 11(2):162–71.

35. Kawahara R, Hamazaki Y, Takeshita H. Effect of REM sleep deprivation on the each seizure stage in feline amygdaloid kindling. Seishin Shinkeigaku Zasshi 1994;96(2):109–21 [in Japanese].

36. Kreuzer P, et al. Reduced intra-cortical inhibition after sleep deprivation: a transcranial magnetic stimulation study. Neurosci Lett 2011;493(3):63–6.

37. Manganotti P, et al. Effects of sleep deprivation on cortical excitability in patients affected by juvenile myoclonic epilepsy: a combined transcranial magnetic stimulation and EEG study. J Neurol Neurosurg Psychiatry 2006;77:56–60.

38. Bennett DR. Sleep deprivation and major motor convulsions. Neurology 1963;13:953–8.

39. Gunderson CH, Dunne PB, Feyer TL. Sleep deprivation seizures. Neurology 1973;23(7):678–86.

40. Rajna P, Veres J. Correlations between night sleep duration and seizure frequency in temporal lobe epilepsy. Epilepsia 1993;34(3):574–9.

41. Frucht MM, et al. Distribution of seizure precipitants among epilepsy syndromes. Epilepsia 2000;41(12): 1534–9.

42. Malow BA, et al. Sleep deprivation does not affect seizure frequency during inpatient video-EEG monitoring. Neurology 2002;59(9):1371–4.

43. Badawy RA, et al. Sleep deprivation increases cortical excitability in epilepsy: syndrome-specific effects. Neurology 2006;67(6):1018–22.

44. Touchon J, Baldy-Moulinier M, Billiard M, et al. Sleep organization and epilepsy. Epilepsy Res Suppl 1991;2:73–81.

45. Bazil CW, Castro LH, Walczak TS. Reduction of rapid eye movement sleep by diurnal and nocturnal seizures in temporal lobe epilepsy. Arch Neurol 2000;57(3):363–8.

46. Barreto JR, Fernandes RM, Sakamoto AC. Correlation of sleep macrostructure parameters and idiopathic epilepsies. Arq Neuropsiquiatr 2002;60(2-B): 353–7.

47. Hofstra WA, Gordijn MC, van Hemert-van der Poel JC, et al. Chronotypes and subjective sleep parameters in epilepsy patients: a large questionnaire study. Chronobiol Int 2010;27(6):1271–86.

48. Zanzmera P, Shukla G, Gupta A, et al. Markedly disturbed sleep in medically refractory compared to controlled epilepsy - a clinical and polysomnography study. Seizure 2012;21(7):487–90.

49. Kaleyias J, Cruz M, Goraya JS. Spectrum of polysomnographic abnormalities in children with epilepsy. Pediatr Neurol 2008;39(3):170–6.

50. Pereira AM, Bruni O, Ferri R, et al. The impact of epilepsy on sleep architecture during childhood. Epilepsia 2012;53(9):1519–25.

51. Larson AM, Ryther RC, Jennesson M, et al. Impact of pediatric epilepsy on sleep patterns and behaviors in children and parents. Epilepsia 2012;53(7): 1162–9.

52. Manni R, Politini L, Sartori I, et al. Daytime sleepiness in epilepsy patients: evaluation by means of the Epworth sleepiness scale. J Neurol 2000; 247(9):716–7.

53. Malow BA, Bowes RJ, Lin X. Predictors of sleepiness in epilepsy patients. Sleep 1997;20(12):1105–10.

54. Chen NC, Tsai MH, Chang CC, et al. Sleep quality and daytime sleepiness in patients with epilepsy. Acta Neurol Taiwan 2011;20(4):249–56.

55. Giorelli AS, Neves GS, Venturi M, et al. Excessive daytime sleepiness in patients with epilepsy: a subjective evaluation. Epilepsy Behav 2011;21(4):449–52.

56. Krishnan P, Sinha S, Taly AB, et al. Sleep disturbances in juvenile myoclonic epilepsy: a sleep questionnaire-based study. Epilepsy Behav 2012; 23(3):305–9.

57. Hoeppner JB, Garron DC, Cartwright RD. Self-reported sleep disorder symptoms in epilepsy. Epilepsia 1984;25(4):434–7.

58. Vignatelli L, Bisulli F, Naldi I, et al. Excessive daytime sleepiness and subjective sleep quality in patients with nocturnal frontal lobe epilepsy: a case-control study. Epilepsia 2006;47(Suppl 5): 73–7.

59. de Weerd A, de Haas S, Otte A, et al. Subjective sleep disturbance in patients with partial epilepsy: a questionnaire-based study on prevalence and impact on quality of life. Epilepsia 2004;45(11): 1397–404.

60. Haut SR, Katz M, Masur J. Seizures in the elderly: impact on mental status, mood, and sleep. Epilepsy Behav 2009;14(3):540–4.

61. Beghi E. Adverse reactions to antiepileptic drugs: a multicenter survey of clinical practice. Epilepsia 1986;27:323–30.

62. Palm L, Anderson H, Elmqvist D, et al. Daytime sleep tendency before and after discontinuation of antiepileptic drugs in preadolescent children with epilepsy. Epilepsia 1992;33(4):687–91.

63. Wyler AR, Weymuller EA Jr. Epilepsy complicated by sleep apnea. Ann Neurol 1981;9(4):403–4.

64. Vaughn BV, D'Cruz OF, Beach R, et al. Improvement of epileptic seizure control with treatment of obstructive sleep apnoea. Seizure 1996;5(1):73–8.

65. Devinsky O, Ehrenberg B, Barthlen GM, et al. Epilepsy and sleep apnea syndrome. Neurology 1994;44(11):2060–4.

66. Malow BA, Fromes GA, Aldrich MS. Usefulness of polysomnography in epilepsy patients. Neurology 1997;48(5):1389–94.

67. Manni R, Terzaghi M, Arbasino C, et al. Obstructive sleep apnea in a clinical series of adult epilepsy patients: frequency and features of the comorbidity. Epilepsia 2003;44(6):836–40.

68. Jain SV, Simakajornboon S, Shapiro SM. Obstructive sleep apnea in children with epilepsy: prospective pilot trial. Acta Neurol Scand 2012; 125(1):e3–6.

69. Li P, Ghadersohi S, Jafari B. Characteristics of refractory vs. medically controlled epilepsy patients with obstructve sleep apnea and their response to CPAP treatment. Seizure 2012;21(9): 717–21.

70. Chihorek AM, Abou-Khalil B, Malow BA. Obstructive sleep apnea is associated with seizure occurrence in older adults with epilepsy. Neurology 2007;69(19):1823–7.

71. Drake ME. Restless legs with antiepileptic drug therapy. Clin Neurol Neurosurg 1988;90(2):151–4.

72. Newell SA, Drake ME Jr. Sleep apnea and periodic leg movements in epilepsy. Clin Electroencephalogr 1994;25(4):153–5.

73. Chen JT, Garcia PA, Alldredge BK. Zonisamide-induced restless legs syndrome. Neurology 2003; 60(1):147.

74. Langrange AH, et al. Epilepsy Behav 2003;4: 788–92.

75. Yang Z, et al. Epilepsy and narcolepsy-cataplexy in a child. J Child Neurol 2012;27(6):807–10.

76. Manni R, Terzaghi M. REM behavior disorder associated with epileptic seizures. Neurology 2005; 64(5):883–4.

77. Manni R, Terzaghi M, Zambrelli E. REM sleep behaviour disorder in elderly subjects with epilepsy: frequency and clinical aspects of the comorbidity. Epilepsy Res 2007;77(2–3):128–33.

78. Bisulli F, Vignatelli L, Naldi I. Increased frequency of arousal parasomnias in families with nocturnal frontal lobe epilepsy: a common mechanism? Epilepsia 2010;51(9):1852–60.

79. Cortesi F, Giannotti F, Ottaviano S. Sleep problems and daytime behavior in childhood idiopathic epilepsy. Epilepsia 1999;40(11):1557–65.

80. Khatami R, Zutter D, Siegel A. Sleep-wake habits and disorders in a series of 100 adult epilepsy patients–a prospective study. Seizure 2006;15(5): 299–306.

81. Oliveira AJ, Zamagni M, Dolso P. Respiratory disorders during sleep in patients with epilepsy: effect of ventilatory therapy on EEG interictal epileptiform discharges. Clin Neurophysiol 2000;111(Suppl 2): S141–5.

82. Malow BA, Weatherwax KJ, Chervin RD. Identification and treatment of obstructive sleep apnea in adults and children with epilepsy: a prospective pilot study. Sleep Med 2003;4(6):509–15.

83. Hollinger P, Khatami R, Gugger M. Epilepsy and obstructive sleep apnea. Eur Neurol 2006;55(2): 74–9.

84. Vendrame M, Auerbach S, Loddenkemper T, et al. Effect of continuous positive airway pressure treatment on seizure control in patients with obstructive sleep apnea and epilepsy. Epilepsia 2011;52(11): e168–71.

85. Yahyavi-Firouz-Abadi N, Tahsili-Fahadan P, Riazi K, et al. Involvement of nitric oxide pathway in the acute anticonvulsant effect of melatonin in mice. Epilepsy Res 2006;68(2):103–13.

86. Yahyavi-Firouz-Abadi N, Tahsili-Fahadan P, Riazi K, et al. Melatonin enhances the anticonvulsant and proconvulsant effects of morphine in mice: role for nitric oxide signaling pathway. Epilepsy Res 2007;75(2–3):138–44.

87. Ray M, Mediratta PK, Reeta K, et al. Receptor mechanisms involved in the anticonvulsant effect of melatonin in maximal electroshock seizures.

Methods Find Exp Clin Pharmacol 2004;26(3): 177–81.

88. Mevissen M, Ebert U. Anticonvulsant effects of melatonin in amygdala-kindled rats. Neurosci Lett 1998;257(1):13–6.

89. Lapin IP, Mirzaev SM, Ryzov IV, et al. Anticonvulsant activity of melatonin against seizures induced by quinolinate, kainate, glutamate, NMDA, and pentylenetetrazole in mice. J Pineal Res 1998; 24(4):215–8.

90. Malow BA, Edwards J, Marzec M. Effects of vagus nerve stimulation on respiration during sleep: a pilot study. Neurology 2000;55(10):1450–4.

91. Murray BJ, Matheson JK, Scammell TE. Effects of vagus nerve stimulation on respiration during sleep. Neurology 2001;57(8):1523–4.

92. Marzec M, Edwards J, Sagher O, et al. Effects of vagus nerve stimulation on sleep-related breathing in epilepsy patients. Epilepsia 2003;44(7):930–5.

93. Malow BA, Edwards J, Marzec M. Vagus nerve stimulation reduces daytime sleepiness in epilepsy patients. Neurology 2001;57(5):879–84.

94. Ebben MR, Sethi NK, Conto M, et al. Vagus nerve stimulation, sleep apnea, and CPAP titration. J Clin Sleep Med 2008;4(5):471–3.

95. Papacostas SS, Myrianthopoulou P, Dietis A, et al. Induction of central-type sleep apnea by vagus nerve stimulation. Electromyogr Clin Neurophysiol 2007;47(1):61–3.

96. Nagarajan L, Walsh P, Gregory P, et al. Respiratory pattern changes in sleep in children on vagal nerve stimulation for refractory epilepsy. Can J Neurol Sci 2003;30(3):224–7.

97. Alanis-Guevara I, Pena E, Corona T, et al. Sleep disturbances, socieconomic status and seizure control as main predictors of quality of life in epilepsy. Epilepsy Behav 2005;7(3):481–5.

98. Cohen HB, Dement WC. Sleep: suppression of rapid eye movement phase in the cat after electroconvulsive shock. Science 1966;154(3747):396–8.

99. Rondouin G, Baldy-Moulinier M, Passouant P. The influence of hippocampal kindling on sleep organization in cats. Effects of alpha-methylparatyrosine. Brain Res 1980;181(2):413–24.

100. Raol YH, Meti BL. Sleep-wakefulness alterations in amygdala-kindled rats. Epilepsia 1998;39(11): 1133–7.

101. Ayala-Guerrero F, Alfaro A, Martinez C, et al. Effect of kainic acid-induced seizures on sleep patterns. Proc West Pharmacol Soc 2002;45:178–80.

102. Yi PL, Tsai CH, Lin JG, et al. Kindling stimuli delivered at different times in the sleep-wake cycle. Sleep 2004;27(2):203–12.

103. Bastlund JF, Jennum P, Mohapel P, et al. Spontaneous epileptic rats show changes in sleep architecture and hypothalamic pathology. Epilepsia 2005;46(6):934–8.

104. van Luijtelaar G, Bikbaev A. Midfrequency corticothalamic oscillations and the sleep cycle: genetic, time of day and age effects. Epilepsy Res 2007; 73(3):259–65.

105. Alfaro-Rodríguez A, González-Piña R, Arch-Tirado E, et al. Neuro-protective effects of carbamazepine on sleep patterns and head and body shakes in kainic acid-treated rats. Chem Biol Interact 2009;180(3):376–82.

106. Matos G, Tsai R, Baldo MV, et al. The sleep-wake cycle in adult rats following pilocarpine-induced temporal lobe epilepsy. Epilepsy Behav 2010; 17(3):324–31.

107. Legros B, Bazil CW. Effects of antiepileptic drugs on sleep architecture: a pilot study. Sleep Med 2003;4(1):51–5.

108. Sammaritano M, Sherwin A. Effect of anticonvulsants on sleep. Neurology 2000;54(5):16–24.

109. Gigli GL, Placidi F, Diomedi M, et al. Nocturnal sleep and daytime somnolence in untreated patients with temporal lobe epilepsy: changes after treatment with controlled-release carbamazepine. Epilepsia 1997;38(6):696–701.

110. Placidi F, Scalise A, Marciani MG, et al. Effect of antiepileptic drugs on sleep. Clin Neurophysiol 2000;111(Suppl 2):115–9.

111. Foldvary-Schaefer N. Sleep complaints and epilepsy: the role of seizures, antiepileptic drugs and sleep disorders. J Clin Neurophysiol 2002; 19(6):514–21.

112. Placidi F, Marciani MG, Diomedi M, et al. Effects of lamotrigine on nocturnal sleep, daytime somnolence and cognitive functions in focal epilepsy. Acta Neurol Scand 2000;102(2):81–6.

113. Ayala-Guerrero F, Mexicano G, González V, et al. Effect of oxcarbazepine on sleep architecture. Epilepsy Behav 2009;15(3):287–90.

114. Bonanni E, Galli R, Maestri M, et al. Daytime sleepiness in epilepsy patients receiving topiramate monotherapy. Epilepsia 2004;45(4):333–7.

115. Bell C, Vanderlinden H, Hiersemenzel R. The effects of levetiracetam on objective and subjective sleep parameters in healthy volunteers and patients with partial epilepsy. J Sleep Res 2002;11(3):255–63.

116. Cicolin A, Magliola U, Giordano A, et al. Effects of levetiracetam on nocturnal sleep and daytime vigilance in healthy volunteers. Epilepsia 2006;47(1):82–5.

117. Cho YW, Kim do H, Motamedi GK. The effect of levetiracetam monotherapy on subjective sleep quality and objective sleep parameters in patients with epilepsy: compared with the effect of carbamazepine-CR monotherapy. Seizure 2011; 20(4):336–9.

118. Zhou JY, Tang XD, Huang LL, et al. The acute effects of levetiracetam on nocturnal sleep and daytime sleepiness in patients with partial epilepsy. J Clin Neurosci 2011;19:956–60.

119. Coppola G, Iervolino G, Mastrosimone M, et al. Melatonin in wake-sleep disorders in children, adolescents and young adults with mental retardation with or without epilepsy: a double-blind, cross-over, placebo-controlled trial. Brain Dev 2004;26(6):373–6.

120. Gupta M, Aneja S, Kohli K. Add-on melatonin improves sleep behavior in children with epilepsy: randomized, double-blind, placebo-controlled trial. J Child Neurol 2005;20(2):112–5.

121. Elkhayat HA, Hassanein SM, Tomoum HY, et al. Melatonin and sleep-related problems in children with intractable epilepsy. Pediatr Neurol 2010; 42(4):249–54.

122. Uberos J, Augustin-Morales MC, Molina Carballo A. Normalization of the sleep-wake pattern and melatonin and 6-sulphatoxy-melatonin levels after a therapeutic trial with melatonin in children with severe epilepsy. J Pineal Res 2011;50(2):192–6.

# Sleep Movement Disorders and Neurologic Movement Disorders

Carl D. Boethel, MD, FCCP*, Shirley F. Jones, MD, FCCP, James A. Barker, MD, CPE, FCCP

## KEYWORDS

- Movement disorders • Neurologic injury • Epilepsy • Rhythmic movement body disorder
- Somnambulism • Somniloquy

## KEY POINTS

- This article will discuss common sleep movement disorders and neurologic movement disorders.
- Neurologic injury, such as stroke or traumatic brain injury, often markedly alters sleep.
- Sleep movement disorders, including frontal lobe epilepsy, somnambulism, somniloquy, rhythmic movement body disorder, REM behavior disorder, and restless leg syndrome, are discussed.

## INTRODUCTION

In this article we discuss 2 types of movement disorders. First, we briefly discuss common sleep movement disorders and, second, we discuss neurologic movement disorders. Neurologic injury, such as stroke or traumatic brain injury, often markedly alters sleep, and we cover much of that in detail as well.

There are a variety of "things that go bump in the night." These could be roughly lumped into the category of sleep movement disorders. To begin with, epilepsy often arises from sleep and is more common in sleep than in wake. Frontal lobe epilepsy can be difficult to diagnose because stereotypic behaviors can be seen, and, thus, the epilepsy can be mistaken for a parasomnia or even conversion disorder.

Somnambulism, or sleep walking, and somniloquy, or sleep talking, are common events. These are the most common parasomnias. They arise primarily out of stage 3 or slow-wave sleep (SWS). This is extremely common in childhood but still may occur in adulthood.

Rhythmic movement body disorder or bed rocking is an idiopathic disorder that is common in childhood but does occasionally persist in adulthood. A persistent rocking motion or head hitting pillow motion may occur at the beginning of sleep or even throughout the night. Multiple medication attempts have generally been unsuccessful. The use of a water bed may actually be the most effective therapy. Hypnosis has also been tried. Rhythmic movement disorder can be a frontal lobe seizure, so investigation is indicated before assigning this diagnosis.

Restless legs syndrome (RLS) is a common disorder. There are 2 groups of patients. One is an autosomal dominant inherited group, usually with onset early in life such as teenage years. These patients have a creepy, crawly feeling, usually on the legs or sometimes on arms. All 4 extremities can be involved. There is an urge to move, and it is actually quite difficult for these patients to hold still for an entire hour. The second form is associated with iron deficiency. It can also be known to occur after beginning certain medications such as

Division of Pulmonary, Critical Care, and Sleep Medicine, Department of Internal Medicine, Texas A&M Health Science Center-College of Medicine, Scott & White Healthcare, 2401 South 31st Street, Temple, TX 76508, USA
* Corresponding author.
E-mail address: CBOETHEL@sw.org

Sleep Med Clin 7 (2012) 631–642
http://dx.doi.org/10.1016/j.jsmc.2012.10.004
1556-407X/12/$ – see front matter © 2012 Elsevier Inc. All rights reserved.

tricyclic antidepressants. Parkinson's medications are used to treat this disorder but paradoxically can sometimes make it worse. There is a clinical correlate during sleep that is called periodic limb movement disorder. Periodic limb movement disorder can be associated with a number of other sleep disorders, in particular obstructive sleep apnea (OSA). The association with sleep apnea is not well understood. The periodic limb movement disorder is typically in the first third of the night with muscle contractions lasting 0.5 to 5.0 seconds at regular intervals of 40 to 90 seconds. Periodic limb movements are not generally seen during rapid eye movement (REM) sleep. Most experts think that periodic limb movements need to show evidence of an accompanying arousal to be considered clinically significant. In fact, periodic limb movements cannot be staged or counted if they occur within an OSA because there is an association with OSA (which is poorly misunderstood, yet real).

Finally, REM behavior disorder is a fascinating disorder that, again, is closely tied to parkinsonism and is discussed in detail within this article. In brief, REM sleep behavior disorder represents loss of skeletal muscle paralysis such that active movement occurs during REM sleep. Thus, there is a loss of inhibition for this activity. The minimum criteria for diagnosis are the following:

1. Suggestive history with polysomnographic abnormality during REM sleep showing elevated electromyographic (EMG) tone;
2. Documentation of abnormal REM sleep behavior during the polysomnogram (PSG), such as prominent limb or truncal jerking, or vigorous, complex or even violent behavior; and
3. Absence of electroencephalogram (EEG) epileptic form activity.

## SPECIFIC DISORDERS AND THE ASSOCIATED SLEEP MOVEMENT RESPONSE THAT MAY OCCUR
### Stroke

Strokes may occur in a number of discrete loci within the brain and, thus, sequelae vary depending on the lesion. Unfortunately, strokes remain common. Hypersomnia occurs in 22% of patients after an ischemia stroke. Sleep apnea is also common after stroke, occurring in up to 71% of patients after cortical stroke.[1] Insomnia, likewise, is common after stroke.

RLS and increased periodic limb movements of sleep (PLMS) have been reported by numerous investigators to follow stroke. REM sleep behavior disorder, likewise, has been seen to arise after stroke. And, finally, seizures are well known to occur as a new entity in patients following stroke.

In particular, nocturnal frontal lobe epilepsy (NFLE) may occur as a form fruste movement disorder following stroke.[2] NFLE arises from sleep 90% of the time. It now encompasses what had previously been called paroxysmal nocturnal dystonia (PND). PND is now known to be a form of frontal lobe seizure. NFLE can be very difficult to distinguish from parasomnia.

Some useful differentiations include the following:

1. Parasomnia onset is almost always in those younger 10 years and NFLE can begin at any age.
2. There are typically only 1 or 2 parasomnias per night, whereas NFLEs are commonly 3 or 4 per night. This equates to 20 to 40 NFLE episodes per month; whereas parasomnias tend to be less than four per month.
3. Parasomnias usually disappear in adolescence, although they can persistent into adulthood.
4. Episodes are seconds to 3 minutes for NFLE, whereas they are seconds to 30 minutes for parasomnias.
5. NFLEs are highly stereotyped, frequently vigorous. Parasomnias are rarely stereotyped but can be violent.
6. There are no known triggers for NFLE except perhaps for sleep deprivation. Triggers for parasomnias are thought to be stress or emotional trauma.
7. Frankly epileptiform ictal movements are only in 10% of NFLEs, so EEG is not a perfect "gold standard." EEG shows activity plus SWS in parasomnia.
8. Parasomnias are almost always out of stage 3, whereas NFLEs primarily occur in stage 2.

### Medications

Obviously, it will be important to realize that the therapies that we initiate in any setting (outpatient, hospital, or skilled nursing facility/rehabilitation center) may have unexpected consequences. It is extremely common for certain medications to worsen or induce new sleep disorders. RLS can be induced by escitalopram, fluoxetine, L-dopa/carbidopa and pergolide, L-thyroxine, mianserin, mirtazapine, olanzapine, and tramadol. Periodic limb movements of sleep are worsened by this list but may also particularly be worsened by bupropion, citalopram, fluoxetine, paroxetine, sertraline, and venlafaxine.[3]

Of course, it should be remembered that many medications have predictable side effects, that is, haloperidol and droperidol may induce torticollis or parkisonian features.

## Traumatic Brain Injury

Patients with traumatic brain injury (TBI) suffer a variety of sequelae. It is interesting to note that hypocretin falls in many of these patients and then normalizes. Consequently, they may act much like patients with narcolepsy and may require stimulants, such as modafinil or ritalin.[4] Severe hypersomnia is common in patients with TBI. Of course, seizures may also occur in those patients after TBI. Again, care must be used to separate posttraumatic seizures from parasomnias; however, in this particular group a seizure would be much more common than a new-onset parasomnia.[1]

## Multiple Sclerosis

Multiple sclerosis (MS) is an autoimmune demyelinating disease that can have multiple foci and thus can have a wide variety of different clinical presentations. Sleep disorders within patients with MS are estimated to be between 25% and 54%.[5] These may include insomnia, sleep-disordered breathing, circadian rhythm disorder, RLS, narcolepsy, and REM sleep behavior disorder. All of these may arise as complications of the MS-associated plaques, creating specific lesions in the brain. New origin of sleep behavior disorder has been described with an increase of about 10-fold beyond the general age-matched public. Clonazepam has appeared effective in these patients, as it is in idiopathic rapid eye movement sleep behavior disorder (RBD). RLS is likewise common.

## REMEMBER, THE DIAGNOSTIC ACRONYM URGE

1. U: an urge to move the legs, usually associated with unpleasant leg sensations;
2. R: rest induces symptoms;
3. G: getting active (physically and mentally) brings relief;
4. E: evening and nights make symptoms worse.

RLS is about twice more frequent in patients with MS as in the age-matched general population. Also of interest, cytokine levels are increased in MS. Proinflammatory cytokines, such as tumor necrosis factor-alpha, interleukin (IL)-1beta, and IL-6 have some sleep-inducing properties and are common in many disease states.

## Muscular Dystrophy

Myotonic dystrophy type 1 (MD1) is a common adult-onset muscular dystrophy. Obviously, because of the progression of skeletal muscle weakness, MD1 is commonly associated with hypo-ventilation at night, OSA, and respiratory insufficiency (sleep-disordered breathing). Periodic limb movements and RLS are also increased in this population. REM sleep is dysregulated, so these patients may have increased number of sleep-onset REM periods (SOREMP); however, they do not have new-onset narcolepsy. Excessive daytime sleepiness is common in these patients. They are often managed with central nervous system stimulant drugs. Other parasomnias have not been particularly increased in myotonic dystrophy.[6]

## Quadraplegia

Patients with quadriplegia do have disordered sleep, as might be expected. This is primarily OSA and mixed sleep apnea. In addition, they have a prolonged REM latency.[7]

## Cerebellar Ataxias

Cerebellar ataxias are becoming more and more described. They commonly do involve sleep disturbance. In particular, RLS and periodic limb movement disorder are increased. Spinocerebellar ataxia types 1, 2, and 3 are known to do this. There are no good data for Friedreich ataxia, the most common recessive ataxia across the world; however, OSA and mixed apnea are increased in patients with Friedreich ataxia. REM behavior disorder is known to be increased in SCA2 and SCA3.[8]

## SLEEP AND MOVEMENT DISORDERS
### Parkinson Disease

Of all the movement disorders that may be seen by the sleep medicine specialist, the most common is Parkinson disease (PD). This is primarily because most patients with PD complain of some form of disturbed sleep. Tandberg and colleagues[9] reported that approximately two-thirds of all patients with PD suffer from sleep and nocturnal disorders. This was compared with patients with diabetes at 46% and healthy elderly at 33%. The disease is a neurologic disorder characterized by progressive disability of motor function. Common findings include muscle rigidity, resting tremors, and slow movements. The pathophysiology is a neurodegenerative disorder that involves loss of dopaminergic neurons in the substantia nigra; however, it appears that other neurotransmitter systems are not immune to the damage that results from this disease. There is evidence that the serotonergic, cholinergic, orexinergic, and noradrenergic systems are affected as well,[10] and the loss or damage to these neurons probably accounts for some of the sleep-related symptoms these patients experience.

In addition, the most common side effects seen with medications used to treat PD are the development of sleep disturbance and/or daytime sleepiness. Age-related changes in sleep architecture and quality may also play a role in sleep-related dysfunction. Therefore, when encountering a patient with PD, the cause of the patient's complaint may not be so easy to elucidate, and problems with sleep and wakefulness may result from multiple causes. Not only does the disease itself result in sleep pathology, the treatment may worsen or aggravate sleep complaints. To better understand the sleep issues that a patient with PD may have, it is worthwhile to address the disease as it relates to multiple sleep disorders. It should also be noted that Lewy body dementia, progressive supranuclear palsy, and the grouping "neurodegenerative disorders" have all been reported to have these same associated sleep disorders.

## Sleep-Disordered Breathing

With it affecting upward of 2% to 9% of the US population, OSA syndrome has become one of the most common sleep disorders. Multiple studies have shown a prevalence of OSA of 20% to 67% among patients with PD[11]; however, data are mixed on the relationship between the 2 disorders. Patients with PD are likely to snore, and in a series of 86 patients, 72% of the patients snored, and of these patients they had higher complaints of excessive daytime sleepiness.[12–14] Given the higher risk of sleep apnea in REM sleep, the findings of less REM sleep and higher apnea-hypopnea index in patients with PD suggests another mechanism for the sleep-disordered breathing. Most likely, upper airway changes in muscle tone at the level of the glottis lead to increased airway collapsibility. It appears that patients with PD and OSA do not have the same sympathetic response to the obstructive events that control patients with OSA encounter. In a study performed by Valko and colleagues,[15] patients with PD who had OSA and those without OSA had similar levels of heart rate variability, a marker of sympathetic nervous system tone. This was in stark contrast to control patients with OSA who showed greater heart rate variability. Patients with PD and OSA do not appear to have the typical physiologic profile of a patient with OSA.

However, there have been 2 recent studies that show no increased risk of sleep apnea associated with PD. When comparing French patients with PD without sleepiness with age-matched, sex-matched, and body mass index (BMI)-matched control patients without neurologic diseases and with patients with PD with excessive sleepiness, Cochen De Cock and colleagues[16] showed that patients with PD did not have an increased risk of having OSA; however, the control patients were recruited from hospitalized patients, and may have had a higher risk for sleep apnea than the patients with PD. Interestingly, the average BMI in both patient groups was 24. In another study that compared patients after 3 nights of sleep studies with normative data from the Sleep Heart Health Study, there was no increased incidence of sleep apnea in patients with PD.[17] It appears that the data are mixed when determining whether patients with PD are at higher risk of sleep apnea. There do not appear to be any studies that have looked at sleep apnea as a risk factor for PD, and it is unclear if patients suffering from both PD and OSA have a more rapid progression of their parkinson symptoms. Nor are there any population-based studies that test if OSA risk increases as the PD progresses, but with the risk of upper airway collapse and changes in muscle tone, patients should be assessed for a concomitant sleep breathing disorder if they have PD and present with fatigue or snoring.

## REM Sleep Behavior Disorder

Based on the International Classification of Sleep Disorders (ICSD)-2, the minimal criteria to diagnose RBD are as follows:

1. The presence of REM sleep without atonia, defined as sustained or intermittent elevation of submental EMG tone or excessive phasic muscle activity in the limb EMG.
2. At least one of the following:
   a. Sleep related injurious or potentially injurious disruptive behaviors by history.
   b. Abnormal REM behaviors documented on polysomnogram.
3. Absences of epileptiform activity during REM sleep, unless RBD can be clearly distinguished from any concurrent REM sleep-related seizure disorder.
4. Sleep disturbance not better explained by another sleep disorder, medical or neurologic disorder, mental disorder, medication use, or substance use disorder.[18]

Since first identified by Drs Schenck and Mahowald in 1986, RBD has been identified with neurodegenerative disorders, notably PD.[19] Then in 1996, the same investigators reported the development of PD in patients initially diagnosed with idiopathic RBD. Of 29 patients, 38% developed PD symptoms. The RBD symptoms and signs anteceded the development of PD by on average 12 years.[20] Further studies have confirmed similar findings, as one study showed a 10-year risk of development of a neurodegenerative disease on diagnosis of RBD to be 40.6%.[21]

Although history alone can often give enough evidence to suggest a diagnosis of RBD, the use of a polysomnogram is helpful to give a definitive diagnosis. In a study by Frauscher and colleagues[22] that looked at 13 different muscles to localize the best group of muscles to help support a diagnosis of RBD, they found that EMG of the mentalis, flexor digitorum superficialis, and extensor digitorum brevis was superior to the routine polysomnogram (PSG EMG) of mentalis plus left and right tibialis anterior. The use of this 3-muscle montage, known as the SINBAR EMG montage, provided the highest rates of REM sleep phasic EMG activity in subjects with RBD, and there was no difference between idiopathic RBD patients and those with PD. The SINBAR EMG was later validated to detect upward of 94.4% of motor and vocal events occurring with Phasic REM sleep in RBD.[23]

As mentioned previously, the diagnosis usually involves a history of increased muscle activity during REM sleep accompanied by abnormal motor and vocal manifestations. These may include jerking, hitting, punching, and kicking, which can affect the limbs. The facial muscles may reveal grimaces, laughter, and shouting, and, occasionally, patients may even jump or fall out of bed. The first sign of RBD may be the patients presenting with complaints of an accidental laceration from a fall across a nightstand. Physicians should rule out other sleep-related disorders, such as frontal lobe epilepsy and severe sleep apnea, before diagnosing RBD.

RBD is characterized by complex behaviors that correspond with dreams. These patients are not known to engage in behaviors such as eating, drinking, or relieving oneself. There appears to be variable penetrance of the degree to which these behaviors are violent. Some patients present with nonviolent behaviors, such as singing, dancing, whistling, or engaging in daytimelike activities,[24] but the violent behaviors often will be frightening to the bed partner or spouse.

Patients with PD suffer from RBD are more likely to have mild cognitive impairment as opposed to patients with PD without RBD. The patients with PD with RBD scored worse on neuropsychiatric testing than patients with PD without the disease. Since RBD is associated with other neurocognitive disorders, such as lewy body dementia and multisystem atrophy, it is fair to say that RBD predisposes patients with PD to the early signs of dementia.[25,26]

It appears that women are more likely than men to have non-violent RBD manifestations. Relying on the REM Sleep Behavior Disorder Screening Questionnaire, this was apparent in a study done by Bjornara and colleagues[27] that screened 107 patients with PD for symptoms of RBD. Men appeared to have more fights and violent behavior despite a similar representation of the disorder in both sexes. The study did not use polysomnographic data to confirm the diagnosis.

This begs the question, is it necessary to perform a PSG on patients to confirm the diagnosis of RBD? The ICSD-2 recommends a PSG, and a study performed by Eisensehr and colleagues[28] at the University of Munich showed that sleep interview alone was not sufficient to make the diagnosis of RBD in patients with PD. They theorize that factors such as the medications used to treat PD have a beneficial effect on RBD symptoms. Therefore, patients with PD may not manifest the same behaviors as idiopathic RBD patients. Conversely, some of the medications used to treat PD can cause hallucinations, most notably levodopa. Therefore, differentiating the cause of nocturnal behaviors in patients with PD should be done with a thorough history and physical examination enhanced by a polysomnogram.

There are medications that can cause symptoms of RBD to occur. Levodopa can cause hallucinations, but these may occur in the daytime as well as at night. Other medications that have been implicated in causing RBD-like behaviors include tricyclic antidepressants, selective serotonin reuptake inhibitors, serotonin norepinephrine reuptake inhibitors, mirtazapine, and bisoprolol. Other substances that have been noted to cause similar symptoms include alcohol, caffeine, and even chocolate.[29]

Treatment of RBD in patients with PD is the same as all patients who suffer from RBD. The long-acting benzodiazepine clonazepam has been the drug of choice since the original patients were treated in the 1980s. The drug has a half-life of 30 hours, but it is rapidly absorbed over 1 to 4 hours. It is recommended to take the drug 30 minutes before bedtime. Cessation of the drug can cause immediate relapse of RBD symptoms. There are no randomized controlled trials that have looked at treatment of RBD with clonazepam, so use of the medication is based on expert opinion, and case series that have shown a 90% response rate to the drug.[30] Although there are multiple case reports of various medications that have been tried in RBD, other than clonazepam, the only other medication that can be recommended for therapy is melatonin. It appears to improve desynchronization and lacks the side effects that commonly are associated with other therapies.

The efficacy of pramipexole for RBD symptoms is inconclusive. Of 29 patients treated with pramipexole at a dose sufficient to treat their PD, only 13 had a favorable response in RBD symptoms. Thus, one can surmise that there may be other neuropathologic mechanisms involved in the development of RBD in patients with PD.[30]

The primary concern that should be dealt with in these patients when first seen is safety. This includes safety for both the patient and the patient's bed partner. Making the room safe from accidents that may occur while sleeping, such as lacerations caused by hitting furniture or falls that may cause fractures, should be addressed and need to be discussed with the patient and family. A safe environment is key to therapy of all patients with RBD. It is clear that RBD predates PD by upward of 12 years, but it is unfortunate that there are no studies that have looked at the prevention of PD in this patient population. RBD appears to predate the development of PD; however, multisystem atrophy (MSA) and Lewy body dementia are also predated by RBD. So, it is important for any patient presenting with RBD symptoms to have a thorough evaluation and close follow-up.

## Restless Legs Syndrome

RLS is a movement disorder that shares a common pathophysiological pathway with PD. Both show a significant improvement in symptoms when treated with medications that enhance dopamine in the brain. It appears that the two may be related, but it is unclear that RLS predisposes patients to the development of PD over time. Patients with PD do have a higher rate of RLS symptoms in comparison with patients with idiopathic RLS in the general population.[10] In addition, most patients with PD may underreport their symptoms of RLS, as the symptoms may be within the constellation of PD symptoms.[31] Thus, patients with PD may find their RLS symptoms occurring during the daytime and may not find the need to report nocturnal RLS symptoms.

Most patients with RLS symptoms require minimal to modest dosages of dopaminergic agonists to control symptoms at night, whereas the dosages required of patients with PD to control their PD symptoms are much higher and can often elicit the augmentation symptoms (which entail RLS symptoms occurring earlier in the day). Although both disorders respond to treatment with dopaminergic agonists, there appears to be a divergence of pathobiology between the two. Low serum ferritin levels and low substantia nigra iron levels have been observed in patients with RLS.[32] This is opposed to the findings in patients with PD, in which the substantia nigra iron stores appear to be increased.[33]

Periodic limb movements are common in patients with PD, and the movement disorder seems to disrupt sleep as a result, leading to decreased total sleep time, poorer sleep efficiency, and less sleep period time.[34] Another study reported recently in the *Journal of Neurologic Sciences* compared patients with PD with high and low numbers of periodic limb movements. Patients with PD with higher levels of PLMS had increased sleep complaints and poorer quality of life. The data showed that the patients with PD with higher levels had more severe progression of PD. This is despite similar objective sleep measures between the two groups.[35] There appears to be improvement in sleep quality in patients with PD with levodopa and dopaminergic agonists. Hogl and colleagues[36] found that the use of the D1 and D2 receptor agonist cabergoline, when given at bedtime, significantly improved PLMS in patients with PD. Also, these patients had improved movement and motor performance on awakening and improved reports of subjective sleepiness. This is despite the fact that the medication cohort appeared to have worse sleep fragmentation and increased nocturnal arousals and awakenings.

## Insomnia

Insomnia is a common subjective complaint of patients with PD. They will present with either sleep onset or sleep maintenance insomnia, and because of the numerous causes of sleep disturbances in patients with PD, it helps to classify insomnia in these terms. RLS, as mentioned previously, is commonly a comorbidity of PD, and can cause sleep-onset insomnia. A high proportion of patients with PD can present with symptoms of depression, anxiety, nocturnal hallucinations, panic attacks, and other mood disorders, all of which can cause both sleep-onset insomnia and sleep maintenance insomnia. In addition, the medications used to treat PD can worsen sleep. Nocturia has also been implicated as a culprit of sleep maintenance insomnia, although it is difficult to separate its cause from other sleep problems. Because most patients with PD are elderly, age-related sleep changes can cause worsening insomnia. Two recent studies have examined the use of dopaminergic agonists versus placebo to treat sleep disturbances. The EASE-PD study explored the use of extended-release ropinirole versus placebo and showed improvement in PD sleep scale scores.[37] In the CLEOPATRA study, in which the clinical efficacy of pramipexole and transdermal rotigotine in patients with advanced PD was explored, more than 400 patients with advanced PD were evaluated. There was a small but significant improvement in PD sleep scale scores with both pramipexole and the transdermal rotigotine.[38] It is not clear whether the improvements were because of improved sleep or if this was because of improvement in the akinesia and hypokinesia that accompanies PD and can lead to sleep disturbances in these patients.

A recent study examined the relationship between nocturnal hypokinesia, the inability to turn in bed, and sleep quality; 240 patients were studied. On the Parkinson Disease Quality of Life Questionnaire (PDQL), the question was asked, "How often in the last 3 months did you have trouble turning over in bed?" It is then scored on a 5-point Likert scale. Patients were then asked to complete the Pittsburgh Sleep Quality Index (PSQI), which gives a good measure of the various aspects of nocturnal sleep. A low value on the PSQI suggests good sleep. The authors found that 60% of the patients with PD had a PSQI greater than 5, but the patients with nocturnal hypokinesia scored much higher on the PSQI. There appears to be a relationship between sleep maintenance insomnia, sleep disruption, and nocturnal hypokinesia.[39]

In a longitudinal cohort study of patients with PD from Norway conducted over 8 years, 89 patients completed the study of an initial 231 patients. Of those 89, 83% experienced insomnia at 1 or more of the study visits; 20% of the 89 developed insomnia as their disease progressed. The data showed a higher level of depression and insomnia in female patients as opposed to males. In addition, the insomnia appears to occur early and appears to be associated with the duration of the disease.[40]

## Measuring Sleep in Patients with PD

As can be judged from the previous information, sleep disturbances, including sleep apnea, RLS, RBD, and insomnia can all affect patients who suffer from PD. For the practicing sleep clinician, there are a number of tools available that can help to diagnose and aid in treatment of patients with PD with sleep complaints. In addition to the commonly used Epworth Sleepiness Scale, the Berlin Sleep Questionnaire is helpful at determining if a patient is at high risk for OSA. The Epworth sleepiness scale provides a measure of subjective sleepiness based on a scale of 0 to 3. Patients with scores of 10 or greater are considered to be excessively sleepy and in need of further workup. The Berlin Sleep Questionnaire asks a serious of questions pertaining to snoring, apneas, and hypertension.

The Parkinson disease sleep scale (PDSS) is a visual analog scale of 15 questions that was developed to aid clinicians in diagnosing sleep disturbances in patients with PD.[41] The scale was initially written by Dr Chaudhuri, and since its initial release has been revised to the Parkinson Disease Sleep Scale-2 (PDSS-2). This scale has been validated in multiple countries and is a reliable and valid tool for measuring sleep disorders in patients with PD, and it adds to the original PDSS by asking about nocturnal hypokinesia, RLS, sleep apnea, and pain.[42]

To question patients about both nocturnal sleep and daytime sleepiness, the Scales for Outcomes in PD-Sleep Scale (SCOPA-S) is available. It does not give evidence for a potential cause of the sleep disorder as opposed to the PDSS-2, but it does assess daytime sleepiness very well and appears to be valid and reliable at assessing sleep in patients with PD.[43,44]

Overnight PSG is highly recommended in the diagnosis of patients with RBD, as with all other parasomnias. Actigraphy is useful in diagnosing circadian rhythm disorders, and it appears to aid in the diagnosis of sleep disturbance in patients with PD. Along with sleep logs or diaries, actigraphy appears to correlate with the PDSS in patients with PD. Although not many studies have been done that have used actigraphy in patients with PD, it has value in assessing movement disorders in sleep medicine and may aid in diagnosis of sleep disruption and assist in management.

## Treatment and Its Side Effects

The main method of treatment of patients with PD is oral L-dopa and the dopamine agonists. However, these medications may benefit the patient with PD in that the movement symptoms may improve, but they may have side effects that can affect sleep and levels of wakefulness and alertness. In addition, dopamine agonists can cause patients to engage in behaviors that can compromise their quality of life such as the dopaminergic dysfunction syndrome. This disorder causes loss of impulse control and has been associated with uncontrolled shopping, gambling, and sexual infidelity. These behaviors can cause great financial and social loss to patients, so patients should be advised of this side effect whenever starting a dopaminergic agonist.

One can hypothesize that the best way to treat patients with PD is to catch them early and prevent neurodegeneration. One study has looked at this issue. By attempting to find patients with precursor disorders that suggest the development of PD, one can find early patients and hopefully prevent the damage. Hyposmia, loss of smell, and RBD fit these criteria. The rate of development of PD in 2 years is 10% in patients with hyposmia and 40% to 50% in patients with RBD. Rasagiline, a selective monoamine oxidase B inhibitor, was found to show some neuroprotection and delay of onset of need for symptomatic therapy in patients with PD. Transcranial sonography may identify changes in substania nigra echogenicity.[26,45]

## SLEEP IN CHOREA AND DYSTONIAS

Movement disorders can be classified into hypokinetic and hyperkinetic disorders. PD classically encompasses the hypokinetic disorder and is characterized as bradykinesia, akinesia, and rigidity. Disorders of hyperkinesis include tremor, chorea, ballism, dystonia, athetosis, tics, myoclonus, startle, and sterotypies. In this section, we focus on the hyperkinetic movement disorders of chorea and dystonia and their sleep-related issues.

### Definitions

Chorea is a defined as random, irregular, brief, flowing movements. The term chorea is derived from the Greek word choreia, which denotes an ancient circle dance. Choreic movements are seen in a variety of illnesses, which can be further classified into genetic disorders (Huntington), infectious (Syndham chorea, which is seen in children with rheumatic fever), drug-related (seen with use of dopamine agonists), endocrine/metabolic conditions (hyperthyroidism), immunologic disorders (systemic lupus erythematosus), vascular disorders (following stroke), and other conditions (cerebral palsy). Dystonia is distinct from chorea and characterized by sustained muscle contractions that result in twisting and abnormal posturing.[46]

### Huntington Disease and Sleep

Huntington disease (HD) is a rare autosomal dominant neurodegenerative disease with a prevalence of 10 cases per 100,000 individuals. A trinucleotide repeat of the sequence CAG in the gene that encodes for the huntington protein is responsible for the disease. Affected individuals are young to middle age. Most cases develop in patients between 30 and 55 years of age. Cognitive impairment, mood disorders, personality changes, and chorea are manifestations of the disease. Early in the disease, patients may exhibit chorea only; however, as the disease progresses, psychiatric symptoms ensue. Sleep becomes increasingly disrupted. The prevalence of sleep problems in patients with HD is 87.8% according to a survey of community-dwelling patients with HD or their caregivers.[47] These sleep problems were ranked very or moderately important in 61.7% of responders and were significant enough for patients and caregivers to seek help.[47] Frequently reported sleep problems included restless limb movements, periodic jerky movements, waking during the night, sleepy by day, and early wakening.[47] More than half of those surveyed reported choreic movements.[47] The role of sleep and HD is particularly important because the inability of caregivers to cope with nocturnal sleep dysfunction is one of the most common reasons for institutionalization of patients with neurodegenerative disease.[48]

Using PSG, multiple studies report sleep disturbances in patients with HD. Patients have prolonged sleep-onset latency[49,50] increase in the number of awakenings[49] and reduced sleep efficiency.[50,51] Higher degrees of clinical disease impairment correlate with less total sleep time, more time spent awake, and reduced sleep efficiency.[49] Mood disorders of depression, common in HD, are associated with worse sleep quality as measured by the Pittsburgh Sleep Quality Index.[52] There are 64% to 80% of patients who report[51,52] sleep stage composition also differs among patients with HD compared with controls, with higher percentages of "light" N1 sleep and wake[49,51] and REM sleep.[51] However, the decrease in REM sleep is not a reported finding in other studies.[49] Multiple studies report higher sleep spindle density in patients with HD.[49,53] Although it seems that sleep worsens as the disease progresses, these sleep disturbances have not been shown to correlate with the number of CAG repeats. The risk of sleep-disordered breathing does not appear to be increased in patients with HD compared with controls[51,54] but if found, responds well to continuous positive airway pressure with improvements in sleep structure, memory, and daytime hypersomnolence in one report.[55] The prevalence of OSA in HD is understudied and is worthy of further investigation, as sleep-disordered breathing is potentially reversible. Excessive daytime sleepiness based on the Epworth Sleepiness Scale affects between 32% and 50%[51,52] of patients with HD and appears to be more common as the disease progresses. Although sleep-disordered breathing should be considered in this population, excessive daytime sleepiness attributed to side effects of medications, sleep-related movements, parasomnias, circadian rhythm dysfunction, and depression warrant additional thought. Daytime somnolence in HD is associated with comorbid depression[52] and correlates with night time sleep disturbances.[56]

In studies examining circadian rhythms of patients with HD, both advanced[51] and delayed sleep phase[56] have been reported. Delayed sleep phase is associated with depression, lower function, and cognitive performance.[56] In the transgenic R6/2 mouse model of HD, disruptions of sleep wake circadian rhythms became more pronounced compared with wild-type mice once neurodegenerative symptoms appeared.[57] Activity became less defined and more irregular in the R6/2 mouse and was accompanied by abnormal expression of mPer2 mRNA in the suprachiasmatic nucleus.[57] Expression of mBmal1b mRNA was also disrupted compared with wild-type mice.[57] Use of a combination of alprazolam to facilitate sleep and modafinil to facilitate wakefulness in the R6/2 mice improved cognitive function and apathy.[58,59] Effects were more robust with the combination compared with each drug alone.[58] Although these findings have not been verified in human studies, profiles of the circadian rhythm of melatonin in 9 patients with early-stage HD exhibited a delay in the nocturnal rise of melatonin compared with controls.[56] Mean diurnal melatonin levels were inversely associated with motor and functional disability in patients with HD.[56] Further research examining circadian rhythm dysfunction directly at the suprachiasmatic nucleus level in patients with HD is needed. The findings of circadian rhythm dysfunction in this population should prompt studies of the effects of photic and nonphotic therapies to resynchronize/restore the circadian rhythm in this population.

Sleep-related movement disorders such as RLS and periodic limb movements have been reported in patients with HD. Although there is no definite known association between RLS and HD, Evers and Stögbauer[60] described a family in which RLS and HD occurred in several members. In another case report, Savva and colleagues[61] described a typical case of RLS that responded to gabapentin in a patient who developed signs and symptoms of HD 3 years later. Using polysomnography, patients with HD have a significant increase in the number of periodic limb movements, but these are not associated with significant arousals when compared with controls.[51] Based on these findings, it is possible that the A11 dopaminergic system that is involved in the RLS may be involved in the pathology of HD,[61] although this is not proven.

REM sleep behavior disorder is a parasomnia characterized by movements of skeletal muscle during REM sleep. In a single study of 25 patients with HD, 3 patients or 12% had findings of REM sleep behavior disorder, reduction in REM sleep, and prolonged onset of REM sleep.[51] Further studies of the effect of mutant huntington protein on evaluating brain structures involved in REM sleep generation should be performed.

Other disorders of REM sleep generation include narcolepsy, a disorder of which components of REM sleep extend into wakefulness. Narcolepsy is classified as with or without cataplexy. Patients with narcolepsy with cataplexy have a reduction of hypocretin-1 also known as orexin-A levels is the cerebrospinal fluid.[62] A similar finding by Petersen and colleagues[63] shows a loss of hypocretin in a transgenic R6/2 mouse model of HD. In this study, the R6/2 mouse model displayed 72% fewer hypocretin neurons and levels of hypocretin-1 in the cerebrospinal fluid. Translation in human studies unfortunately have not been reproduced, as cerebrospinal fluid hypocretin-1 levels are normal in patients with HD[64,65] and hence is not a biomarker for HD in humans. The reduction in hypocretin-1 in HD may be specific only to the mouse model.[65] In a study of 25 patients with HD, mean sleep latencies based on the multiple sleep latency test were significantly longer in patients with HD compared with patients with narcolepsy.[51] Sleep-onset REM periods were not observed in patients with HD and symptoms of narcolepsy including sleep paralysis, cataplexy, and hypnogogic hallucinations were not reported.[51] It does not appear that dysfunction of the hypocretin/orexin system plays a role in human HD.

### Dystonias and Sleep

In dystonia, involuntary muscle contractions cause twisting and sometimes painful abnormal posturing. Prevalence rates vary widely likely because of underdiagnosis or misdiagnosis. Prevalence data from 1950 to 1982 indicate that there are 34 per million persons with generalized dystonia and 295 per million persons with focal dystonias.[66] Cervical dystonia is the most common focal dystonia.[66] Many types of disorders are recognized as dystonia and can be classified by anatomic distribution of muscles affected, age at onset, and cause of the dystonia. The cause of the dystonia is further classified as primary or secondary. In primary dystonia, no other underlying disorders are found and the involuntary muscle contractions are the sole symptom.[67] In secondary dystonia, the dystonia is due to a hereditary neurologic disorder or and exogenous insult,[46] such as Wilson disease, traumatic brain injury, or medications.[67] Examples of dystonias involving certain anatomic distributions include cervical dystonia and blepharospasm. Dystonia that involves contiguous muscles are termed segmental and include oromandibular dystonia. Multifocal and hemidystonia further describe involved areas. Patients less than 26 years of age have early-onset disease. Although the motor symptoms of dystonia are important for classification, the non-motor symptoms of dystonia, including sleep, are drawing increased interest, as such symptoms may impart negative effects on quality of life.

The literature examining sleep in dystonia is limited. A study using the Pittsburgh Sleep Quality Index indicates that 44% of patients with cervical dystonia and 46% of patients with blepharospasm report impaired sleep quality compared with 20% of controls without known neurologic disorders.[68] In patients who reported impaired sleep, association with cervical dystonia and blepharospasm was reported in only 22% and 13% of patients respectively.[68] Improvements in sleep occurred after treatment with botulinum toxin in nearly 40% of patients with cervical dystonia[68]; 19% of patients met clinical criteria for RLS.[68] Despite impaired quality of sleep, most patients did not self-report sleepiness.[68] Avanzino reported similar findings of higher Pittsburgh Sleep Quality Index scores indicating poor sleep in 98 patients with cervical dystonia and blepharospasm compared with controls.[69] However, in patients with cervical dystonia, rates of depression were high and confounded any effect of cervical dystonia on sleep quality.[69] High rates of depression in dystonia are supported in additional studies.[68,70] Higher scores in sleep latency, duration, and efficiency suggest problems with insomnia.[69] Interestingly, sleep quality did not correlate with severity of dystonia.[69] It is unknown whether a separate mechanistic effect of dystonia on sleep exists. Limitations to these studies are the use of survey instruments that do not necessarily correlate with PSG measures of sleep.[71,72]

Using PSG in 10 patients with cervical dystonia, blepharospasm, and oromandibular dystonia, patients had reduced sleep efficiencies, increase in wake after sleep onset, and stage 1 and stage 2 of sleep and reductions in slow wave sleep and REM compared with reference values.[73] Similarly, Jankel reported reduced sleep efficiency, prolonged sleep onset, and an increase in stage 2 sleep with an additional finding of changes in spindle activity.[74] The number of muscle spasms decreased as sleep progresses.[73,75]

## SUMMARY AND RECOMMENDATIONS

Patients with chorea and dystonia suffer from sleep-related problems. While the exact etiology of the sleep disturbance is unclear, sleep quality can be poor. Recognition of comorbid mood disorders, such as depression, sleep-related breathing disorders, parasomnias, sleep-related movement disorders, and circadian rhythm dysfunction is important. Future research should focus on the pathophysiology of the disease and its relation to sleep modulation, examine sleep specific treatment on comorbid disease and symptoms, and their effects on quality of life in patients and their caregivers.

## REFERENCES

1. Dyken JE, Afifi AK, et al. Sleep-related problems in neurologic diseases. Chest 2012;141(2):528–44.
2. Derry C. Nocturnal frontal lobe epilepsy vs parasomnias. Sleep Dis 2012;14:451–63.
3. Hoque R, Chesson AL Jr. Pharmacologically Induced/exacerbated restless legs syndrome, periodic limb movements of sleep, and REM behavior disorder/REM sleep without atonia: literature review, qualitative scoring, and comparative analysis. Sleep 2010;6(1):79–83.
4. Anderson K. Sleep disturbance and neurological disease. Sleep Dis 2011;11:271–4.
5. Brass SD, Duquette P, Proulx-Therrien J, et al. Sleep disorders in patients with multiple sclerosis. Sleep Med Rev 2012;1:121–9.
6. Dauvilliers YA, Laberge L. Myotonic dystrophy type 1, daytime sleepiness and REM sleep dysregulation. Sleep Med Rev 2012;1:1–7.
7. Berlowitz DJ, Spong J, et al. Relationships between objective sleep indices and symptoms in a community sample of people with tetraplegia. Arch Phys Med Rehabil 2012;93:1246–52.
8. Pedroso JL, Braga-Neto P, et al. Sleep disorders in cerebellar ataxias. Arq Neuropsiquiatr 2011;69(2-A): 253–7.
9. Tandberg E, Larsen JP, et al. A community based study of sleep disorders in patients with Parkinson's disease. Mov Disord 1998;13(6):895–9.
10. Suzuki K, Miyamoto M, et al. Sleep disturbances associated with Parkinson's disease. Parkinsons Dis 2011;2011:1–10 Article ID 219056.

11. Lelieveld I, Muller M, et al. The role of serotonin in sleep disordered breathing associated with Parkinson disease: a correlative [11C]DASB PET Imaging study. PLoS One 2012;7(7):e40166.
12. Braga-Neto P, da Silva-Junior FP, et al. Snoring and excessive daytime sleepiness in Parkinson's disease. J Neurol Sci 2004;217(1):41–5.
13. Hogl B, Seppi K, et al. Increased daytime sleepiness in Parkinson's disease: a questionnaire survey. Mov Disord 2003;18(3):319–23.
14. Maria B, Sophia S, et al. Sleep breathing disorders in patients with idiopathic Parkinson's disease. Respir Med 2003;97(10):1151–7.
15. Valko P, Hauser S, Werth E, et al. Heart rate variability in patients with idiopathic Parkinson's disease with and without obstructive sleep apnea syndrome. Parkinsonism Relat Disord 2012;18:525–31.
16. De Cock VC, Abouda M, et al. Is obstructive sleep apnea a problem in Parkinson's disease? Sleep Med 2010;11:247–52.
17. Trotti L, Bliwise D. No increased risk of obstructive sleep apnea in Parkinson's disease. Mov Disord 2010;25(13):2246–9.
18. American Academy of Sleep Medicine. International classification of sleep disorders, 2nd ed.: diagnostic and coding manual. Westchester (IL): American Academy of Sleep Medicine; 2005.
19. Schenck C, Bundlie S, et al. Chronic behavioral disorders of human REM sleep: a new category of parasomnia. Sleep 1986;9(2):293–308.
20. Schenck C, Bundlie S, et al. Delayed emergence of parkinsonian disorder in 38% or 29 older men initially diagnosed with idiopathic rapid eye movement sleep behavior disorder. Neurology 1996;46:388–93.
21. Postuma R, Gagnon J, et al. Quantifying the risk of neurodegenerative disease in idiopathic REM sleep behavior disorder. Neurology 2009;72(15):1296–300.
22. Frauscher B, Iranzo A, et al. Quantification of electromyographic activity during REM sleep in multiple muscles in REM sleep behavior disorder. Sleep 2008;31(5):724–31.
23. Iranzo A, Frauscher B, et al. Usefulness of the SINBAR electromyographic montage to detect the motor and vocal manifestations occurring in REM sleep behavior disorder. Sleep Med 2011;12:284–8.
24. Ouidette D, De Cock VC, et al. Nonviolent elaborate behaviors may also occur in REM sleep behavior disorder. Neurology 2009;72:551–7.
25. Gagnon JF, Vendette M, et al. Mild cognitive impairment in rapid eye movement sleep behavior disorder and Parkinson's disease. Ann Neurol 2009;66(1):39–47.
26. Postuma R, Lang A, et al. Caffeine for treatment of Parkinson's disease. Neurology 2012;79:651–8.
27. Bjornara K, Dietrichs E, et al. REM sleep behavior disorder in Parkinson's disease—Is there a gender difference? Parkinsonism Relat Disord 2012. Available at: http://dx.doi.org/10.1016/j.parkreldis.2012.05.027. Accessed October 12, 2012.
28. Eisensehr I, v Lindeiner H, et al. REM sleep behavior disorder in sleep-disordered patients with versus without Parkinson's disease: is there a need for polysomnography? J Neurol Sci 2001;186:7–11.
29. Frenette E. REM sleep behavior disorder. Med Clin North Am 2010;94:593–614.
30. Aurora RN, Zak R, et al. Best practice guide for the treatment of REM sleep behavior disorder (RBD). J Clin Sleep Med 2010;6(1):85–95.
31. Ondo W, Vuong K, et al. Exploring the relationship between Parkinson disease and restless leg syndrome. Arch Neurol 2002;59(3):421–4.
32. Connor J, Boyer P, et al. Neuropathological examination suggests impaired brain iron acquisition in restless legs syndrome. Neurology 2003;61:301–9.
33. Morris C, Edwardson J. Iron histochemistry of the substantia nigra in Parkinson's disease. Neurodegeneration 1994;3(4):277–82.
34. Wetter T, Pollmacher T. Restless legs and periodic limb movements in sleep syndromes. J Neurol 1997;244(Suppl 1):S37–45.
35. Covassin N, Neikrug A, et al. Clinical correlates of periodic limb movements in sleep in Parkinson's disease. J Neurol Sci 2012;316(1):131–6.
36. Hogl B, Rothdach A, et al. The effect of cabergoline on sleep, periodic leg movements in sleep, and early morning motor function in patients with Parkinson's disease. Neuropsychopharmacology 2003;28:1866–70.
37. Pahwa R, Stacy M, et al. Ropinirole 24 hour prolonged release randomized, controlled study in advanced Parkinson's disease. Neurology 2007;68(14):1108–15.
38. Poewe W, Rascol O, et al. Efficacy of pramipexole and transdermal rotigotine in advanced Parkinson's disease: a double-blind, double-dummy, randomised controlled trial. Lancet Neurol 2007;6(6):513–20.
39. Louter M, Munneke M, et al. Nocturnal hypokinesia and sleep quality in Parkinson's disease. J Am Geriatr Soc 2012;60(6):1104–8.
40. Gjerstad M, Wentzel-Larsen T, et al. Insomnia in Parkinson's disease: frequency and progression over time. J Neurol Neurosurg Psychiatry 2007;78:476–9.
41. Chaudhuri K, Pal S, DiMarco A, et al. The Parkinson's disease sleep scale: a new instrument for assessing sleep and nocturnal disability in Parkinson's disease. J Neurol Neurosurg Psychiatry 2002;73:629–35.
42. Trenkwalder C, Kohnen R, et al. Parkinson's disease sleep scale—validation of the revised version PDSS-2. Mov Disord 2011;26(4):644–52.
43. Martinez-Martin P, Visser M, et al. SCOPA-Sleep and PDSS: two scales for assessment of sleep disorder in Parkinson's disease. Mov Disord 2008;23(12):1681–8.

44. Diederich N, McIntyre D. Sleep disorders in Parkinson's disease: many causes, few therapeutic options. J Neurol Sci 2012;314:12–9.

45. Antonini A. The conundrum of neuroprotection in Parkinson's disease. Lancet Neurol 2011;10:396–7.

46. Geyer HL, Bressman SB. The diagnosis of dystonia. Lancet Neurol 2006;5:780–90.

47. Taylor N, Bramble D. Sleep disturbance and Huntingdon's disease. Br J Psychiatry 1997;171:393.

48. Bianchetti A, Scuratti A, Zanetti O, et al. Predictors of mortality and institutionalization in Alzheimer disease patients 1 year after discharge from an Alzheimer dementia unit. Dementia 1995;6:108–12.

49. Wiegand M, Möller AA, Lauer CJ, et al. Nocturnal sleep in Huntington's disease. J Neurol 1991;238:203–8.

50. Hansotia P, Wall R, Berendes J. Sleep disturbances and severity of Huntington's disease. Neurology 1985;35:1672–4.

51. Arnulf I, Nielson J, Lohmann E, et al. Rapid eye movement sleep disturbances in Huntington's disease. Arch Neurol 2008;65:482–8.

52. Videnovic A, Leurgan S, Fan W, et al. Daytime somnolence and nocturnal sleep disturbances in Huntington disease. Parkinsonism Relat Disord 2009;15:471–4.

53. Emser W, Brenner M, Stobere T, et al. Changes in nocturnal sleep in Huntington's and Parkinson's disease. J Neurol 1988;235:177–9.

54. Bollen EL, Den Heijer JC, Ponsioen C, et al. Respiration during sleep in Huntington's chorea. J Neurol Sci 1998;84:63–8.

55. Banno K, Hobson DE, Kryger MH. Long-term treatment of sleep breathing disorder in a patient with Huntington's disease. Parkinsonism Relat Disord 2005;11:261–4.

56. Aziz NA, Anguelova GV, Marinus J, et al. Sleep and circadian rhythm alterations correlate with depression and cognitive impairment in Huntington's disease. Parkinsonism Relat Disord 2010;345:350.

57. Morton AJ, Wood NI, Hastings MH, et al. Disintegration of the sleep-wake cycle and circadian timing in Huntington's disease. J Neurosci 2005;25:157–63.

58. Pallier PN, Morton AJ. Management of sleep/wake cycles improves cognitive function in transgenic mouse model of Huntington's disease. Brain Res 2009;1279:90–8.

59. Aziz NA, Pijl H, Frölich M, et al. Delayed onset of the diurnal melatonin rise in patients with Huntington's disease. J Neurol 2009;256:1961–5.

60. Evers S, Stögbauer F. Genetic association of Huntington's disease and restless legs syndrome? A family report. Mov Disord 2003;18:225–7.

61. Savva E, Schnorf H, Burkhard RP. Restless legs syndrome: an early manifestation of Huntington's disease? Acta Neurol Scand 2009;119:274–6.

62. Mignot E, Lammers GJ, Ripley B, et al. The role of cerebrospinal fluid hypocretin measurement in the diagnosis of narcolepsy and other hypersomnias. Arch Neurol 2002;59:1553–62.

63. Petersen A, Gil J, Maat-Schieman ML, et al. Orexin loss in Huntington's disease. Hum Mol Genet 2005; 14:39–47.

64. Meier A, Molenhauer B, Cohrs S, Rodenbeck A, et al. Normal hypocretin-1 (orexin-A) levels in the cerebrospinal fluid of patients with Huntington's disease. Brain Res 2005;1063:201–3.

65. Gaus SE, Ling L, Mignot E. CSF hypocretin levels are normal in Huntington's disease patients. Sleep 2005;28:1607–8.

66. Nutt JG, Muenter MD, Aronson A, et al. Epidemiology of focal and generalized dystonia in Rochester, Minnesota. Mov Disord 1988;3:188.

67. Hanson M. Use of chemodenervation in dystonic conditions. Cleve Clin J Med 2012;79:S25–9.

68. Paus S, Gross J, Moll-Müller M, et al. Impaired sleep quality and restless legs syndrome in idiopathic focal dystonia: a case controlled study. J Neurol 2011;258:1835–40.

69. Avanzino L, Martino D, Marchese R, et al. Quality of sleep in primary focal dystonia: a case control study. Eur J Neurol 2010;17:576–81.

70. Miller KM, Okun MS, Fenandez HF, et al. Depression symptoms in movement disorders: comparing Parkinson's disease, dystonia, and essential tremor. Mov Disord 2007;22:666–72.

71. Buysse DJ, Reynolds CF, Monk TH, et al. The Pittsburgh Sleep Quality Index: a new instrument for psychiatric practice and research. Psychiatry Res 1989;28:193–213.

72. Olson LG, Cole MF, Ambrogetti A. Correlations among Epworth sleepiness scale scores, multiple sleep latency tests and psychological symptoms. J Sleep Res 1998;7:248–53.

73. Sforza E, Montagna P, Defazio G, et al. Sleep and cranial dystonia. Electroencephalogr Clin Neurophysiol 1991;79:166–9.

74. Jankel WR, Allen RP, Nedermeyer E, et al. Polysomnographic findings in dystonia musculorum deformans. Sleep 1983;6:281–5.

75. Lobbezoo F, Thu Thon M, Rémillard G, et al. Relationships between sleep, neck muscle activity and pain in cervical dystonia. Can J Neurol Sci 1996; 23:285–90.

# Sleep Disorders in Spinal Cord Injury

Richard J. Castriotta, MD[a],*, Mark C. Wilde, PsyD[b],
Sandeep Sahay, MD[c]

## KEYWORDS

- Spinal cord injury • Hypoventilation • Sleep-disordered breathing • Sleep apnea • Insomnia
- Circadian rhythm disorder • Melatonin • Restless legs

## KEY POINTS

- Pathophysiological changes after spinal cord injury predispose to hypoventilation and obstructive sleep apnea, both of which are very common after SCI.
- SCI may result in circadian rhythm disorders due to disruption of pathways controlling melatonin and body temperature.
- SCI patients have multiple reasons for insomnia, including pain, psychological distress, restless legs and periodic limb movements in REM and NREM sleep.

## INTRODUCTION

At present, there are approximately 270,000 people living with spinal cord injury (SCI) in the United States, with an additional 12,000 new cases each year.[1] The average age at injury has increased from 28.7 years in 1979 to 41 years since 2005.[1] Respiratory problems are the major cause of morbidity and mortality in these patients[2–4] and these are worsened by the physiology of sleep and especially rapid eye movement (REM) sleep.[5] It is estimated that 56.6% of patients with SCI have cervical cord lesions with partial or complete tetraplegia,[1] which impairs the neuronal control of breathing.[5,6] The most important forms of sleep-disordered breathing in patients with SCI are sleep-related hypoventilation and obstructive sleep apnea (OSA), but there are also a number of nonrespiratory sleep problems that are common. These include circadian rhythm disorders, insomnia, restless legs syndrome, and periodic limb movements in sleep. Sleep disorders are underrecognized in patients with SCI, in part because many sleep-related respiratory problems are without symptoms, and in part because many nonrespiratory sleep disturbances are not generally investigated during neurorehabilitation; however, recent literature suggests an increased prevalence of sleep disorders in this group of patients.[7–9] In the able-bodied population, sleep disorders are known to cause a multitude of problems, such as hypertension, dyslipidemia, cardiac arrhythmias, and neurocognitive impairment.[10] Similarly, in patients with SCI, sleep-disordered breathing leads to neurocognitive impairment adversely affecting neurorehabilitation.[11]

## NEURAL CONTROL OF RESPIRATION

All respiratory muscles are paralyzed with SCI above C3. The main inspiratory muscle is the diaphragm, innervated by the phrenic nerve at

Disclosures: None of the authors have any conflicts of interest to disclose.
[a] Division of Pulmonary and Sleep Medicine, University of Texas Medical School at Houston, 6431 Fannin Street, MSB 1.274, Houston, TX 77030, USA; [b] Department of Physical Medicine and Rehabilitation, University of Texas Medical School at Houston, 6431 Fannin Street, Houston, TX 77030, USA; [c] Division of Pulmonary and Sleep Medicine, University of Texas Medical School at Houston, 6431 Fannin Street, Houston, TX 77030, USA
* Corresponding author.
E-mail address: Richard.J.Castriotta@uth.tmc.edu

C3 to C5. Expiratory muscle function is performed by the abdominal and lateral intercostal muscles innervated at T1 to T12. These are important in generating adequate cough and airway clearance. The neurons present in the pre-Bötzinger complex and the neurons in the parafacial respiratory group in the ventrolateral medulla generate the automatic rhythm and project it to the ventral respiratory group located ventrolateral to the nucleus ambiguous of the medulla.[12–14] This contains the inspiratory and expiratory bulbospinal neurons. The respiratory depressant effects of opioids are brought about by acting on pre-Bötzinger complex neurons expressing neurokinin-1 receptors, and these effects are magnified in deep, non–rapid eye movement (NREM) sleep.[15] The pathways from the ventral respiratory group go downward and synapse with the phrenic nerve lower motor neurons in the ventral horn of the spinal cord at C3, C4, and C5 levels, which innervate the diaphragm (in humans).[16,17] Thus, SCI even below the phrenic nerve nuclei may adversely affect respiratory muscles in the thorax and abdomen. Even though the decussation of these descending tracts causing bilateral innervation of the phrenic nerve nuclei has been demonstrated in animal models, this has not been definitively confirmed in humans.[6] Unilateral disruption of the pre-Bötzinger complex leads to impaired breathing during sleep but not while awake,[18] a sort of Ondine curse.

## PHYSIOLOGIC CHANGES IN RESPIRATION DURING SLEEP

SCI leads to a series of pathophysiological alterations causing impaired ventilation, which worsens during sleep, in part because of a normally lower hypoxic and hypercapnic ventilatory drive during sleep. During NREM sleep, in healthy adults, the minute ventilation ($V_E$) is lowered by 0.4 to 1.5 L/min with a mean reduction in $V_T$ by 132 mL,[19] which leads to an increase in $Pco_2$ by 3 to 7 torr.[20] In REM sleep, hypercapnic respiratory drive is decreased by 70% compared with wakefulness, so that hypoventilation related to REM sleep may be common in predisposed individuals.[21] The hypoxic ventilatory drive is also decreased by 40% in NREM sleep as compared with wakefulness and further decreased by another 50% during REM sleep.[22] In phasic REM sleep, alveolar ventilation is reduced by 10% to 25% as compared with wakefulness.[21] Thus, in patients with SCI, ventilatory impairment can be expected to worsen in sleep, especially during REM sleep.

## SLEEP-DISORDERED BREATHING AND SPINAL CORD INJURY

In patients with SCI, central control of respiratory muscles may be lost. The intercostal and abdominal muscles are paralyzed in quadriplegic patients, and the diaphragm is impaired in those with lesions at C5 or above. This leads to altered mechanics of the chest and abdominal wall with a reduction in vital capacity, maximum breathing capacity, functional residual capacity, expiratory reserve volume, peak inspiratory and expiratory flow rates, inspiratory capacity, total lung capacity, and rib cage and chest wall compliance accompanied by an increase in diaphragmatic and abdominal wall compliance.[23–26] This results in a restrictive ventilatory defect with normal diffusing capacity but impaired gas exchange with mild hypoxemia and hypercapnia in the stable waking state. In addition to the increased work of breathing and impaired lung mechanics, hypoventilation during sleep in quadriplegic patients may be facilitated by a blunted ventilatory drive.[25,27,28] The prevalence of hypercapnia in these patients increases over time.[29] This is important, because the average 40-year-old patient with SCI with tetraplegia who survives the first 24 hours can now be expected to live for another 20 years or more, and this would be 35 to 40 years for a 20-year-old.[1] In patients with low cervical cord lesions, ventilatory function depends largely on the inspiratory capacity of the diaphragm. The intercostal and abdominal muscle contribution is lost and changes in tone or spasms in these muscles may have a detrimental effect. Measured lung function remains permanently well below predicted and would render such patients more susceptible to the effects of hypoventilation and apnea. Patients with high spinal cord lesions have adequate ventilation in their chronic stable state of immobility, they have difficulty responding to the need for increasing ventilation in circumstances such as sepsis and pneumonia, which are now the most frequent causes of death in this population.[1] A study of C5 quadriplegic patients demonstrated blunting of ventilatory response to breathing 5% carbon dioxide.[25] Many of these patients also have increased upper airway resistance owing to an increase in neck circumference[30] and an increase in body mass index.[31] When added to the baseline restrictive ventilatory mechanics and physiologic changes during sleep, this addition to the work of breathing may lead to worsening alveolar hypoventilation and respiratory decompensation during sleep. There is also a high risk of nocturnal hypoxemia in those with C4 to C6 lesions.[32,33] All of the factors that predispose patients with SCI to alveolar hypoventilation and hypoxemia are heightened during sleep and even more so during REM sleep.

These may lead to overt OSA with cardiovascular consequences, such as hypertension, cardiac dysfunction, and heart failure. The prevalence of OSA in SCI is very high (**Table 1**). Estimates range from a low of 15% in selected nonobese Swedish patients with complete or incomplete cervical cord injury[31] to a high of 83% in Australians with acute tetraplegia who were 13 weeks from injury.[34] That number subsequently fell to 62% of the cohort at 52 weeks. This high prevalence was also seen in the most recent prospective longitudinal study[7] of acute SCI (T12 and above), in which OSA was seen as early as 7 weeks after injury and persisted in 75% of patients 4 to 6 months after injury. This group had an average age of 34.0 ± 12.3 years and body mass index (BMI) of 23.6 ± 4.1 kg/m². There was no correlation with BMI, neck circumference, American Spinal Injury Association (ASIA) impairment, or oxygen saturation nadir. Patients were not overtly symptomatic, with average Epworth sleepiness scores of 6.0 ± 3.8. The overall prevalence of OSA in chronic, stable patients with SCI (1–37 years from injury) appears to be 40% to 63%.[30,33–38] Most of these studies used a Respiratory Disturbance Index (RDI) of 15 or more apneas and hypopneas per hour of study or sleep as the criterion for the diagnosis of OSA, so that these would be considered moderate to severe sleep apnea. Although none of the usual risk factors seem to be important in patients with SCI early after injury,[7,34] that does not appear to be the case when they are evaluated later. In patients with chronic SCI, the incidence of OSA correlates with age, BMI, neck circumference, and time after injury.[30,36,37] Indeed one way of moderating the risk of developing OSA for patients with SCI might

be to attempt to avoid excessive weight gain. In general, patients with SCI and OSA are asymptomatic,[34,36,37] although some of those with an RDI greater than 40 may express complaints of daytime sleepiness.[37] Sudden onset of life-threatening delayed apnea can occur weeks after SCI, with risk factors consisting of diffuse cord lesions, bradycardia, and prior transient respiratory distress.[39]

Nonobstructive hypoventilation may occur in SCI. Many people with SCI take medications to suppress muscle spasms, such as benzodiazepines and baclofen, which can depress the central nervous system. Medications that have a depressant effect on the central nervous system have been shown to increase the frequency and severity of sleep-disordered breathing.[40,41] There is also evidence that sleep apnea is associated with cognitive disturbances in subjects with SCI.[42] Sajkov and colleagues[43] have demonstrated that neuropsychological variables (such as verbal attention and concentration, immediate and short-term memory, cognitive flexibility, internal scanning, and working memory) were significantly correlated with measures of sleep hypoxia. Therefore, the presence of sleep apnea may be significant in subjects with SCI. Significant neurocognitive dysfunction could have a major negative impact on quality of life in this group of patients with severe physical restrictions. Additionally, impairment of cognitive tasks may also adversely affect these subjects' rehabilitation. Even in patients who have no OSA-related complaints, it is important to treat sleep-disordered breathing because of the associated risks of mortality and morbidity. In the general population, an apnea-hypopnea index (AHI) or RDI of 30 or more resulted in a threefold risk of mortality and fivefold risk of cardiovascular mortality over an 18-year period.[44]

## MANAGEMENT OF HYPOVENTILATION AND SLEEP APNEA IN SCI

Some patients with SCI with high cervical lesions will require tracheostomy and positive pressure ventilation. This mode of treatment will overcome both hypoventilation and OSA, but is more costly than noninvasive methods and is more frequently associated with episodes of pneumonia and hospitalization.[1,45] Many patients with SCI, however, may be optimally managed with noninvasive positive pressure ventilation (NPPV),[46–48] and this is perceived by patients and caregivers to lead to less discomfort and better appearance, speech, and swallowing.[49] Many will require assisted ventilation only during sleep, especially during

**Table 1**
**Prevalence of OSA in SCI**

| Author, Year | Number of Subjects | % OSA |
|---|---|---|
| Short et al,[35] 1992 | 22 | 45.5 |
| McEvoy et al,[30] 1995 | 40 | 27.5 |
| Klefbeck et al,[33] 1998 | 28 | 15 |
| Burns et al,[36] 2000 | 20 | 40 |
| Stockhammer et al,[37] 2002 | 50 | 62 |
| Berlowitz et al,[34] 2005 | 30 | 60–83 |
| Leduc et al,[38] 2007 | 51 | 53 |
| Tran et al,[7] 2010 | 16 | 73 |

REM sleep.[50] For those requiring NPPV for sleep-related hypoventilation, this will also be an effective treatment for concomitant OSA if appropriately titrated to this end by adequately raising the expiratory positive airway pressure beyond the critical pressure ($P_{crit}$) to prevent upper airway collapse. An alternative to NPPV for hypoventilation is diaphragmatic pacing via bilateral phrenic nerve stimulation.[51–56] This can be used only if both phrenic nerves are viable.[52] This can be evaluated with phrenic nerve conduction studies[57] demonstrating conduction velocities of 14 ms[54] or less or visual descent of the diaphragm of 3 or more under fluoroscopy.[58] Care should be taken to use only the minimal current necessary to obtain results and to have the patient undergo a slow conditioning process to avoid burnout and damage to the phrenic nerves and diaphragm.[55] If diaphragmatic pacing is used, it should be noted that this does not provide any protection from OSA, so polysomnography should be performed to determine if these patients might require additional treatment for OSA. Recent refinements of NPPV, such as averaged volume-assured pressure support, have been used for other causes of hypoventilation[59,60] and need to be further evaluated in SCI. Titration guidelines for NPPV in the management of hypoventilation have been recently published.[61] NPPV should not be used in those with inadequate expiratory muscle function (peak cough flow <160 L/min), facial abnormalities preventing a good mask fit, or those unable to protect their airway.[62]

The mainstay of treatment for OSA in patients with SCI remains continuous positive airway pressure (CPAP), and its use is common in this population.[31] CPAP has been shown to improve sleep architecture, oxygen saturation, and daytime sleepiness in patients with SCI and OSA.[63] CPAP, however, is inadequate for management of hypoventilation.[64] In patients with SCI and OSA, adherence to CPAP therapy depends largely on the presence or absence of daytime complaints and perceived benefit. In one Swiss study,[37] of those patients with SCI who manifested long-term CPAP adherence, 91% had daytime complaints, which improved with CPAP. Of those who refused CPAP, only 1 of 15 had daytime complaints. A proper interface between CPAP and patient is crucial to long-term adherence. Among the patients who discontinued CPAP after a few weeks, 80% did so because of mask discomfort.[37] Patients with SCI with OSA require significantly lower levels of CPAP at any given apnea-hypopnea index (AHI) or RDI than able-bodied patients with OSA, and there is no correlation between AHI and effective CPAP level.[8] The role of auto-titrating positive airway pressure (APAP) in this population is unclear. This modality has been used predominantly in uncomplicated OSA without comorbidities, such as hypoventilation and hypoxemia. There is moderate strength of evidence that APAP and CPAP have similar treatment effects for such uncomplicated patients with OSA in the able-bodied population,[65] but no studies in patients with SCI. Bilevel positive airway pressure may be required when there is concomitant sleep-related hypoventilation, but has no advantage over CPAP in simple OSA.[66]

## Melatonin, Body Temperature, and Circadian Rhythm Disruption in Cervical SCI

The normal circadian rhythm in humans involves the secretion of melatonin by the pineal gland, which increases as darkness begins and reaches a peak in the middle of the night. The mirror image of this would be the core body temperature, which reaches its normal peak in late afternoon and has a nadir in the early morning about 2 hours before awakening. Both of these may be disrupted in cervical SCI. The neural pathways for endogenous production of melatonin pass from the suprachiasmatic nucleus in the hypothalamus through the cervical spinal cord and superior cervical ganglion and back to the pineal gland.[67,68] In cervical SCI (C4–C7) with tetraplegia, it has been shown that the normal evening increase in melatonin secretion is obliterated.[69–71] This is not seen in thoracic SCI. The disrupted melatonin secretion has been shown to cause reduced sleep duration and sleep efficiency, a doubling of time awake after sleep onset and prolonged latency to REM sleep in patients with cervical SCI compared with healthy individuals and those with thoracic SCI.[72] The sleep disruption may in part be a result of disruption in the circadian regulation of core body temperature because of disrupted afferent and efferent sensory information below the lesion with consequent impact on circadian core body temperature or because of the role of melatonin in decreasing core temperature and increasing peripheral temperature. Tetraplegic patients have been shown to have a disturbed circadian core body temperature rhythm with a 5-hour advance in circadian trough time, significantly higher mean nocturnal core body temperature, and a period length shortened from the normal 24.0 to 16.5 hours.[73] The retino-pineal neural pathway for melatonin production runs along very closely to the oculosympathetic pathway descending from the hypothalamus through the cervical spinal cord and then up to the superior ganglion with sympathetic innervation of the ispsilateral face and eye. Lesions to this pathway cause oculosympathetic paresis. Because the 2 pathways are so close, both are often affected together in high cervical SCI. It has been shown that bilateral oculosympathetic paresis in patients with cervical SCI is predictive of absent nocturnal melatonin production.[74] Treatment of circadian rhythm disruption and difficulty sleeping in SCI with melatonin may have additional benefits because of its effectiveness as an antioxidant and free radical scavenger. Multiple animal studies have produced promising results for the use of melatonin in SCI.[75–78] Use of melatonin for treatment of circadian rhythm disorders must be directed by the type of problem. For correction of advanced sleep phase (going to sleep too early), melatonin (0.5–5.0 mg) may be administered around dawn. For those with delayed sleep phase (unable to sleep until very late), melatonin may be administered around dusk.[79] It is important for all patients with SCI, even those with lower (thoracic) lesions, to keep a clear-cut light/dark schedule with plenty of light during the day and darkness at night. It is especially important to have blue light during the day and avoid blue light at night to avoid further suppression of melatonin.[80]

## Restless Legs and Periodic Limb Movements in SCI

Ekbom syndrome or restless legs syndrome (RLS) is a sensorimotor disorder characterized by uncomfortable feelings in the legs with an irresistible urge to move them to bring relief. According to the 2003 National Institutes of Health consensus,[81] the essential criteria for diagnosis are[1] an urge to move the legs with uncomfortable/unpleasant sensations,[2] which begin or worsen at rest and inactivity,[3] are partially or totally removed by movement,[4] and are worse (or only) in the evening or at night. The diagnosis may be made clinically without the need for sleep testing. These symptoms may cause considerable discomfort and result in sleep-onset insomnia. Clear-cut RLS has been recently described in patients with cervical (ASIA A) SCI.[82] All 8 of a randomly selected group of patients with SCI aged 18 to 40 years had RLS. An earlier study on patients with T7 to T12 SCI described RLS, but this was based on the presence of periodic limb movements.[83] Some patients with SCI and RLS may be misdiagnosed as having neuropathic pain or infralesional spastic syndrome. Such patients respond poorly to the usual antispastic drugs (eg, baclofen), tricyclic antidepressants, or drugs such as gabapentin and pregabalin, but in one study, such patients with SCI responded

well to pramipexole in doses of 0.09 to 0.72 mg per day.[84] Prior studies have shown an association of RLS with coronary artery disease and cardiovascular disease,[85] but this has recently been refuted in a large prospective study.[86] The treatment of choice for Ekbom syndrome are dopaminergic agents, such as pramipexole and ropinirole. Pramipexole has been used successfully in patients with SCI for RLS for up to 49 months without problems.[84] Long-term use of pramipexole for RLS in the able-bodied population has been associated with the need for increasing doses, problems with augmentation, sleepiness (including sleep attacks), and impulse control disorders.[87]

Periodic limb movements in sleep (PLMS) are slow, stereotypical, rhythmic limb movements during sleep that are diagnosed by objective criteria by monitoring limb electromyogram on polysomnography.[88,89] They may be an asymptomatic polysomnographic finding, or be a cause of sleep-maintenance insomnia, nonrefreshing sleep, or daytime sleepiness. When accompanied by associated symptoms, the term periodic limb movement disorder may be used.[88] In most of the published studies on PLMS and SCI, the diagnosis was made using a PLM Index (PLMI) of 5 PLMs per hour, based on older criteria,[90] but current guidelines use a PLMI of 15 PLMs per hour in adults and 5 PLMs per hour in children.[88] Most (84%) patients with RLS also have PLMS (by the older criteria),[91] so that PLMS is now considered part of RLS and serves as corroborative evidence for the diagnosis of Ekbom syndrome. There are many people with asymptomatic PLMS without RLS, however, and the significance of PLMS in these circumstances is not clear. PLMS may occur because of myelopathy and have been documented in SCI,[82,92] with PLMs occurring in both REM and non-REM sleep.[93,94] PLMS in able-bodied patients usually occurs only during non-REM sleep. PLMS has been produced in a rat model of T9-level spinal cord injury[95] and was accompanied by reduced sleep efficiency.[95] Although PLMS in SCI, like RLS, responds to dopaminergic agents,[96] there is ample evidence that an equivalent reduction in PLMs can be achieved with physical activity alone.[83,96,97]

## INSOMNIA

Insomnia, which is characterized by difficulties with sleep onset, maintenance, and/or subjective complaints of nonrestorative sleep, is a common problem that can present as a stand-alone problem but is frequently associated with other medical and psychiatric disorders.[98] As with many medical conditions, insomnia has been found to have a higher rate in SCI than in the general population. According to one questionnaire study, patients with SCI had greater difficulty with sleep initiation and maintenance as well as less-restorative sleep than the healthy population.[99] The SCI group had a higher frequency of snoring, slept more hours, and napped more frequently than the healthy population. The culprits cited were voiding problems, spasms, pain, and parasthesias. No differences were found between the groups on alcohol intake, although the SCI group's use of sleeping pills, tobacco, and coffee/tea was significantly higher. In another study, the Medical Outcomes Study Sleep Scale was administered to 620 patients with SCI and the results compared with normative samples of chronically ill persons and healthy individuals.[100] The investigators found that the SCI group reported significantly greater overall sleep problems than the 2 normative comparison groups with the magnitude of these effects being medium to large ($d = 0.50$ and $0.63$) according to Cohen effect size guidelines.[101] They also found that the SCI group reported greater sleep disturbance, more snoring, fewer hours of sleep per night, less-restorative sleep, and greater daytime sleepiness than the other 2 groups. They reported that age of the patients with SCI was negatively associated with the number of sleep complaints and that duration of SCI was not significantly associated with sleep difficulties.

One of the problems with the studies discussed previously is that no effort was made to examine sleeping problems in SCI, excluding the potential influence of sleep-disordered breathing (SDB). In a Department of Veterans Affairs study, 821 patients with SCI were mailed a questionnaire probing dysfunctional sleep or insomnia during the past year along with a number of demographic and other characteristics.[9] The investigators were careful to exclude patients with a diagnosis of OSA or multiple sclerosis with spinal involvement. They found that 49% of the sample complained of sleep dysfunction. Those with sleep complaints were found to be typically younger and greater proportions were smokers; had problems with alcohol, hypertension, asthma, or chronic obstructive pulmonary disease; and problematic weight gain. Thus, although it is entirely conceivable that some of the complaints reported in the studies discussed previously may have been attributable to SDB; there is likelihood that insomnia is a significant presenting sleep complication in patients with SCI without SDB.

Aside from alcohol and tobacco consumption and other medical problems, psychological sequelae from SCI could be associated with insomnia in SCI. Mood and anxiety disorders by themselves and comorbid mood and anxiety disorders are associated with severe insomnia complaints.[102] Depression appears to be common in the SCI population. In one study of 947 patients with SCI using the Patient Health Questionnaire-9 Depression Scale, 50% reported at least some degree of depression, ranging from mild to severe, with a prevalence of probable major depression of 23%.[103] However, there was also a high lifetime prevalence of psychiatric conditions in the depressed group of 60% compared with 28% for the nondepressed group, suggesting that premorbid psychiatric conditions were contributory in some cases. A Portuguese study evaluated 65 patients with SCI within the first 6 weeks and last 6 weeks of their rehabilitation stay with the Symptom Checklist 90-R, Eysenck Personality Inventory, and Coping Assessment Scale.[104] The investigators found psychopathological scores consistent with depression in 57% of patients at evaluation 1 and 40% of patients at evaluation 2, as well as those consistent with anxiety in 30% of patients at the first evaluation and 18% at evaluation 2. These changes from time 1 to time 2 were statistically significant only for anxiety and not for depression. The investigators also make note of a high prevalence of sleep problems. More research into the links between insomnia and psychological distress in SCI is needed. Also, care should be taken to remove the potential influence of SDB by excluding patients with OSA and related conditions. Finally, only one of the studies mentioned previously inquired about premorbid psychiatric status. Premorbid psychiatric status should be evaluated carefully in future studies, as it is likely to have an influence on adjustment to a later disease.

Along with emotional distress, pain seems to play a role in promoting abnormal sleep in SCI. In one study, 77 men with SCI completed a battery of standardized questionnaires, interviews, and physical examinations.[105] In this sample, 75% of the sample reported chronic pain. Of this group, 49% reported that pain "sometimes" caused difficulties with sleep initiation whereas 10% reported that pain "always" caused difficulties with sleep onset. Twenty-four percent "sometimes" required pain medications to sleep whereas 6% "always" used medication for sleep promotion. Thirty-eight percent reported that pain "sometimes" resulted in being awakened from sleep whereas 4% reported that this was "always" the case. In addition, chronic pain was associated with more depressive symptoms and more perceived stress. In a questionnaire study, 217 patients with chronic pain answered questions regarding the how often pain interfered with life activities including sleep.[106] In this study, 77% of patients with SCI reported significant interference in daily activities because of pain, including sleep. Specifically, 38% reported that pain frequently interfered with sleep onset (3–7 nights per week), whereas 20% experienced difficulties with sleep onset 1 to 2 times per week. Forty percent of patients with SCI with pain reported that it interfered with sleep maintenance 3 to 7 nights per week, whereas 16% reported difficulties with sleep maintenance 1 to 2 nights per week. High average pain intensity and the use of more pain descriptors was associated with sleep onset problems, whereas older age, higher pain intensity, and anxiety were associated with complaints of poor sleep maintenance. A cross-sectional questionnaire study comparing patients with SCI without pain (26%), with intermittent pain (22%), and with continuous pain (52%) according to the visual analog scale (VAS) found that the persons with continuous pain reported the poorest quality of sleep on the Basic Nordic Sleep Questionnaire along with the most intense self-reported anxiety and depression on the Hospital Anxiety and Depression scale.[107] Anxiety, pain intensity, and depression were the main predictors of sleep quality in this study. Based on prior research on the relation between melatonin release and abnormal diurnal rhythms in some patients with SCI, as well as independent links between melatonin, pain, and depression, the investigators put forward the hypothesis that melatonin may play a role as a modulator for pain, sleep, and emotional distress in patients with SCI. The studies cited previously demonstrate that pain is an important factor in sleep disruption and quality in patients with SCI; however, it appears that emotional distress in the form of anxiety and depression also play a significant role and may act as moderator variables in determining the impact of pain on sleep.

Insomnia appears to be a significant problem in patients with SCI, even when other sleep disorders and the effect of SDB is controlled for. A number of factors seem to be contributory and may function together in simple and complex ways to promote insomnia. These include pain, psychological distress, alcohol use, tobacco consumption, voiding problems, parasthesias, and other medical complications. More research is needed to elucidate the relationship between these multiple factors, their interrelationships, and potential contributions to insomnia in SCI to ensure effective treatment to improve daytime functioning and ultimately improve functional independence.

## REFERENCES

1. National Spinal Cord Injury Statistical Center. Spinal cord injury: facts and figures at a glance. Birmingham (AL): University of Alabama at Birmingham, National Spinal Cord Injury Statistical Center; 2012. Available at: www.nscisc.uab.edu/Public Documents/.Feb2012.pdf. Accessed September 18, 2012.

2. Lemons VR, Wagner FC Jr. Respiratory complications after cervical spinal cord injury. Spine (Phila Pa 1976) 1994;19:2315–20.

3. DeVivo MJ, Krause JS, Lammertse DP. Recent trends in mortality and causes of death among persons with spinal cord injury. Arch Phys Med Rehabil 1999;80:1411–9.

4. Aarabi B, Harrop JS, Tator CH, et al. Predictors of pulmonary complications in blunt traumatic spinal cord injury. J Neurosurg Spine 2012;17:38–45.

5. Castriotta RJ, Murthy JN. Hypoventilation after spinal cord injury. Semin Respir Crit Care Med 2009;30(3):330–8.

6. Zimmer MB, Nantwi K, Goshgarian HG. Effect of spinal cord injury on the respiratory system: basic research and current clinical treatment options. J Spinal Cord Med 2007;30:319–30.

7. Tran K, Hukins C, Geraghty T, et al. Sleep-disordered breathing in spinal cord-injured patients: a short-term longitudinal study. Respirology 2010; 15:272–6.

8. Le Guen MC, Ciotulli PA, Berlowitz DJ. Continuous positive airway pressure requirements in patients with tetraplegia and obstructive sleep apnoea. Spinal Cord 2012. http://dx.doi.org/10.1038/sc.2012.57.

9. LaVela SL, Burns SP, Goldstein B. Dysfunctional sleep in persons with spinal cord injuries and disorders. Spinal Cord 2012;50:682–5. http://dx.doi.org/10.1038/sc.2012.31.

10. Punjabi NM. The epidemiology of adult obstructive sleep apnea. Proc Am Thorac Soc 2008;5:136–43.

11. Redline S, Strohl KP. Recognition and consequences of obstructive sleep apnea hypopnea syndrome. Clin Chest Med 1998;19:1–19.

12. Smith JC, Ellenberger HH, Ballanyi K, et al. Pre-Botzinger complex: a brainstem region that may generate respiratory rhythm in mammals. Science 1991;254:726–9.

13. Onimaru H, Homma I. A novel functional neuron group for respiratory rhythm generation in the ventral medulla. J Neurosci 2003;23:1478–86.

14. Feldman JL, Del Negro CA. Looking for inspiration: new perspectives on respiratory rhythm. Nat Rev Neurosci 2006;7:232–42.

15. Montandon G, Qin W, Liu H, et al. PreBötzinger complex neurokinin-1 receptor-expressing neurons mediate opioid-induced respiratory depression. J Neurosci 2011;31:1292–301.

16. Hollinshead WH, Keswani NH. Localization of the phrenic nucleus in the spinal cord of man. Anat Rec 1956;125:683–99.

17. Routal RV, Pal GP. Location of the phrenic nucleus in the human spinal cord. J Anat 1999;195(Pt 4): 617–21.

18. McKay LC, Feldman JL. Unilateral ablation of pre-Botzinger complex disrupts breathing during sleep but not wakefulness. Am J Respir Crit Care Med 2008;178:89–95.

19. Bulow K. Respiration in wakefulness in man. Acta Physiol Scand Suppl 1963;209:1–110.

20. Douglas NJ, White DP, Pickett CK, et al. Respiration during sleep in normal man. Thorax 1982;37: 840–4.

21. Douglas NJ, White DP, Weil JV, et al. Hypercapnic ventilatory response in sleeping adults. Am Rev Respir Dis 1982;126:758–62.

22. Douglas NJ, White DP, Weil JV, et al. Hypoxic ventilatory response decreases during sleep in normal men. Am Rev Respir Dis 1982;125:286–9.

23. Bergofsky EH. Mechanism for respiratory insufficiency after cervical cord injury; a source of alveolar hypoventilation. Ann Intern Med 1964;61: 435–47.

24. Haas F, Axen K, Pineda H, et al. Temporal pulmonary function changes in cervical cord injury. Arch Phys Med Rehabil 1985;66:139–44.

25. Estenne M, De Troyer A. The effects of tetraplegia on chest wall statics. Am Rev Respir Dis 1986; 134:121–4.

26. McCool FD, Tzelepis GE. Dysfunction of the diaphragm. N Engl J Med 2012;366:932–42.

27. Manning HL, Brown R, Scharf SM, et al. Ventilatory and PO.1 response to hypercapnia in quadriplegia. Respir Physiol 1992;89:97–112.

28. Lin KH, Wu HD, Chang CW, et al. Ventilatory and mouth occlusion pressure responses to hypercapnia in chronic tetraplegia. Arch Phys Med Rehabil 1998;79:231–9.

29. Bach JR, Wang TG. Pulmonary function and sleep disordered breathing in patients with traumatic tetraplegia: a longitudinal study. Arch Phys Med Rehabil 1994;75:279–84.

30. McEvoy RD, Mykytyn I, Sajkov D, et al. Sleep apnoea in patients with quadriplegia. Thorax 1995;50:613–9.

31. Burns SP, Kapur V, Yin KS, et al. Factors associated with sleep apnea in men with spinal cord injury: a population-based case-control study. Spinal Cord 2001;39:15–22.

32. Flavell H, Marshall R, Thornton AT, et al. Hypoxia episodes during sleep in high tetraplegia. Arch Phys Med Rehabil 1992;73:623–7.

33. Klefbeck B, Sternhag M, Weinberg J, et al. Obstructive sleep apneas in relation to severity of spinal cord injury. Spinal Cord 1998;36:621–8.

34. Berlowitz DJ, Brown DJ, Campbell DA, et al. A longitudinal evaluation of sleep and breathing in the first year after cervical spinal cord injury. Arch Phys Med Rehabil 2005;86:1193–9.

35. Short DJ, Stradling JR, Williams SJ. Prevalence of sleep apnea in patients over 40 years of age with spinal cord lesions. J Neurol Neurosurg Psychiatry 1992;55:1031–6.

36. Burns SP, Little JW, Hussey JD, et al. Sleep apnea syndrome in chronic spinal cord injury: associated factors and treatment. Arch Phys Med Rehabil 2000;81:1334–9.

37. Stockhammer E, Tobon A, Michel F, et al. Characteristics of sleep apnea syndrome in tetraplegic patients. Spinal Cord 2002;40:286–94.

38. Leduc BE, Dagher JH, Mayer P, et al. Estimated prevalence of obstructive sleep apnea-hypopnea syndrome after cervical cord injury. Arch Phys Med Rehabil 2007;88:333–7.

39. Lu K, Lee TC, Liang CL, et al. Delayed apnea in patients with mid- to lower cervical spinal cord injury. Spine 2000;25:1332–8.

40. Taasan VC, Block AJ, Boysen PG, et al. Alcohol increases sleep apnea and oxygen desaturation in asymptomatic men. Am J Med 1981;71: 240–5.

41. Dolly FR, Block AJ. Effect of flurazepam on sleep-disordered breathing and nocturnal oxygen desaturation in asymptomatic subjects. Am J Med 1982;73:239–43.

42. Montplaisir J, Bedard MA, Richer F, et al. Neurobehavioural manifestations in obstructive sleep apnea syndrome before and after treatment with continuous positive airway pressure. Sleep 1992; 15(Suppl 6):S17–9.

43. Sajkov D, Marshall R, Walker P, et al. Sleep apnoea related hypoxia is associated with cognitive disturbances in patients with tetraplegia. Spinal Cord 1998;36:231–9.

44. Young T, Finn L, Peppard PE. Sleep-disordered breathing and mortality: eighteen-year follow-up of the Wisconsin Sleep Cohort. Sleep 2008;31: 1071–8.

45. Bach JR, Intintola P, Alba AS, et al. The ventilator-assisted individual: cost analysis of institutionalization vs rehabilitation and in-home management. Chest 1992;101:26–30.

46. Bach JR. Alternative methods of ventilatory support for the patient with ventilatory failure due to spinal cord injury. J Am Paraplegia Soc 1991;14:158–74.

47. Bach JR, Alba AS. Management of chronic alveolar hypoventilation by nasal ventilation. Chest 1990;97: 52–7.

48. Bach JR. New approaches in the rehabilitation of the traumatic high level quadriplegic. Am J Phys Med Rehabil 1991;70:13–9.

49. Bach JR. A comparison of long-term ventilatory support alternatives from the perspective of the patient and care giver. Chest 1993;104:1702–6.

50. Steier J, Jolley CJ, Seymour J, et al. Sleep-disordered breathing in unilateral diaphragm paralysis or severe weakness. Eur Respir J 2008;32:1479–87.

51. Glenn WW, Hogan JF, Phelps ML. Ventilatory support of the quadriplegic patient with respiratory paralysis by diaphragm pacing. Surg Clin North Am 1980;60:1055–78.

52. Glenn WW, Hogan JF, Loke JS, et al. Ventilatory support by pacing of the conditioned diaphragm in quadriplegia. N Engl J Med 1984;310:1150–5.

53. Glenn WW, Phelps ML. Diaphragm pacing by electrical stimulation of the phrenic nerve. Neurosurgery 1985;17:974–84.

54. Glenn WW, Sairenji H. Diaphragm pacing in the treatment of chronic ventilatory insufficiency. In: Roussos C, Macklem P, editors. The thorax: lung biology in health and disease. New York: Marcel Dekker; 1985. p. 1407–40.

55. Elefteriades JA, Quin JA, Hogan JF, et al. Long-term follow-up of pacing of the conditioned diaphragm in quadriplegia. Pacing Clin Electrophysiol 2002;25:897–906.

56. Hirschfeld S, Exner G, Luukkaala T, et al. Mechanical ventilation or phrenic nerve stimulation for treatment of spinal cord injury-induced respiratory insufficiency. Spinal Cord 2008;46:738–42.

57. Alshekhlee A, Onders RP, Syed TU, et al. Phrenic nerve conduction studies in spinal cord injury: applications for diaphragmatic pacing. Muscle Nerve 2008;38:1546–52.

58. Shaw RK, Glenn WW, Hogan JF, et al. Electrophysiological evaluation of phrenic nerve function in candidates for diaphragm pacing. J Neurosurg 1980;53:345–54.

59. Storre JH, Seuthe B, Fiechter R, et al. Average volume-assured pressure support in obesity hypoventilation: a randomized crossover trial. Chest 2006;130:815–21.

60. Ambrogio C, Lowman X, Kuo M, et al. Sleep and non-invasive ventilation in patients with chronic respiratory insufficiency. Intensive Care Med 2009;35:306–13.

61. Berry RB, Chediak A, Brown LK, et al. Best clinical practices for the sleep center adjustment of noninvasive positive pressure ventilation (NPPV) in stable chronic alveolar hypoventilation syndromes. J Clin Sleep Med 2010;6:491–509.

62. Bach JR. Continuous noninvasive ventilation for patients with neuromuscular disease and spinal cord injury. Semin Respir Crit Care Med 2002;23:283–92.

63. Biering-Sorensen M, Norup PW, Jacobsen R, et al. Treatment of sleep apnoea in spinal cord injured patients. Paraplegia 1995;33:271–3.

64. Guilleminault C, Philip P, Robinson A. Sleep and neuromuscular disease: bilevel positive airway pressure by nasal mask as a treatment for sleep disordered breathing in patients with neuromuscular disease. J Neurol Neurosurg Psychiatry 1998;65:225–32.

65. Ip S, D'Ambrosio C, Parel K, et al. Auto-titrating versus fixed continuous positive airway pressure for the treatment of obstructive sleep apnea: a systematic review with meta-analysis. Syst Rev 2012;1(1):1–24.

66. Kakkar RK, Berry RB. Positive airway pressure treatment for obstructive sleep apnea. Chest 2007;132:1057–72.

67. Claustrat B, Brun J, Chazot G. The basic physiology and pathophysiology of melatonin. Sleep Med Rev 2005;9:11–24.

68. Pandi-Penmal SR, Smits M, Spencew W, et al. Dim light melatonin onset (DLMO): a tool for the analysis of circadian phase in human sleep and chronobiological disorders. Prog Neuropsychopharmacol Biol Psychiatry 2007;31:1–11.

69. Zeitzer JM, Ayas NY, Shea SA, et al. Absence of detectable melatonin, preservation of cortisol, thyrotropin rhythms in tetraplegia. J Clin Endocrinol Metab 2000;85:2189–96.

70. Gezici AR, Karakas A, Ergun H, et al. Rhythms of serum melatonin in rats with acute spinal cord injury at the cervical and thoracic regions. Spinal Cord 2010;48:10–4.

71. Verheggen RJ, Jones H, Nyakin J, et al. Complete absence of evening melatonin increase in tetraplegics. FASEB J 2012;26:3059–64.

72. Scheer FA, Zeitzer JM, Ayas NT. Reduced sleep efficiency in cervical spinal cord injury; association with abolished night time melatonin secretion. Spinal Cord 2006;44:78–81.

73. Thijssen DH, Eijsvogels TM, Hesse M, et al. The effects of thoracic and cervical spinal cord lesions on the circadian rhythm of core body temperature. Chronobiol Int 2011;28:146–54.

74. Zeitzer JM, Ayas NT, Wu AD, et al. Bilateral oculosympathetic paresis associated with loss of nocturnal melatonin secretion in patients with spinal cord injury. J Spinal Cord Med 2005;28:55–9.

75. Samantaray S, Das A, Thakore NO, et al. Therapeutic potential of melatonin in traumatic central nervous system injury. J Pineal Res 2009;47:134–42.

76. Park K, Lee Y, Park S, et al. Synergistic effect of melatonin on exercise-induced neuronal reconstruction and functional recovery in spinal cord injury animal model. J Pineal Res 2010;48:270–81.

77. Hong Y, Palaksha KJ, Park K, et al. Melatonin plus exercise-based neurorehabilitative therapy for spinal cord injury. J Pineal Res 2010;49:201–9.

78. Park S, Lee SK, Park K, et al. Beneficial effects of endogenous and exogenous melatonin on neural reconstruction and functional recovery in an animal model of spinal cord injury. J Pineal res 2012;52: 107–19.

79. Bjorvatn B, Pallesen S. A practical approach to circadian rhythm sleep disorders. Sleep Med Rev 2009;13:47–60.

80. Phipps-Nelson J, Redman JR, Schlangen LJ, et al. Blue light exposure reduces objective measures of sleepiness during prolonged nighttime performance testing. Chronobiol Int 2009;26:891–912.

81. Allen R, Picchietti D, Hening W, et al. Restless legs syndrome: diagnostic criteria, special considerations and epidemiology. A report from the restless legs syndrome diagnosis and epidemiology workshop at the National Institutes of Health. Sleep Med 2003;4:101–19.

82. Telles SC, Alves RC, Chadi G. Periodic limb movements during sleep and restless legs syndrome in patients with ASIA A spinal cord injury. J Neurol Sci 2011;303:119–23.

83. DeMello MT, Lauro FA, Silva AC, et al. Incidence of periodic limb movements and of the restless legs syndrome during sleep following acute physical activity in spinal cord injury subjects. Spinal Cord 1996;34:294–6.

84. Nilsson S, Levi R, Nordström A. Treatment-resistant sensory motor symptoms in persons with SCI may be signs of restless legs syndrome. Spinal Cord 2011;49:754–6.

85. Winkelman JW, Shahar E, Sharief I, et al. Association of restless legs syndrome and cardiovascular disease in the Sleep Heart Health Study. Neurology 2008;70:35–42.

86. Winter AC, Schürks M, Glynn RJ. Restless legs syndrome and risk of incident cardiovascular disease in women and men: a prospective cohort study. BMJ Open 2012;2(2):e000866.

87. Lipford MC, Silber MH. Long-term use of pramipexole in the management of restless legs syndrome. Sleep Med 2012. http://dx.doi.org/10.1016/j.sleep.2012.08.004. pii: S1389–9457(12)00314-0.

88. International classification of sleep disorders, 2nd edition: diagnostic and coding manual. Westchester (IL): American Academy of Sleep Medicine; 2005. p. 182–6.

89. Zucconi M, Ferri R, Allen R, et al. The official World Association of Sleep Medicine (WASM) standards for recording and scoring periodic limb movements in sleep (PLMS) and wakefulness (PLMW) developed in collaboration with a task force from the International Restless Legs Study Group (IRLSSG). Sleep Med 2006;7:175–83.

90. Coleman RM. Periodic limb movements in sleep (nocturnal myoclonus) and restless legs syndrome. In: Guilleminault C, editor. Sleeping and waking disorders: indications and techniques. Menlo Park (CA): Addison-Wesley; 1982. p. 265–95.

91. Michaud M, Pacquet J, Lavigne G, et al. Sleep laboratory diagnosis of restless legs syndrome. Eur Neurol 2002;48:108–13.

92. Lee MS, Choi YC, Lee SH, et al. Sleep-related periodic limb movements associated with spinal cord lesions. Mov Disord 1996;11:719–22.

93. Yokota T, Hirose K, Tanabe H, et al. Sleep-related periodic limb movements (nocturnal myoclonus) due to spinal cord lesion. J Neurol Sci 1991;104: 13–8.

94. Dickel MJ, Renfrow SD, Moore PT, et al. Rapid eye movement sleep periodic leg movements in patients with spinal cord injury. Sleep 1994;17: 733–78.

95. Esteves AM, deMello MT, Lancellotti CLP, et al. Occurrence of limb movement during sleep in rats with spinal cord injury. Brain Res 2004;1017: 32–8.

96. De Mello MT, Esteves AM, Tufik S. Comparison between dopaminergic agents and physical exercise as treatment for periodic limb movements in patients with spinal cord injury. Spinal Cord 2004; 42:218–21.

97. De Mello MT, Silva AC, Rueda AD, et al. Correlation between K complex, periodic leg movements (PLM), and myoclonus during sleep in paraplegic adults before and after an acute physical activity. Spinal Cord 1997;35:248–52.

98. Brown WD. Insomnia: prevalence and daytime consequences. In: Lee-Choing TL, editor. Sleep medicine essentials. Hoboken (NJ): Wiley Blackwell; 2009. p. 23–6.

99. Biering-Sorensen F, Biering-Sorensen M. Sleep disturbances in the spinal cord injured: an epidemiological questionnaire investigation, including a normal population. Spinal Cord 2001;39:505–13.

100. Jensen MP, Hirsh AT, Molton IR, et al. Sleep problems in individuals with spinal cord injury: frequency and age effects. Rehabil Psychol 2009; 54:323–51.

101. Cohen J. Statistical power analysis for the behavioral sciences. 2nd edition. Hillsdale (NJ): Lawrence Erlbaum Associates; 1988.

102. Soehner AM, Harvey AG. Prevalence and functional consequences of severe insomnia symptoms in mood and anxiety disorders: results from a nationally representative sample. Sleep 2012; 35:1367–75.

103. Fann JR, Bombaardier CH, Richards JS, et al. Depression after spinal cord injury: comorbidities, mental health service use and adequacy of treatment. Arch Phys Med Rehabil 2011;92: 352–60.

104. Dias de Carvalho SA, Andrade MJ, Tavares MA, et al. Spinal cord injury and psychological response. Gen Hosp Psychiatry 1998;20:353–9.

105. Rintala DH, Loubser PG, Castro J, et al. Chronic pain in a community based sample of men with spinal cord injury: prevalence, severity, and relationship with impairment, disability, handicap, and subjective well-being. Arch Phys Med Rehabil 1998;79:604–14.

106. Widerstrom-Noga EG, Felipe-Cuervo E, Yezierski RP. Chronic pain after spinal cord injury: interference with sleep and daily activities. Arch Phys Med Rehabil 2001;82:1571–7.

107. Norrbrink Budh C, Hultling C, Lundeberg T. Quality of sleep in individuals with spinal cord injury: a comparison between patients with and without pain. Spinal Cord 2005;43:85–95.

# Relevance of Chronobiology to the Research and Clinical Practice of Neurorehabilitation

Francesco Portaluppi, MD, PhD[a],*,
Michael H. Smolensky, PhD[b], Erhard Haus, MD[c],
Fabio Fabbian, MD[a]

## KEYWORDS

- Circadian rhythm • Rest-activity cycle • Shift work • Mental performance • Physical performance
- Fatigue • Neurorehabilitation

## KEY POINTS

- Chronobiology is the study of endogenous biological rhythms and the mechanisms of biological time-keeping in health and disease.
- Circadian rhythms affect patients' mental and physical capabilities and stamina, thereby potentially affecting reaction to physical and cognitive retraining depending on timing.

## INTRODUCTION

Observations of predictable-in-time (eg, 24-hour and seasonal) variations in biology and pathophysiology date back to Hippocrates; however, their scientific study did not commence until the seventeenth century. Thus, chronobiology, the study of biological rhythms and the mechanisms of biological time-keeping in health and disease, is a relatively new science, with applications to medicine and therapeutics being rather recent developments.[1] The purpose of this article is to communicate the relevance of this rapidly developing field to the (1) research and clinical practice of neurorehabilitation and (2) work schedules, performance, and well-being of medical personnel caring for institutionalized neurologic patients. Because the length of this contribution to this special issue is limited and because in-depth description of the principles and definitions of chronobiology is beyond the scope of this article, relevant concepts and terminology of chronobiology

are introduced without specific citation to the original works. Specific references are cited for the latest developments; general background information on the field, if desired, can be found in comprehensive textbooks of chronobiology (eg, Refs.[2,3]).

## ESSENTIALS OF CHRONOBIOLOGY

A *biological rhythm* is a self-sustaining oscillation of endogenous origin defined by the characteristics of period, level, amplitude, and phase.

*Period* is the duration of time required to complete an entire cycle of the biological rhythm. The spectrum of biological rhythms is broad, with periods being as short as a second or so to as long as a year. The highest magnitude of variability (see "amplitude" below) of most functions is shown by rhythms of about 24 hours, termed *circadian*, and it is these rhythms that have been most explored for their relevance to activities of everyday life and clinical medicine.

[a] Department of Clinical and Experimental Medicine, Hypertension Center, University Hospital S. Anna, University of Ferrara, Corso Giovecca 203, Ferrara I-44121, Italy; [b] Department of Biomedical Engineering, The University of Texas at Austin, 808 Lakewood Hills Terrace, Austin, TX 78732, USA; [c] Department of Laboratory Medicine & Pathology, HealthPartners Medical Group, Regions Hospital, 640 Jackson Street, St Paul, MN 55, USA
* Corresponding author. Corso Giovecca 203, Ferrara I-44121, Italy.
*E-mail address:* prf@unife.it

Sleep Med Clin 7 (2012) 655–666
http://dx.doi.org/10.1016/j.jsmc.2012.08.005
1556-407X/12/$ – see front matter © 2012 Elsevier Inc. All rights reserved.

*Level* is the baseline, that is, mean value of a rhythm of a given period, around which predictable-in-time variation is manifested.

*Amplitude* is a measure of the magnitude of the predictable-in-time variability ascribable specifically to biological rhythmicity. Many rhythms are of high amplitude, accounting for 50% or more of the total variability observed during the time period. Amplitudes of rhythms may change, for example, with aging, in disease, by medications, and according to work pattern (shift work).

*Phase* refers to the clocking of specific features, such as peak and trough, of a rhythm relative to a reference point of a given time scale, for example, in the case of circadian rhythms, local midnight, or time since awakening from the major sleep span.

Circadian rhythms are controlled by an inherited *master clock* network composed of the (1) paired suprachiasmatic nuclei (SCN) situated in the hypothalamus, and (2) pineal gland through the 24-hour pattern in the synthesis and secretion of the hormone melatonin. Rhythmic activities in the SCN of the so-called clock genes of *Per1*, *Per2*, *Per3*, *Bmal*, *Clock*, and *Cry*, and their gene products comprise the central time-keeping mechanism. The transcription factors CLOCK and BMAL1 form the positive loop of the 24-hour cycle, driving the expression of *Per1*, *Per2*, *Cry1*, and *Cry2*, plus a variety of clock-controlled genes via E-box sequences in their promoters. PER and CRY proteins constitute the negative loop of the cycle, feeding back on the transcriptional activity of CLOCK:BMAL1. The combined duration of the positive and negative loops is approximately 24 hours and gives rise to the body's so-called circadian time structure (CTS). The precision of the period of CTS is achieved via posttranslational modulation of the clock proteins by cyclic environmental time cues, the most important being the 24-hour environmental light-dark cycle. The biological time-keeping system also includes *peripheral circadian clocks* found in cells, tissues, and organs that are regulated and coordinated by the master SCN clock.

Proper phasing of individual circadian rhythms to meet expected environmental and societal demands, that is, to attain optimal external synchronization of the CTS, is achieved by ambient time cues termed *zeitgebers* (English: time givers and synonymous with the terms of *synchronizers* and *entraining agents*), the light-dark cycle being most powerful under ordinary circumstances. Others especially important time cues for humans include meal schedule, and cyclic social phenomena and routines. Features of the natural light-dark cycle vary predictably over 24 hours,

month, and year; in addition to overall light exposure, the spectral composition of light exposure varies over the day and year, which may constitute entraining information for the CTS.[4] In human beings, the central circadian clock network relies on the ambient (natural and/or artificial) daily light-dark cycle to titrate its period to exactly 24 hours and to determine phase so as to best meet the cyclic (ie, predictable-in-time) demands of the immediate environment. Thus, the timing of the peaks and troughs of circadian rhythms is quite predictable from one day to the next in the majority of people who adhere to a fairly regular routine of activity in light/sleep in darkness. Light is considered the most potent synchronizer of the human circadian system and exerts many non–image-forming effects, including those that affect brain function. The synchronizing effect is mediated in part by intrinsically photosensitive retinal ganglion cells that express the photopigment melanopsin. The spectral sensitivity of melanopsin is greatest for the blue light wavelength of approximately 480 nm. It must be emphasized that sleep in darkness/activity in light and other environmental synchronizers are not the source or cause of rhythms; rather, they serve only as time cues to entrain the period and phase of genetically constituted circadian clock mechanisms and the 24-hour oscillations they drive.

Human beings, because of the genetics of their inherited circadian clock, age, sex, lifestyle, or disease, differ in their biological preference for the clock times of sleep and wakefulness. *Chronotype* refers to the time-preference of sleep and activity of individuals and associated minor, but nonetheless significant, differences in the exact circadian phasing of the CTS. Three different chronotypes can be distinguished using validated questionnaires. Morning types, commonly referred to as *larks*, are most alert and efficient in the morning. Larks express strong preference for early morning waking times and early evening bedtimes, as early as 04:00 and 19:00 to 21:00, respectively, in extreme morning types. Evening types, commonly referred to as *owls*, are most alert and efficient late in the day and at night. Owls express strong preference for late-night bedtimes and late morning or afternoon waking times, as late as 02:00 to 04:00 and midday or later, respectively, in extreme evening types. The remaining intermediate types constitute the vast majority, perhaps 70% to 85%, of the population. With reference to the CTS of intermediate types, the clock-time phasing of circadian rhythms, for example, body temperature, cortisol, and melatonin, of extreme morning types is likely to be advanced on average by approximately 2 hours, whereas that of extreme evening types is likely to be delayed on average by approximately 2 hours. The CTS of morning and intermediate chronotypes in most cases shows good internal synchronization, with phasing adjusted to the circadian sleep-wake rhythm. However, in extreme owls, the CTS may be disrupted and desynchronized because of too great a conflict between the environmental light-dark cycle and societal, school, and work synchronizer schedules versus the endogenous biological-clock–driven preference for very late sleep and activity timings.

Different personality traits have been linked to the different chronotypes. For example, morning types typically score significantly higher than evening and intermediate types on conscientiousness, whereas evening types tend to score higher on impulsivity and risk-taking than morning types.[5] Although no causal relationship has been demonstrated between evening preference and depression, investigations suggest functional associations between mood adjustment and biological clock systems that regulate diurnal preference, with evening preference related to increased susceptibility to mood disorders.[6] If this is true, evening types might show lower motivation, conscientiousness, and adherence to rehabilitation programs.

Individuals who have suffered significant head/brain trauma often exhibit significant sleep and wake abnormalities; in actuality they may be a consequence of an altered circadian sleep-wake rhythm, manifesting as an extreme evening chronotype orientation (often termed delayed sleep phase disorder), irregular/fragmented, or even free-running (non–24-hour) sleep-wake cycle.[7,8] As an illustration, a recent study of epilepsy patients found this neurologic condition (independent of the seizure timing pattern) to affect chronotype behavior and subjective sleep parameters; epileptic patients were found to be more morning oriented, have an earlier mid-sleep time, and longer sleep duration on free (nonscheduled leisure) days.[9] Relevant to neurorehabilitation programs are patient complaints and symptoms of these often unrecognized sleep-wake circadian rhythm disorders that are interpreted as sleep-onset insomnia, but which are seldom satisfactorily resolved by sleep medications alone. Properly timed bright-light therapy or special pharmacotherapy to reset the circadian clock, for example, circadian timed melatonin, is warranted.[10] It is worthy of mention that evening chronotype patients are likely to be poorly receptive to neurorehabilitative interventions when timed too early in the day, but to be optimally responsive when timed in the afternoon. The situation may be reversed in morning chronotypes, because they are likely to be less fatigued when undergoing procedures in the morning than in the afternoon.

An important concept of chronobiology is *phase response*: difference of effect, advance or delay of the staging of individual circadian rhythms or the entire CTS, elicited by environmental time signals, medications, or other agents. The phase and period of circadian clocks and rhythms are maintained from day to day by entraining cues provided by the onset and offset times of the natural environmental photoperiod, or in the case of institutionalized patients the artificial lights-on/lights-off (dark) cycle. Of relevance to patient care is the fact that even a single brief exposure of ordinarily diurnally active human beings to artificial light of sufficient intensity (greater than dim light intensity), late at night or during the early sleep (dark) span, can cause phase delay of the CTS of up to approximately 1 hour in the ensuing 24-hour period, whereas exposure to the same identical artificial light signal very early in the morning, before sunrise and before the end of the nocturnal sleep span, can cause phase advance of the CTS by approximately 1 hour. By contrast, identical light exposure during the middle of the day, when the ambient environment is normally brightly lit, results in no alteration of circadian phase. Altogether, phase response represents an aspect of the adaptive plasticity of the CTS, that is, the ability of the body clock to adjust its internal timing in response to perceived external clues (most importantly light signals). While this attribute is of great importance to the adjustment of the CTS of employees to night shift work and of travelers rapidly displaced by jet aircraft across several time zones, the immediate effects of light at night (LAN) signals in hospital, rehabilitation, and recuperative home settings can be quite disruptive to the CTS of patients and staff, with potential risk of compromised metabolic, physical, and cognitive rhythms and abilities.[11,12]

The phase, and sometimes even exact period, of circadian rhythms, and thus organization of the CTS, in those who are employed in rotating shift work, those who have recently traveled across multiple time zones, or those who have a variable rest-activity routine, are less predictable than those who maintain a relatively consistent routine of sleep in darkness/activity in light. The activity in light/sleep in darkness routine determines when the peak and trough of circadian rhythms occur with reference to the 24-hour time scale. It also determines, qualitatively and quantitatively, the responses to diagnostic tests, and efficacy and safety of therapeutic interventions according to their timing. A very simple example may be enlightening in this respect. Bilirubin is a common laboratory test used in clinical medicine and is known to be associated with the sleep pattern even in healthy individuals. Much lower circadian variation of serum bilirubin levels is measured in healthy individuals with normal night sleep than in those with sleep acutely displaced to the daytime hours.[13] Hence, bilirubin sampling should be restricted to standard (usually morning) hours, and proper consideration should be given to the individual's rest-activity schedule to avoid misinterpretation of the intraindividual variation. Even variations in body temperature during and after physical exercise differ according to circadian timing.[14]

## RELEVANCE OF SLEEP-WAKE CYCLES

Twin studies demonstrate that similar genes are important for diurnal preference and sleep quality.[15] A large study of an elderly population, whose rest-activity pattern was assessed by wrist actigraphy, demonstrated that disruption of the rest-activity cycle and earlier acrophase timing are associated with modestly higher all-cause and cardiovascular disease-related mortality rates.[16] Different factors are known to influence morningness-eveningness, biological rhythms, and sleep-wake cycles, including social habits. In women, morningness is predicted by pregnancy and presence of children and their age; children exert strong influence on their mother's lifestyle and sleep-wake rhythm, far beyond the first months of life.[17]

Rotating shift and permanent night-work arrangements are known to compromise sleep. Entering shift work (with or without night shifts) from day work increases the risk of experiencing difficulties falling asleep, whereas leaving shift work for day work reduces this risk.[18] Early-morning shift start times are associated with sleep deprivation, feelings of not being well rested, and undue daytime fatigue when not compensated with earlier bedtimes.[19] Moreover, working outside the regular daytime hours is strongly associated with elevated risk of accidents while driving; night work is the most disruptive, as it is associated with insufficient sleep during the designated rest span and excessive sleepiness and sleep attacks during the span of activity, again with increased risk of accidents while driving as a consequence.[20] In fact, sleep deprivation (by increasing the time spent awake) is associated with decreased alertness and increased fatigue, as well as negative effects on performance, even for a simple task such as throwing darts at a target.[21] These considerations apply also to competitive athletes, whose individual rest-activity schedules, including daytime napping, may be helpful, especially during the stressful training and rehearsal experienced before performances.[22] Night shift workers may try to overcome sleepiness and fatigue by napping. However, awakening from naps of too long duration may result in the phenomenon of sleep inertia, that is, an acute carry-over effect of reduced alertness, even in the absence of self-reported sleepiness, additionally compromising performance and mood, with possible dangerous implications for occupational safety.[23] Moreover, significant increases in work-related injury risk with decreasing usual daily self-reported sleep hours and increasing weekly work hours, independent of industry, occupation, type of pay, sex, age, education, and body mass, have been demonstrated.[24] Finally, at northern latitudes, socioeconomic factors have been reported to exert significant influence on sleep length, with climatic conditions reported to significantly influence the CTS. Residing at the more northerly latitudes for long periods is associated with sleep disturbances and internal desynchronization of the CTS, which in children and teenagers have been associated with poor school achievement and psychological problems, and exacerbation of certain chronic diseases in the elderly.[25]

A recent study investigated possible effects of sleep quality and chronotype on severity of depressive symptoms and suicide risk in patients with depressive disorder and in healthy controls.[26] Poor sleep quality and depression symptom severity significantly predicted the onset of major depression. Morningness was found to be a significant relief factor after onset of major depression. Although sleep variables of chronotypes and their sleep quality did not significantly predict suicide ideation after controlling for depressive symptoms in patients with major depression, suicide ideation and poor sleep quality, in general, were found to be antecedents of depression symptom severity in patients with major depression and also in healthy controls. Based on these findings, it seems that complex interrelationships exist between chronotype, sleep quality, depression, and suicide ideation.

## RELEVANCE OF DISTURBANCE AND DISRUPTION OF CIRCADIAN TIME STRUCTURE

Integrity of the CTS is critical for efficient biological and cognitive functioning, and maintenance of health and well-being. Millions of people annually are exposed to transient (several days' duration) disruption of their sleep-wake cycle and CTS, either relatively infrequently by rapid travel across multiple time zones or chronically at regular intervals when working rotating or permanent night-shift schedules. The consequent disruption of the CTS typically results in a set of acute and transient symptoms during the several days of adjustment to the new activity/rest cycle and differently timed environmental synchronizers, including the light/dark, social, and meal cycles, among others. These "jet-lag" symptoms, so called even though they occur in nontravelers as a consequence of rotating between day and night work shifts, include fatigue and sleepiness, difficulty in initiating and maintaining sleep, cognitive and physical deficits, changed mood (melancholy/anxiety), altered appetite, and disrupted digestive track function with digestive complaints.

Night and rotating shift workers experience disruption of the CTS and several or all of the aforementioned symptoms to some degree with each rotation between day and night work, which occurs at regular (typically weekly or shorter) intervals. Repetition of these biological insults over one's shift-work career poses health risks, such as sleep/mood disorder, metabolic syndrome and obesity, peptic ulcer disease, hypertension, and coronary heart disease, plus an elevated risk of breast and colorectal cancer in women and prostate cancer in men.[27–32] LAN exposure during night shifts inhibits melatonin production and secretion, and disrupts the CTS.[30,33] Melatonin is a hormone produced only during the darkness of night by the pineal gland under the control of the circadian clock, and its synthesis is suppressed both by natural and artificial LAN. As an indolamine, melatonin acts as a potent scavenger of free oxygen radicals that can damage DNA and cause cancer.[34] In fact, preliminary studies indicate alteration of DNA methylation, including changes in methylation of Alu repetitive elements and gene-specific methylation of promoters of interferon-$\gamma$ and tumor necrosis factor $\alpha$, may mediate some of the negative effects of shift work on human health.[35] In addition, recent data suggest the *Per1* clock gene exerts tumor-suppressor activity that diminishes cancer proliferation and tumor growth, but only at specific times of day.[36] In women, chronic, long-term LAN exposure in the sleep environment has been linked to increased risk of breast cancer.[37] In men, long-term LAN exposure has also been linked with increased risk of prostate cancer. A recently published study involving data from 164 countries found that the risk of prostate cancer was 110% greater in the highest compared with the lowest LAN-exposed countries; however, this finding may be due, at least in part, to various confounding factors also

linked to the risk of prostate cancer.[38] Shift work is also related to higher prevalence of depressed mood than is day work, particularly in male employees, while male and female employees show an opposite trend in depressed mood in relation to the number of working hours per week.[39] Night work is also a significant predictor of weight gain,[40] because activity and eating patterns are altered, as are the circadian rhythms that regulate appetite and energy balance. The appetite-regulating hormones of acylated ghrelin and leptin are suppressed after energy expenditure in the form of exercise during the day shift, whereas they are increased after identical effort (same level of exercise) during the night shift.[41] Working fixed 12-hour night shifts is associated with increased risk for central obesity and arterial hypertension among female workers.[42] Moreover, female workers seem to recover from cardiac stress on the first off-day following a night shift, but they do not completely recover from the increased vascular stress as quickly.[43] Substantiation of these and other risks to the maintenance of normal physiologic and biochemical states and, more concerning, the health of career shift workers supports the integrity of the CTS as a most important aspect of well-being, and again indicates that need for refinement of working-time arrangements. These data also reinforce the concept that therapeutic interventions for neurorehabilitation and for other patients must avoid disturbance of the circadian time-keeping system. Although further research is necessary to better understand the relationship between circadian disruption, LAN, and cancer risk, evidence is mounting that (1) LAN is disruptive to the CTS of patients and their biological and cognitive status, and (2) LAN plus night shift work is disruptive and potentially detrimental to the work efficiency and long-term well-being of personnel involved in neurorehabilitation and other types of patient care. Shift workers may also experience difficulties in job performance related to problems of reconciling work and nonwork activities; as such, this conflict may be mitigated by designing and implementing effective preventive actions at the workplace.[44] The reverse relationship is also true: work-family conflict affects the adjustment of employees, particularly male employees, to atypical work schedules and working hours.[45]

## CIRCADIAN RHYTHMS OF PHYSICAL AND MENTAL PERFORMANCE

Physical and mental performances vary substantially over the 24 hours of circadian rhythms; thus, an individual's mental and physical abilities may differ substantially during the course of the waking span. Greatest reactivity to a given amount of uninterrupted physical exercise occurs within the first 2 hours after waking from nighttime sleep, whereas lowest reactivity occurs late at night, 18 to 20 hours after waking.[46,47] On the other hand, intermittent exercise mediates greater postexercise hypotension compared with a single continuous bout of equivalent work, and this protocol-dependent difference is greatest in the afternoon; therefore, a bout of afternoon exercise occasionally interrupted with short rest periods is recommended for lowering blood pressure acutely.[48] These notions are important when planning exercise schedules for retraining or rehabilitation purposes in persons at increased cardiovascular risk, in whom too great reactivity might trigger acute events.

Circadian patterning of cognitive performance is demonstrable at various levels, commencing in childhood, although often confined to more demanding tasks tapping input-related and central cognitive processes.[49] Interindividual variability is also present, primarily in the form of morningness-eveningness, but not to the extent of hampering generalizations about the population as a whole.[50] For instance, the precision of performing a visually guided tracking task is specific according to time of day, being best in the afternoon and worst around 04:00, although interindividual differences are clearly present; half the subjects of one study maintained fairly stable performance over time, whereas the other half showed clear circadian rhythmicity in tracking precision and delay.[51] Higher cognitive functions also show circadian modulation, For example, language performance displays an internally generated circadian rhythmicity, with optimal time for parsing language found early in the day, 3 to 6 hours after the habitual wake time, around 10:00 to 13:00 in ordinarily diurnally active persons.[52] Similarly, physical performance of diurnally active healthy subjects usually is best in the late afternoon (when time of awakening and breakfast consumption are standardized), closely in phase with the circadian rhythm of body temperature.[53] The circadian rhythms of alertness and cognitive performance are phased approximately 1 hour earlier than the core body temperature (CBT) rhythm, while the rhythm of fatigue is phased approximately 1 h earlier than the inverse of the CBT rhythm.[21] Also, maximal muscle power, but not fatigability, in nonpatient samples is greater during repeated cycling sprints performed in the afternoon than morning.[54] Hence, being less efficient in the early morning than afternoon potentially exposes people to elevated risk of accident and injury at this time of the day.[55]

These notions seem crucial to the research and clinical practice of neurorehabilitation, because different inferences deriving from circadian rhythms are of importance in the implementation and evaluation of training/retraining and rehabilitation programs. Neurobehavioral and neuromuscular functions are affected by circadian phase and duration of prior wakefulness (**Box 1**), with an established significant effect of circadian phase on muscle strength.[56,57] Circadian variations similar to those of physical and mental activity, each with an afternoon peak, are observed in anaerobic power output,[58] adenosine triphosphate–phosphocreatine, anaerobic and aerobic metabolism, all types of muscle contractions (eccentric, isometric, concentric), nerve conduction velocity, joint suppleness, muscular blood flow, glycogenolysis and glycolysis, as well as cycles in ambient temperature and other environmental variables may contribute to the observed temporal variation in physical performance during the wake span.[59] However, the diurnal variation in strength performance can be blunted by a repeated resistance training protocol routinely executed in the morning, whereas optimal adaptations to resistance training (muscle hypertrophy and strength increases) are likely to occur more readily when the resistance training is routinely done in the late afternoon. Thus, strength performance without time-of-day–specific training is likely to elicit the typical diurnal pattern as well as resistance training adaptations.[59] Hence, training times should coincide with expected times of performance (a notion particularly useful for athletes), because individuals may experience greater hypertrophy and strength gains when resistance training protocols are individually designed with reference to one's CTS, including

---

**Box 1**
**Circadian rhythm importance in rehabilitation programs**

Circadian variations are observed in:

Anaerobic power output

Adenosine triphosphate–phosphocreatine

Anaerobic and aerobic metabolism

Muscle contractions (eccentric, isometric, concentric)

Nerve conduction velocity

Joint suppleness

Muscular blood flow

Glycogenolysis

chronotype (a notion with obvious implication for rehabilitation programs).

Both cognitive (ie, mental imagery) and motor (ie, laterality) states of human behavior are modulated by circadian rhythms.[60] Different tasks are associated with different best times of day of performance with each under different oscillatory control, whose phasing is adjusted at different rates related to change in the sleep/wake synchronizer schedule. The mechanisms underlying differences in both memory and nonmemory tasks seem to be based essentially on changes in the strategy used by the nervous system for information processing rather than changes in the capacity for information storage. The quality of any type of physical or mental performance depends on the effective coordination of many physiologic systems showing circadian rhythms, for example, nervous, neuroendocrine, energy, and cardiovascular, as well as time into the awake span (time since awakening from sleep as an index of accumulating fatigue) and amount of rapid eye movement sleep in the previous rest period.[61] The central mechanism underlying such circadian periodicity appears to be a combination of mechanisms, one correlating with the sleep-wake 24-hour cycle and the other correlating with the body-temperature circadian cycle.

Using magnetic resonance to observe these phenomena at the neural level,[62] it is possible to demonstrate time-of-day–related variations activity of brain regions linked to the orienting attentional system (left parietal lobe, left and right frontal eye fields), suggesting that the involuntary, exogenous (bottom-up) mechanism of attention is more vulnerable to circadian and fatigue factors than the voluntary (top-down) mechanism, which appear to be maintained at the same functional level during the day. Both internal and external stimuli can influence the oscillatory mechanisms of cognitive and motor states. Therefore, the quality of performance depends on the time of day and degree of preservation of the normal CTS. For example, better types of performances are observed in the morning for activities dependent on short-term memory, whereas afternoon and evening are optimal for tasks involving long-term memory, and significant decrements relative to peak performance are found at other times of the day. For this reason, all activities that depend on performance, including training and rehabilitation programs, must give proper consideration to pertinent circadian rhythms. Alteration or even desynchronization of the individual's CTS because of atypical exposure to environmental time cues, such as artificial LAN or an abnormal sleep-wake cycle,[63] may interfere with one's ability to perform optimally, both physically and mentally. In patients, this is in addition to decrements in performance that result from brain and neuromuscular trauma. In night employees, mounting fatigue may contribute to deterioration of work capacity at the end of due shift, leading to a decrease in the general stability of performance and an increase in errors.[64]

On the other hand, the CTS can be re-entrained to normal using several external cues (eg, sleep and exercise regimes, bright-light timing, meal timing, and in some cases drug-administration schedules), the success of which implies full knowledge on their physiologic impact on the CTS. In this respect, more research is warranted to improve our understanding as to how the circadian system modulates mental and physical performance, and to assess the relationships of common clinical concepts such as "fitness" and "fatigue" to the physiologic CTS.[65] In keeping with this body of knowledge are the observations that during the early hours of the morning, maintenance technicians are at heightened risk of "absent-minded" errors involving failures to execute action plans as intended.[66]

## CIRCADIAN RHYTHMS IN THE MANIFESTATION AND SEVERITY OF DISEASE

Patients undergoing neurorehabilitation, especially elderly ones, are likely to have developed one or more coexisting chronic medical conditions. Knowledge of their 24-hour patterning is of value in understanding how to best optimize patient care and neurorehabilitative interventions (**Fig. 1**). As recently reviewed by the authors,[67] exacerbation of, for example, gout, gallbladder, renal, fibromyalgia, and peptic ulcer disease, is most frequent late at night or in the initial hours of the usual sleep span. Acute pulmonary edema, congestive heart failure, vagotonic atrial fibrillation, claudication of the legs, bronchial asthma, chronic obstructive pulmonary disease, atopic dermatitis, restless legs syndrome, and periodic limb movement disorder manifest or worsen nocturnally.[68–74] Symptoms of allergic rhinitis, acute or upper respiratory infectious disease, and rheumatoid arthritis either are most intense overnight or in the morning. Risk of migraine headache, angina pectoris, ventricular arrhythmia, acute myocardial infarction, sudden cardiac death, ischemic and hemorrhagic stroke, fatal pulmonary embolism, and hypertensive crises is greatest in the morning, as are the symptoms and crises of certain other cardiovascular disease conditions, such as adrenergic fibrillation, aortic aneurysm rupture, third-degree atrial-ventricular

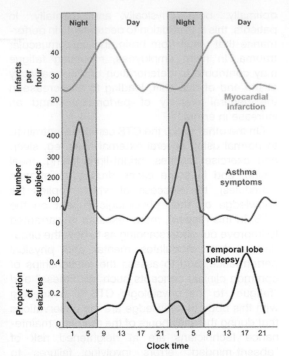

**Fig. 1.** The day/night patterns of disease severity. Results of 3 epidemiologic studies demonstrating robust day/night patterns of disease severity for myocardial infarction (*top panel*), asthma (*middle panel*), and temporal lobe seizures (*bottom panel*). The disease severity for myocardial infarction broadly peaks around 10 AM. The disease severity for asthma sharply peaks around 4 AM. The disease severity for temporal lobe seizures peaks around 5 PM. Data are double plotted to emphasize rhythmicity. (*Data from* Muller JE. Circadian variation and triggering of acute coronary events. Am Heart J 1999;137(4 Pt 2):S1–8; Dethlefsen U, Repgas R. Ein neues therapieprinzip bei nachtlichen asthma. Clin Med 1985;80:44; and Pavlova MK, Shea SA, Bromfield EB. Day/night patterns of focal seizures. Epilepsy Behav 2004;5(1):44–9.)

heart block, and acute arterial limb occlusion. Symptoms of depression are most severe in the morning, as are cravings for alcohol and tobacco by dependent patients, whereas those of osteoarthritis worsen during the course of daily activity, typically being most intense in the afternoon and evening. Intraocular pressure of glaucoma is highest during sleep, and certain seizure disorders manifest only during the nighttime, being triggered by specific sleep stages and/or transitions between sleep and wakefulness. Knowledge of the time patterns of coexisting medical conditions of neurorehabilitation patients is of great relevance, first in regard of the appropriate timing of pharmacotherapy (as chronotherapies: timing medications to circadian rhythms to optimize desired benefit and/or to modulate or avoid

adverse effects) and second to devise optimal individualized neurorehabilitation programs through appropriate timings during the day.

## RELEVANCE OF THE CTS TO THE THERAPEUTIC RESPONSE TO MEDICATIONS

The biological time when medications are administered may affect their pharmacokinetics (PK) and pharmacodynamics (PD), no matter their route of delivery. Chronopharmacology is the study of the manner and extent to which the PK and PD of medications are affected by endogenous biological rhythms, and also how the timing of medications affects biological time-keeping and CTS, that is, period, level, amplitude, and phase (**Fig. 2**).

Chronokinetics refers to dosing-time (ie, biological rhythm) differences in the absorption, distribution, metabolism, and elimination of medications. Such patterns are revealed by, for example, administration-time differences in PK parameters of various types and classes of therapeutic agents, including time to peak concentration, peak height, elimination rate, volume of distribution, and area under the time-concentration curve. These differences result from circadian rhythms in gastrointestinal pH affecting drug dissolution plus circadian rhythms in gastric emptying, motility, and blood flow affecting the rate, and sometimes amount,

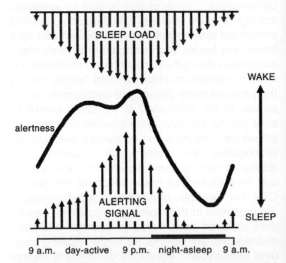

**Fig. 2.** Illustration of the opponent processes model. Sleep load is thought to increase during waking and to decrease during sleep. Sleep load is thought to influence sleepiness, whose influence is opposed by an alerting signal generated by the circadian pacemaker. The heavy line symbolizes the resulting course of alertness as a function of time of day (after Ref.[44]). (*From* Beersma DG, Gordijn MC. Circadian control of the sleep-wake cycle. Physiol Behav 90(2–3):190–5; with permission.)

of drug absorption. Circadian rhythms in hepatic blood flow and enzyme activity affect drug biotransformation and metabolism, while hepatic and kidney rhythms, for example in bile function and flow and renal glomerular filtration and tubular function, affect drug elimination. Many examples of dosing-time differences in the PK of commonly prescribed medications can be found in previously published reviews.[75–77]

Chronodynamics refers to dosing-time (ie, rhythm-dependent) differences in the effects of medications that cannot be attributed to their PK. Such administration-time differences result from rhythms in free-to-bound drug fraction, number and conformation of drug-specific receptors, second-messenger and ion-channel dynamics, and rate-limiting steps in metabolic pathways. Beneficial and adverse effects of medications both may vary significantly according to their administration time. Many examples of chronodynamics can be cited. One is the differential anticoagulant effect during the 24 hours of constant-rate infusion of standard (non–low molecular weight) heparin on patients with deep vein thrombosis.[78,79] The effect may be too great overnight, posing a risk of hemorrhage, whereas in the morning it may be subtherapeutic, risking aggravation of the medical condition. Another example concerns synthetic corticotherapy for inflammatory conditions. Single 4-hour methylprednisolone (MP) infusion at a rate of 660 µg/h between midnight and 04:00, the approximate trough time of the circadian rhythm of cortisol in day-active persons, results in profound adrenal suppression. In comparison, MP infusion, even at twice the dose, that is, as an 8-hour infusion, between 08:00 and 16:00 causes no adrenal suppression. Finally, 4-hour MP infusion commencing either at 04:00 or 16:00 results in an intermediate level of adrenal suppression.[80] These and other findings indicate that morning (once-a-day) dosing of tablet corticotherapy is associated with best patient tolerance, that is, absence of plasma cortisol suppression and optimal therapeutic benefit. Other examples, given the large number of people worldwide diagnosed with hypertension (eg, an estimated 63 million in the United States and 163 million in China), are the differential ingestion-time–dependent effects of blood pressure–lowering monotherapies, including angiotensin-converting enzyme inhibitors, angiotension receptor blockers, calcium-channel blockers, β-blockers, α-blockers, and loop diuretics.[81] The effects of such hypertension medications have been found to be significantly enhanced when routinely taken at bedtime rather than in the morning. Taken together, these and numerous other studies[82] indicate that the circadian time when medications are administered, regardless of the route of administration, can be critical in determining the extent of both their beneficial and adverse effects.

## SUMMARY

The major goals of this article relative to neurorehabilitation are to stimulate new research into (1) the chronobiology of neurologic conditions and their therapy as a means of improving patient management and outcomes, and (2) work schedules to enhance well-being and productivity of involved health care workers. Chronobiology has been little investigated for its relevance to neurorehabilitation; nonetheless, findings of patient investigations involving a broad spectrum of other medical conditions suggest the field is likely to play a strong role in improving the management and therapy for patients with neurologic deficits. The mood, motivation, tolerance for, and therapeutic benefit of cognitive and physical retraining all can vary in a predictable manner during the 24 hour as a result of the staging of the multitude of rhythms that comprise the CTS. Primary and secondary neurologic deficits may disrupt the CTS, manifesting as altered sleep-wake cycling, melancholy/depression, and extreme fatigue/poor stamina, which may be unknowingly worsened by unnatural, inappropriate, and illogical LAN coupled with poorly lit daytime ambient conditions of patient housing. The CTS also has been shown to influence the PK and PD of most classes of medications. Thus, poorly chosen times to administer medications, both for neurologic and coexisting acute and chronic medical conditions, can compromise the extent of desired outcomes, magnify adverse effects, and perhaps interfere with neurorehabilitation. Brain trauma itself may result in disruption of the CTS, which may interfere with the success of physical and cognitive retraining programs. In certain circumstances, patients can benefit from resynchronization of their CTS, either by use of properly timed bright-light therapy or physiologic melatonin dosing at optimal circadian times, resulting in better tolerance to and effects of interventions. The work schedule of health care personnel may also be disruptive to their CTS. Day-work schedules that commence too early in the morning or rotating and night shift work arrangements can result in undue fatigue with risk of less than optimal work performance and patient management. Relevant investigations of circadian rhythm are warranted to improve both patient outcomes and the working-time arrangements and welfare of neurorehabilitation employees.

## REFERENCES

1. Lemmer B. Discoveries of rhythms in human biological functions: a historical review. Chronobiol Int 2009;26:1019–68.
2. Foster RG, Kreitzman L. Rhythms of life. New Haven (CT): Yale University Press; 2004.
3. Touitou Y, Haus E. Biologic rhythms in clinical and laboratory medicine. Heidelberg (Germany): Springer Verlag; 1992.
4. Thorne HC, Jones KH, Peters SP, et al. Daily and seasonal variation in the spectral composition of light exposure in humans. Chronobiol Int 2009;26:854–66.
5. Tonetti L, Fabbri M, Natale V. Relationship between circadian typology and big five personality domains. Chronobiol Int 2009;26:337–47.
6. Kitamura S, Hida A, Watanabe M, et al. Evening preference is related to the incidence of depressive states independent of sleep-wake conditions. Chronobiol Int 2010;27:1797–812.
7. Ayalon L, Borodkin K, Dishon L, et al. Circadian rhythm sleep disorders following mild traumatic brain injury. Neurology 2007;68:1136–40.
8. Carter KA, Lettieri CJ, Pena JM. An unusual cause of insomnia following IED-induced traumatic brain injury. J Clin Sleep Med 2010;6:205–6.
9. Hofstra WA, Gordijn MC, Van Hemert-Van Der Poel JC, et al. Chronotypes and subjective sleep parameters in epilepsy patients: a large questionnaire study. Chronobiol Int 2010;27:1271–86.
10. Dodson ER, Zee PC. Therapeutics for circadian rhythm sleep disorders. Sleep Med Clin 2010;5:701–15.
11. Haus E, Smolensky M. Biological clocks and shift work: circadian dysregulation and potential long-term effects. Cancer Causes Control 2006;17:489–500.
12. Reinberg A, Smolensky MH. Night and shift work and transmeridian space flights. In: Touitou Y, Haus E, editors. Biologic rhythms in clinical and laboratory medicine. Heidelberg (Germany): Springer Verlag; 1992. p. 243–55.
13. Larsson A, Hassan M, Ridefelt P, et al. Circadian variability of bilirubin in healthy men during normal sleep and after an acute shift of sleep. Chronobiol Int 2009;26:1613–21.
14. Morris C, Atkinson G, Drust B, et al. Human core temperature responses during exercise and subsequent recovery: an important interaction between diurnal variation and measurement site. Chronobiol Int 2009;26:560–75.
15. Barclay NL, Eley TC, Buysse DJ, et al. Diurnal preference and sleep quality: same genes? A study of young adult twins. Chronobiol Int 2010;27:278–96.
16. Paudel ML, Taylor BC, Ancoli-Israel S, et al. Rest/activity rhythms and mortality rates in older men: MrOS Sleep Study. Chronobiol Int 2010;27:363–77.
17. Leonhard C, Randler C. In sync with the family: children and partners influence the sleep-wake circadian rhythm and social habits of women. Chronobiol Int 2009;26:510–25.
18. Akerstedt T, Nordin M, Alfredsson L, et al. Sleep and sleepiness: impact of entering or leaving shiftwork—a prospective study. Chronobiol Int 2010;27:987–96.
19. Akerstedt T, Kecklund G, Selen J. Early morning work—prevalence and relation to sleep/wake problems: a national representative survey. Chronobiol Int 2010;27:975–86.
20. Ohayon MM, Smolensky MH, Roth T. Consequences of shiftworking on sleep duration, sleepiness, and sleep attacks. Chronobiol Int 2010;27:575–89.
21. Edwards BJ, Waterhouse J. Effects of one night of partial sleep deprivation upon diurnal rhythms of accuracy and consistency in throwing darts. Chronobiol Int 2009;26:756–68.
22. Fietze I, Strauch J, Holzhausen M, et al. Sleep quality in professional ballet dancers. Chronobiol Int 2009;26:1249–62.
23. Kubo T, Takahashi M, Takeyama H, et al. How do the timing and length of a night-shift nap affect sleep inertia? Chronobiol Int 2010;27:1031–44.
24. Lombardi DA, Folkard S, Willetts JL, et al. Daily sleep, weekly working hours, and risk of work-related injury: US National Health Interview Survey (2004-2008). Chronobiol Int 2010;27:1013–30.
25. Borisenkov MF, Perminova EV, Kosova AL. Chronotype, sleep length, and school achievement of 11- to 23-year-old students in northern European Russia. Chronobiol Int 2010;27:1259–70.
26. Selvi Y, Aydin A, Boysan M, et al. Associations between chronotype, sleep quality, suicidality, and depressive symptoms in patients with major depression and healthy controls. Chronobiol Int 2010;27:1813–28.
27. Esquirol Y, Bongard V, Mabile L, et al. Shift work and metabolic syndrome: respective impacts of job strain, physical activity, and dietary rhythms. Chronobiol Int 2009;26:544–59.
28. Lin YC, Hsiao TJ, Chen PC. Persistent rotating shift-work exposure accelerates development of metabolic syndrome among middle-aged female employees: a five-year follow-up. Chronobiol Int 2009;26:740–55.
29. Padilha HG, Crispim CA, Zimberg IZ, et al. Metabolic responses on the early shift. Chronobiol Int 2010;27:1080–92.
30. Stevens RG, Hansen J, Costa G, et al. Considerations of circadian impact for defining 'shift work' in cancer studies: IARC Working Group Report. Occup Environ Med 2011;68:154–62.
31. Suwazono Y, Dochi M, Oishi M, et al. Shiftwork and impaired glucose metabolism: a 14-year cohort study on 7104 male workers. Chronobiol Int 2009;26:926–41.

32. Wirtz A, Nachreiner F. The effects of extended working hours on health and social well-being– a comparative analysis of four independent samples. Chronobiol Int 2010;27:1124–34.

33. Grundy A, Sanchez M, Richardson H, et al. Light intensity exposure, sleep duration, physical activity, and biomarkers of melatonin among rotating shift nurses. Chronobiol Int 2009;26:1443–61.

34. Kantermann T, Roenneberg T. Is light-at-night a health risk factor or a health risk predictor? Chronobiol Int 2009;26:1069–74.

35. Bollati V, Baccarelli A, Sartori S, et al. Epigenetic effects of shiftwork on blood DNA methylation. Chronobiol Int 2010;27:1093–104.

36. Yang X, Wood PA, Ansell CM, et al. The circadian clock gene Per1 suppresses cancer cell proliferation and tumor growth at specific times of day. Chronobiol Int 2009;26:1323–39.

37. Kloog I, Portnov BA, Rennert HS, et al. Does the modern urbanized sleeping habitat pose a breast cancer risk? Chronobiol Int 2011;28:76–80.

38. Kloog I, Haim A, Stevens RG, et al. Global co-distribution of light at night (LAN) and cancers of prostate, colon, and lung in men. Chronobiol Int 2009;26:108–25.

39. Driesen K, Jansen NW, Kant I, et al. Depressed mood in the working population: associations with work schedules and working hours. Chronobiol Int 2010;27:1062–79.

40. Tanaka K, Sakata K, Oishi M, et al. Estimation of the benchmark duration of shiftwork associated with weight gain in male Japanese workers. Chronobiol Int 2010;27:1895–910.

41. Morris CJ, Fullick S, Gregson W, et al. Paradoxical post-exercise responses of acylated ghrelin and leptin during a simulated night shift. Chronobiol Int 2010;27:590–605.

42. Chen JD, Lin YC, Hsiao ST. Obesity and high blood pressure of 12-hour night shift female clean-room workers. Chronobiol Int 2010;27:334–44.

43. Lo SH, Lin LY, Hwang JS, et al. Working the night shift causes increased vascular stress and delayed recovery in young women. Chronobiol Int 2010;27:1454–68.

44. Camerino D, Sandri M, Sartori S, et al. Shiftwork, work-family conflict among Italian nurses, and prevention efficacy. Chronobiol Int 2010;27:1105–23.

45. Jansen NW, Mohren DC, Van Amelsvoort LG, et al. Changes in working time arrangements over time as a consequence of work-family conflict. Chronobiol Int 2010;27:1045–61.

46. Atkinson G, Leary AC, George KP, et al. 24-hour variation in the reactivity of rate-pressure-product to everyday physical activity in patients attending a hypertension clinic. Chronobiol Int 2009;26:958–73.

47. Shiotani H, Umegaki Y, Tanaka M, et al. Effects of aerobic exercise on the circadian rhythm of heart rate and blood pressure. Chronobiol Int 2009;26:1636–46.

48. Jones H, Taylor CE, Lewis NC, et al. Post-exercise blood pressure reduction is greater following intermittent than continuous exercise and is influenced less by diurnal variation. Chronobiol Int 2009;26: 293–306.

49. Van Der Heijden KB, De Sonneville LM, Althaus M. Time-of-day effects on cognition in preadolescents: a trails study. Chronobiol Int 2010;27:1870–94.

50. Clarisse R, Le Floc'h N, Kindelberger C, et al. Daily rhythmicity of attention in morning- vs. evening-type adolescents at boarding school under different psychosociological testing conditions. Chronobiol Int 2010;27:826–41.

51. Jasper I, Roenneberg T, Haussler A, et al. Circadian rhythm in force tracking and in dual task costs. Chronobiol Int 2010;27:653–73.

52. Rosenberg J, Pusch K, Dietrich R, et al. The tick-tock of language: is language processing sensitive to circadian rhythmicity and elevated sleep pressure? Chronobiol Int 2009;26:974–91.

53. Bougard C, Bessot N, Moussay S, et al. Effects of waking time and breakfast intake prior to evaluation of physical performance in the early morning. Chronobiol Int 2009;26:307–23.

54. Racinais S, Perrey S, Denis R, et al. Maximal power, but not fatigability, is greater during repeated sprints performed in the afternoon. Chronobiol Int 2010;27: 855–64.

55. Bougard C, Moussay S, Gauthier A, et al. Effects of waking time and breakfast intake prior to evaluation of psychomotor performance in the early morning. Chronobiol Int 2009;26:324–36.

56. Jasper I, Haussler A, Baur B, et al. Circadian variations in the kinematics of handwriting and grip strength. Chronobiol Int 2009;26:576–94.

57. Sargent C, Ferguson SA, Darwent D, et al. The influence of circadian phase and prior wake on neuromuscular function. Chronobiol Int 2010;27:911–21.

58. Lericollais R, Gauthier A, Bessot N, et al. Time-of-day effects on fatigue during a sustained anaerobic test in well-trained cyclists. Chronobiol Int 2009;26: 1622–35.

59. Hayes LD, Bickerstaff GF, Baker JS. Interactions of cortisol, testosterone, and resistance training: influence of circadian rhythms. Chronobiol Int 2010;27: 675–705.

60. Gueugneau N, Papaxanthis C. Time-of-day effects on the internal simulation of motor actions: psychophysical evidence from pointing movements with the dominant and non-dominant arm. Chronobiol Int 2010;27:620–39.

61. Darwent D, Ferguson SA, Sargent C, et al. Contribution of core body temperature, prior wake time, and sleep stages to cognitive throughput performance during forced desynchrony. Chronobiol Int 2010;27:898–910.

62. Marek T, Fafrowicz M, Golonka K, et al. Diurnal patterns of activity of the orienting and executive

attention neuronal networks in subjects performing a Stroop-like task: a functional magnetic resonance imaging study. Chronobiol Int 2010;27:945–58.

63. Martinez-Nicolas A, Ortiz-Tudela E, Madrid JA, et al. Crosstalk between environmental light and internal time in humans. Chronobiol Int 2011;28: 617–29.

64. Valdez P, Ramirez C, Garcia A, et al. Circadian and homeostatic variation in sustained attention. Chronobiol Int 2010;27:393–416.

65. Greubel J, Nachreiner F, Dittmar O, et al. The validity of the fatigue and risk index for predicting impairments of health and safety under different shift schedules in the context of risk assessments. Chronobiol Int 2010;27:1149–58.

66. Hobbs A, Williamson A, Van Dongen HP. A circadian rhythm in skill-based errors in aviation maintenance. Chronobiol Int 2010;27:1304–16.

67. Smolensky MH, Siegel RA, Haus E, et al. Biological rhythms, drug delivery, and chronotherapeutics. In: Siepmann J, Siegel RA, Rathbone MJ, editors. Advances in drug delivery technology. Heidelberg (Germany): Springer Verlag; 2012. p. 359–443.

68. Manfredini R, Boari B, Portaluppi F. Morning surge in blood pressure as a predictor of silent and clinical cerebrovascular disease in elderly hypertensives. Circulation 2003;108:e72–3.

69. Manfredini R, Gallerani M, Portaluppi F, et al. Circadian variation in the onset of acute critical limb ischemia. Thromb Res 1998;92:163–9.

70. Manfredini R, Boari B, Bressan S, et al. Influence of circadian rhythm on mortality after myocardial infarction: data from a prospective cohort of emergency calls. Am J Emerg Med 2004;22:555–9.

71. Portaluppi F, Hermida RC. Circadian rhythms in cardiac arrhythmias and opportunities for their chronotherapy. Adv Drug Deliv Rev 2007;59:940–51.

72. Portaluppi F, Lemmer B. Chronobiology and chronotherapy of ischemic heart disease. Adv Drug Deliv Rev 2007;59:952–65.

73. Portaluppi F, Cortelli P, Buonaura GC, et al. Do restless legs syndrome (RLS) and periodic limb movements of sleep (PLMS) play a role in nocturnal hypertension and increased cardiovascular risk of renally impaired patients? Chronobiol Int 2009;26:1206–21.

74. Smolensky MH, Hermida RC, Castriotta RJ, et al. Role of sleep-wake cycle on blood pressure circadian rhythms and hypertension. Sleep Med 2007;8: 668–80.

75. Bruguerolle B. Chronopharmacokinetics. Current status. Clinical Pharmacokinetics 1998;35:83–94.

76. Lemmer B, Bruguerolle B. Chronopharmacokinetics—are they clinically relevant? Clinical Pharmacokinetics 1994;26:419–27.

77. Reinberg A, Smolensky MH. Circadian changes of drug disposition in man. Clinical Pharmacokinetics 1982;7:401–20.

78. Decousus H. Chronobiology in hemostasis. In: Touitou Y, Haus E, editors. Biologic rhythms in clinical and laboratory medicine. Heidelberg (Germany): Springer Verlag; 1992. p. 554–65.

79. Decousus HA, Croze M, Levi FA, et al. Circadian changes in anticoagulant effect of heparin infused at a constant rate. Br Med J (Clin Res Ed) 1985; 290:341–4.

80. Angeli A. Circadian ACTH-adrenal rhythm in man. Chronobiologia 1974;1(Suppl 1):253–70.

81. Smolensky MH, Hermida RC, Ayala DE, et al. Administration-time-dependent effects of blood pressure-lowering medications: basis for the chronotherapy of hypertension. Blood Press Monit 2010;15:173–80.

82. Portaluppi F, Tiseo R, Smolensky MH, et al. Circadian rhythms and cardiovascular health. Sleep Med Rev 2012;16:151–66.

# Sleep Hypoventilation in Patients with Neuromuscular Diseases

Madeleine M. Grigg-Damberger, MD[a],*,
Lana K. Wagner, MD[b], Lee K. Brown, MD[b]

## KEYWORDS

- Sleep hypoventilation • Neuromuscular disorders • Bilevel positive pressure ventilation
- Duchenne muscular dystrophy • Amyotrophic lateral sclerosis • Myotonic dystrophy

## KEY POINTS

- Sleep-disordered breathing, especially sleep-related hypercapnic hypoventilation, is common in patients with neuromuscular disorders (NMD).
- Appropriate timing of nocturnal positive pressure ventilation (NPPV) initiation as well as management of challenges related specifically to NPPV use in NMD are essential.
- A proactive approach is needed when managing the care of these patients, including close follow-up and assessment, serial monitoring of lung function, and frequent titration of their NPPV settings.
- Other potential disruptors of sleep should be identified and treated, and ventilation should be maximized by addressing scoliosis, malnutrition, and infections.

Increasing numbers of patients with neuromuscular disorders (NMD) are prescribed assisted nocturnal ventilation for sleep-related chronic alveolar hypoventilation, which has resulted in improved health, prolonged survival, and increased quality of life for them.[1–4] Most patients with NMD who require nocturnal assisted ventilation are now first prescribed bilevel positive pressure devices, which augment spontaneous breaths and may deliver timed backup breaths when required. These devices incorporate separately adjustable inspiratory positive airway pressure (IPAP) and expiratory positive airway pressure (EPAP) bilevel positive airway pressure-spontaneous/timed (BPAP-S/T), with EPAP promoting a patent upper airway and IPAP providing ventilator assistance in the form of pressure support (PS) (PS = IPAP – EPAP).[5–14] Successful nocturnal noninvasive positive pressure ventilation (NPPV) in NMD depends on selecting the

appropriate patient, interface, ventilator, and pressure settings but also the skills of the prescribing clinician, patient motivation, and family/caregiver support.[5] Sleep specialists can diagnose and treat these patients more comfortably with better understanding of their disorders and special needs.

The most common form of chronic sleep-disordered breathing (SDB) in patients with NMD is alveolar hypoventilation that typically first develops during rapid eye movement (REM) sleep. The diaphragm is the major muscle for inspiration awake and asleep. Patients with NMD who have significant diaphragmatic weakness depend on intercostal and accessory respiratory muscles to assist the weakened diaphragm. Because these muscles are inhibited during REM sleep, hypoventilation first appears during REM sleep. Weak cough reflexes, kyphoscoliosis, impaired central respiratory control, restrictive pulmonary disease,

Conflicts of interest: None to declare for any of these authors.
a University of New Mexico School of Medicine, MSC10 5620, One University of NM, Albuquerque, NM 87131-0001, USA; b Division of Pulmonary, Critical Care, and Sleep Medicine, University of New Mexico School of Medicine, 1101 Medical Arts Avenue NE, Building #2, Albuquerque, NM 87102, USA
* Corresponding author.
E-mail address: mgriggd@salud.unm.edu

Sleep Med Clin 7 (2012) 667–687
http://dx.doi.org/10.1016/j.jsmc.2012.09.001
1556-407X/12/$ – see front matter © 2012 Elsevier Inc. All rights reserved.

obesity, malnutrition, macroglossia, and medication effects further predispose, when present, to SDB in NMD. Secondary lung disease can develop in patients with NMD predisposing them to hypoventilation during sleep earlier than would be expected. Weak pharyngeal muscles impair deglutition and predispose patients with NMD to aspiration; weak cough reflexes further compound the effects of aspiration, leading to atelectasis, recurrent pneumonias, and the possible development of pulmonary fibrosis and bronchiectasis.

Nocturnal or sleep-related hypoventilation is defined in the second edition of the *International Classification of Sleep Disorders* as an increase in $Paco_2$ greater than 45 mm Hg or disproportionately increased relative to awake levels.[15] Chronic hypoventilation is defined in the National Institute for Health and Clinical Excellence's (NICE) guidelines as the presence of dyspnea, morning headache, daytime hypersomnolence, and/or one of the following: (1) forced vital capacity (FVC) less than 50% of predicted value, (2) a $Paco_2$ of 45 mm Hg or more, and/or (3) nocturnal oxyhemoglobin desaturation (arterial oxyhemoglobin saturation ($SaO_2$) <88% for 5 consecutive minutes).[16] Sleep-induced hypoxemia is defined as an oxyhemoglobin saturation less than 90% for 5 minutes or more with a nadir of less than 85% or more than 30% of the total sleep time with saturation less than 90%. As defined in the American Academy of Sleep Medicine's (AASM) sleep scoring guidelines for polysomnography (PSG), sleep-related hypoventilation in children is confirmed when $Pco_2$ is more than 50 mm Hg for 25% or more of the total sleep time and in adults as a 10 mm Hg or more increase in $Pco_2$ in sleep compared with wakefulness.[17]

## SYMPTOMS AND SIGNS SUGGESTIVE OF SLEEP HYPOVENTILATION IN NMD

Complaints of orthopnea (difficulty breathing supine) in the absence of congestive heart failure suggest diaphragmatic weakness and increase the likelihood that sleep hypoventilation will be found on PSG. Sleep hypoventilation is likely on overnight PSG in patients who have paradoxic breathing awake while lying supine. The abdomen normally moves out during inspiration as the diaphragm descends and displaces the abdominal contents; supine chest/abdominal paradox is present when the abdomen flattens or moves inward during inspiration because the accessory muscles of inspiration creating negative intrathoracic pressure that pulls the weakened diaphragm superiorly. Paradoxic breathing while supine is not obvious until the diaphragmatic strength is less than 25% of normal. Sleep hypoventilation is likely to be found in patients with NMD who have paradoxic breathing supine and/or have a 25% or more decrease in their FVC supine compared with sitting. Other symptoms and signs that should be considered red flags warning of sleep-related hypoventilation in slowly progressive NMD are summarized in **Table 1**.[18–20] However, it

**Table 1**
**Red flags for SDB in patients with NMD**

| Symptoms | Signs |
|---|---|
| Breathlessness when sleeping supine, bending or standing in water | Paradoxic breathing supine |
| New onset of frequent nocturnal awakenings (>3 per night), difficulty awakening in morning, frequent nightmares, sweating, or complaints of disturbed sleep | Soft voice, cannot finish a sentence because of dyspnea |
| Early morning or nocturnal headaches | Ineffective cough |
| Decreased stamina and endurance without increased weakness | Rapid shallow breathing and tachypnea awake |
| Shallow, noisy, or labored breathing | Quiet breath sounds with little/no air movement in lung bases |
| Tachypnea or cyanosis when sleeping | $SpO_2$ <91% at rest, awake, seated, and breathing room air |
| Daytime tiredness or generalized fatigue | Tachypnea supine and/or with exercise |
| Apnea, gasps, or snorts when sleeping | Use of accessory inspiratory and abdominal expiratory muscles to breathe when awake |
| Cough during or after eating or drinking | |

*Abbreviation:* $SpO_2$, pulse arterial oxygen saturation.

is important to note that patients with NMD with only mild limb weakness can, nevertheless, suffer from severe sleep hypoventilation, particularly patients who have mitochondrial or other metabolic myopathies that can predispose to respiratory muscle fatigue[21–24] or individuals with myotonic dystrophy in whom myotonia of the tongue and diaphragm delays muscle relaxation, thereby impairing ventilation.[25]

PSG is indicated in patients with NMD who have symptoms suggestive of sleep-related hypoventilation (morning headache, fatigue, orthopnea, or dyspnea) or in asymptomatic patients with daytime hypercapnia or significant defects on pulmonary function tests (PFTs). Patients with NMD can also have obstructive SDB, especially those who have bulbar weakness, and is often heralded by snoring or daytime sleepiness. All too often, patients with NMD fail to endorse sleep/wake complaints; in part, this may be explained by the fact that once confined to wheelchairs, they have little to tax them. Earlier studies have shown that sleep/wake symptoms poorly predict which patients with NMD will have SDB, even when using a structured sleep questionnaire.[18–20,26]

However, Steier and colleagues[27] (2011) developed a self-administered multiple-choice questionnaire containing 5 questions screening for diaphragm weakness (**Table 2**). They found that a score of 5 or more of 10 points correctly discriminate NMD with respiratory muscle weakness from normal controls and patients with obstructive sleep

apnea (OSA), with a sensitivity of 86%, a specificity of 89%, a positive predictive value of 69%, and a negative predictive value of 96%. However, the investigators cautioned that comorbidities that have symptoms that also vary with body position, such as heart failure, could alter diagnostic accuracy of the questionnaire.

## PULMONARY PREDICTORS OF SLEEP HYPOVENTILATION IN PATIENTS WITH NMD

Abnormalities in PFTs may help to predict which patients with NMD are most likely to have sleep-related hypoventilation.[28–31] Sleep hypoventilation is likely to be found in patients with NMD exhibiting one or more of the following: (1) an FVC less than 50% predicted (<60% if they are obese, have concomitant pulmonary disease, and/or kyphoscoliosis); (2) paradoxic breathing supine; (3) a 25% or more decrease in FVC from sitting to supine; (3) oxyhemoglobin saturation awake less than 91% breathing room air; (4) daytime hypercapnia (Paco$_2$ >45 mm Hg [>6 kPa]); (5) an oxyhemoglobin saturation (SpO2) of less than 88% for 5 or more consecutive minutes on nocturnal pulse oximetry; and/or (6) a maximal inspiratory pressure (MIP) of less than 40 cm H$_2$O.[29–31] Most guidelines for managing assisted ventilation in patients with NMD encourage serial monitoring of lung function for all such patients when possible.[30,31]

One study found the sensitivity of an inspiratory vital capacity (IVC) less than 40% of predicted for

---

**Table 2**
**A self-administered questionnaire to screen for diaphragm weakness and SDB in NMD (SiNQ-5)**

Dear Patient,
The following questions may help us to decide whether you may have disordered breathing during sleep-related to muscle weakness. Please circle the most appropriate answer to each question.
Thank you for your cooperation.

| Do you feel breathless, if | | | |
|---|---|---|---|
| you lie down? (eg, on your bed) | Yes (2) | Sometimes (1) | No (0) |
| you bend forward? (eg, to tie your shoelaces) | Yes (2) | Sometimes (1) | No (0) |
| you swim in water or lay in a bath? | Yes (2) | Sometimes (1) | No (0) |
| Have you changed your position when in bed? | Yes (2) | No (0) | |
| Have you noticed a change in your sleep (waking more, getting up, poor quality sleep)? | Yes (2) | No (0) | |

Numbers in parentheses represent scores.
   Steier and colleagues developed and validated this self-administered 5-question multiple-choice questionnaire to screen patients with NMD for SDB.[27] The questions are targeted to identify diaphragmatic weakness. A score of more than 5 out of 10 points in the SiNQ-5 had a had a sensitivity of 86.2%, a specificity of 88.5%, a positive predictive value of 69.4%, and a negative predictive value of 95.5% to identify NMD with combined SDB. The investigators caution that comorbidities, such as heart failure, that have symptoms influenced by posture could alter diagnostic accuracy.
   *Abbreviation:* SiNQ-5, Sleep-Disordered Breathing in Neuromuscular Disease Questionnaire-5.
   *From* Steier J, Jolley CJ, Seymour J et al. Screening for sleep-disordered breathing in neuromuscular disease using a questionnaire for symptoms associated with diaphragm paralysis. Eur Respir J 2011;37(2):400–5; with permission.

sleep hypoventilation was more than 90% and the specificity 88% in 49 children and adolescents with NMD.[32] Another found that sleep hypoventilation was likely on overnight PSG in 27 children with congenital and acquired limb muscle dystrophies who had an FVC less than 40% predicted but also in children with IVC less than 60% predicted who were obese, had concomitant lung disease, or had an acute respiratory infection.[33] A recent prospective study of 48 children and adolescents with progressive NMD noted the presence of scoliosis, and an FVC less than 70% or a forced expiratory volume in 1 second ($FEV_1$) less than 65% predicted that sleep hypoventilation would be found on their overnight PSG.[34]

## PARTICULAR NMD OFTEN REFERRED TO SLEEP SPECIALISTS

Probably the 3 most common NMDs referred to sleep specialists are Duchenne muscular dystrophy (DMD), type 1 myotonic dystrophy (DM1), and amyotrophic lateral sclerosis (ALS). It behooves sleep specialists to become knowledgeable at evaluating and treating SDB in these patients.

### DMD

DMD and milder forms of it (intermediate and Becker muscular dystrophy) are caused by a genetic mutation in the short arm of chromosome 21 (Xp21.2) in the dystrophin gene and are now termed dystrophinopathies.[35–38] Dystrophinopathies occur almost exclusively in males, with an incidence of 1 in 3500.[39] Mutations (usually deletions) in the dystrophin gene lead to progressive skeletal and cardiac muscle degeneration that culminates in loss of independent ambulation at variable ages, depending on the severity of the mutation, typically by 13 years of age in those with DMD, 13 to 16 years of age in intermediate muscular dystrophy, and approximately 16 years of age in Becker muscular dystrophy.[37] If left untreated, respiratory, cardiac, and orthopedic complications emerge; without intervention the mean age of death is 19 years.[37]

However, patients with DMD are now surviving into their 40s because of more common use of BPAP-S/T once sleep hypoventilation develops, aggressive use of mechanically assisted cough devices, aggressive treatment of respiratory infections, avoidance of malnutrition, and transition to around-the-clock assisted ventilation as their FVC decreases.[18,36,37] Two other treatment strategies are also contributing to increasing longevity in DMD: long-term treatment with oral glucocorticosteroids and cardioprotective medications.

Ishikawa and colleagues[40] (2011) compared survival in 3 groups of patients with DMD; all 56 patients that were untreated before 1984 died at a mean age of 19 + 3 years, 21 (88%) out of 24 treated with tracheotomy from 1984 to 1991 died at a mean of 28 + 8 years of age (3 still living), whereas 50% of 88 patients using continuous noninvasive ventilation (NIV) died with a mean age of death of 39.6 years. The investigators concluded that NIV, mechanically assisted cough, and cardioprotective medication can result in more favorable outcomes and better survival in comparison with invasive treatment.

Long-term treatment with oral glucocorticoids (prednisone in the United States, deflazacort in Europe and Canada) has changed the natural history of dystrophinopathies. Early randomized clinical trials showed corticosteroid therapy for 6 months improved muscle strength in patients with DMD.[41,42] Chronic oral corticosteroid therapy has been shown in multiple studies to prolong ambulation by 2 to 5 years, preserve cardiopulmonary function, stabilize pulmonary function variables, improve cardiac function, delay the need for assisted ventilation, reduce the risk of progressive scoliosis (and consequent surgery), and increase survival and quality of life in patients with DMD.[42–47] These findings have led to practice parameters recommending that boys with DMD who are older than 5 years of age should be offered treatment with prednisone (0.75 mg/kg/d, maximum dose: 40 mg) as soon as plateauing or decline in motor skills are noted.[48] Weight gain, decreased height, and often asymptomatic cataracts are common adverse effects of corticosteroids in DMD. Excessive weight gain contributes to SDB in DMD; practice guidelines recommend that if patients with dystrophinopathies gain more than 20% over estimated normal weight for height over a 12-month period, their prednisone dosage should be decreased from 0.75 to 0.5 mg/kg/d, and further reduced to 0.3 mg/kg/d after 3 to 4 months if excessive weight gain continues.[48]

Sleep medicine specialists are occasionally asked to evaluate young boys with DMD who snore and have enlarged tonsils. Overnight PSG in younger boys (mean age of 8 years) with DMD often shows only OSA. Tonsillectomy (and adenoidectomy) often resolves the OSA. Sleep hypoventilation in males with DMD mostly begins after they become wheelchair dependent and their kyphoscoliosis (a consequence of weak paraspinal muscles) accelerates. Boys with DMD at an in-between age (after the prevalence of adenotonsillar hypertrophy and OSA has declined, which are most common at a young age, but before the increased likelihood of sleep hypoventilation when wheelchair bound) can develop acute respiratory failure during a serious respiratory infection. In this middle period, expiratory muscles weaken before inspiratory muscles, resulting in only modest impairment that may be clinically silent.

## ALS

ALS is the most severe form of motor neuron disease (MND) and the third most common neurodegenerative disease of adults. The average age of onset of ALS is 55 to 60 years and it affects 5 to 7 people per 100 000. Most survive 2 to 4 years after the onset of symptoms; 50% survive 30 months, less than 10% beyond 10 years.[49] Progressive degeneration of both the upper and lower motor neurons occurs in ALS. Upper motor signs include spasticity, hyperreflexia, extensor toe responses, and emotional lability; weakness, atrophy, fasciculations, hyporeflexia, and muscle cramps are manifestations of lower motor involvement. Dysarthria, dysphagia, fatigability, and respiratory insufficiency are usually caused by a combination of lower and upper motor neuron degeneration.[50]

Many patients with ALS are living longer than before. Increasing use and prescription of BPAP-S/T (and gastrostomy) have been cited as major reasons for longer survival. The number of patients with ALS prescribed BPAP-S/T has increased 2 to 4 times from 16% to 21% 6 to 10 years ago to 51% to 73% of patients within the last 5 years.[51,52] A postal survey of NPPV in MND was conducted on 612 UK patients referred over 12 months; 444 were treated (73%), a marked increase in the number of patients referred (2.6 fold) and using (3.4 fold) NPPV.[53] Monitoring of respiratory function remains suboptimal, and uncontrolled oxygen administration is sometimes used inappropriately before the terminal phase.

Patients with ALS who have severe bulbar dysfunction[4] and/or frontotemporal dementia (FTD)[54] are less likely to tolerate BPAP-S/T and have poorer survival times. Excessive salivation and the inability to close the mouth in patients with ALS with severe bulbar dysfunction contributes to their often poor tolerance of the nasal or oronasal masks. Sialorrhea in these individuals can be lessened by tricyclic antidepressants and ultrasound-guided submandibular injection of botulinum toxin.[55]

ALS was once thought to be limited to the motor system, but we now recognize that ALS is often associated with frontotemporal cognitive changes that range from mild to profound FTD.[54] Caregivers are more likely to report symptoms of FTD in patients with ALS with greater respiratory impairment and treating them with NPPV reversed some reports of cognitive symptoms.[56] Unfortunately, impaired executive function in patients with ALS lessens the likelihood that they will accept BPAP-S/T.[57]

Some patients with ALS choose to extend their life using mechanical ventilation via tracheostomy.[58–61] A recent study evaluated how patients with ALS decide about using assisted ventilation.[62] The investigators found that patients (and their caregivers) made a sharp distinction between BPAP (which they viewed as a means to relieve symptoms of respiratory failure) and invasive mechanical ventilation (taking over their breathing and saving their life when they would otherwise die). Willingness to use assisted ventilation was influenced by gradual familiarization with the equipment and its benefits, fears about respiratory distress, how use of it could impact on daily life, how death caused by respiratory failure occurs, and how they can choose to stop assisted ventilation if and when they wish to die. Clinicians need to have these discussions early and often in patients with progressive NMD.

One study found that most patients with ALS survive less than a year,[58] or a mean of 21 months following tracheostomy.[59] Recent studies report the circumstances in which invasive home mechanical ventilation and palliative care are discontinued in patients with end-stage ALS who perceive a loss of meaning in life.[63–65] Patients are given deep sedation using high-dose morphine and diazepam before disconnecting the ventilator, a technique also used by others.[64] Evidence-based guidelines for managing ALS were published in 2012 by the European Federation of Neurologic Societies and warrant review.[16] Guidelines for the assessment of respiration are shown in **Fig. 1**.

## Myotonic Dystrophies

DM1 is the most common adult-onset muscular dystrophy and is caused by an expansion of a CTG repeat in the DMPK gene, which codes for myotonic dystrophy protein kinase. DM1 is a multisystem disorder characterized by myotonia (delayed muscle relaxation following contraction), skeletal muscle weakness, cataracts, early balding, insulin resistance, cardiac conduction abnormalities, and SDB leading to progressive respiratory failure. Patients with DM1 have a greater susceptibility to SDB (and a greater variety of primary sleep disorders) compared with any other neuromuscular disorder.[19,26,66–71] OSA, sleep-related hypoventilation, restless legs syndrome, periodic limb movement disorder, and

## Assessment pathway

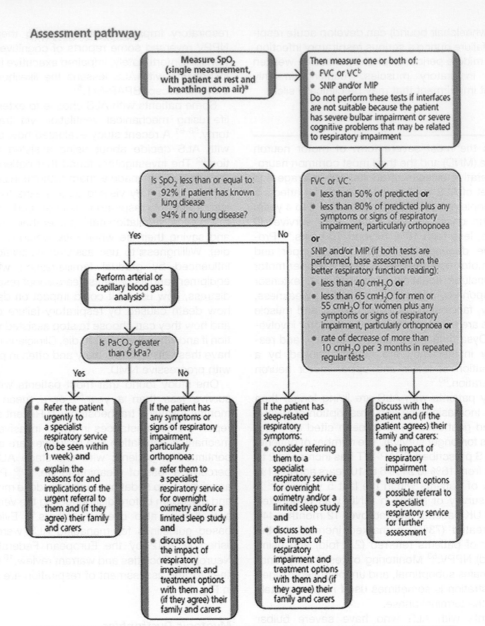

**Fig. 1.** Assessment Pathway from NICE guidelines for managing respiration in ALS. The NICE guidelines for treating ALS endorse NIPPV to improve survival and quality of life (QOL) in patients with ALS. Control of symptoms, such as sialorrhoea, inspissated mucus, emotional lability, cramps, spasticity, and pain, should be attempted. Percutaneous endoscopic gastrostomy feeding improves nutrition and QOL, and gastrostomy tubes should be placed before respiratory insufficiency develops. Noninvasive positive-pressure ventilation also improves survival and QOL. Maintaining patients' ability to communicate is essential. During the course of the disease, every effort should be made to maintain patient autonomy. Advance directives for palliative end-of-life care should be discussed early with patients and caregivers, paying particular respect to patients' social and cultural background. FVC, forced vital capacity; VC, vital capacity; SNIP, sniff test; MIP, maximum inspiratory pressure. *From* National Institute for Health and Clinical Excellence (2010). CG 105 Motor neurone disease: the use of non-invasive ventilation in the management of motor neurone disease. Reproduced with permission. This information was accurate at the time of this publication. Please consult the NICE website at www.nice.org.uk/guidance/CG105 for the most current guideline.

central nervous system hypersomnia unrelated to the SDB are seen in DM1.[68] Most often, sleep-related hypoventilation is the predominant (or only) form of SDB in many types of NMD, but OSA is actually quite common in DM1. OSA was present in 22 (55%) out of 40 young adults with DM1 (mean age 23 + 3 years) without sleep/wake complaints; sleep hypoventilation was additionally found in 4 out of 22 patients with OSA and periodic breathing in 5.[67] Another study found OSA in 14 and central sleep apnea in 3 out of 17 young patients with DM1 without excessive daytime sleepiness (EDS) or other sleep/wake complaints recruited from neurology or pulmonary clinics.[19,67]

Patients with DM1 are extremely sensitive to hypnotics and general anesthesia; many first present when they have difficulty breathing on their own following surgery. Such cases illustrate how patients with DM1 can have severe diaphragmatic and intercostal muscle weakness despite only mild limb weakness. Myotonia of their diaphragm and tongue can also contribute to earlier respiratory failure in patients with DM1 than would usually be predicted. Patients with DM1 can also demonstrate severe sleep hypoventilation with normal PFTs and arterial blood gases while awake.

A great variety of SDB patterns are seen on overnight PSG in patients with DM1: (1) prolonged periods of shallow breathing, periodic breathing, alveolar hypoventilation, and nonapneic desaturations especially during REM sleep; (2) apneas or hypopneas are often absent unless patients snore and/or are obese; (3) when present, apneas are central in type with or without a Cheyne-Stokes pattern; and (4) more irregular breathing patterns awake and during lighter non–REM (NREM) sleep typically disappear during NREM 3 sleep.

Patients with DM1 can also have severe daytime sleepiness, which can develop years before the weakness appears (even in prepubertal childhood). Hypersomnia in patients with DM1 is often first seen before sleep disordered breathing develops, and often persists after the sleep disordered breathing has been treated. Hypersomnia in DM1 unrelated to sleep disordered breathing is thought to related to some dysfunction in the central nervous system (i.e., a central hypersomnia).[26,69,70,72] Yu and colleagues[26] (2011) compared PSG and multiple sleep latency test parameters in 40 consecutive adults with DM1 with 40 age- and sex-matched controls. Eighty percent of the patients with DM1 reported EDS, 31% had Epworth scores greater than 10 but only 13% had objective sleepiness (mean sleep latency <8 minutes). Higher apnea and central apnea indexes, and a greater proportion of

patients with severe apnea/hypopnea syndrome, were found in DM1 compared with controls. Far more sleep-onset REM periods (SOREMPs) were found in the patients with DM1 compared with controls: 1 and 2 SOREMPs were present in 48% and 33% of patients with DM1, whereas only 1 control had a single SOREMP. Compared with controls, patients with DM1 also had (1) higher percentages of NREM 3 and REM sleep; (2) periodic limb movements (PLMs) awake and during NREM and REM sleep; (3) PLMs that were more likely to cause arousals; (4) higher REM density; and (5) REM sleep without atonia or excessive phasic electromyographic (EMG) activity in REM sleep.[26] Another case-control study found 33% of 157 patients with DM1 endorsed EDS and best correlated with the severity of their muscular impairment.[69] Central hypersomnia in some patients with DM1 responds (at least subjectively) to treatment with modafinil.[73–75] NMDs at the greatest risk for SDB are shown in **Box 1**.

---

**Box 1**
**NMD at greatest risk for SDB**

*Myopathies*

- DMD
- Myotonic dystrophies
- Congenital myopathies
- Acid maltase deficiency (Pompe disease)
- Carnitine palmityl transferase deficiency
- Limb-girdle muscular dystrophy
- Polymyositis with pulmonary fibrosis
- Mitochondrial myopathies
- Facioscapulohumeral muscular dystrophy

*Anterior horn cell diseases*

- ALS
- Postpolio syndrome
- Spinal muscular atrophy types 1 and 2

*Peripheral nerve disorders*

- Guillain-Barré syndrome
- Critical illness neuropathy
- Diphtheria
- Porphyria

*Neuromuscular junction disorders*

- Myasthenia gravis
- Botulism
- Pharmacologic neuromuscular blockade

## POLYSOMNOGRAPHIC FINDINGS IN PATIENTS WITH NMD

Initially, sleep-related hypoventilation may only be observed during REM sleep in patients with NMD. Sleep hypoventilation in NREM sleep tends to appear later, with progressive decline in FVC and other pulmonary function measurements. A seminal study by Ragette and colleagues[76] (2002) found that hypoventilation occurred only during REM sleep in 42 patients with primary myopathies when their IVC was less than 40%, during both NREM and REM sleep when the IVC were less than 30%, and respiratory failure when the IVC was less than 25% of predicted. In the authors' experience and that of others, patients whose baseline $SpO_2$ was less than 91% awake are likely to have sleep hypoventilation on overnight PSG.

Apnea-hypopnea indexes in patients with significant sleep hypoventilation can be surprisingly low (**Table 3**). Patients with moderate to severe sleep hypoventilation can have no apneas or hypopneas but only hypercapnia with or without hypoxemia (**Fig. 2**). It is important to note that if PSG is performed with supplemental oxygen, oxyhemoglobin desaturation may not be observed despite hypercapnia. Moreover, the few apneas or short hypopneas that are present may only be seen during REM sleep. Most often these are central events (**Fig. 3**), less often central or mixed, and rarely obstructive apneas. Breathing is often shallow (low tidal volumes), and snoring is uncommon. Early on, periods of tachypnea may be observed during NREM 3 sleep (**Fig. 4**). Because respiration during NREM 3 sleep is under metabolic control, breathing during this stage is particularly regular, often even appearing normal. Patients with severe REM sleep-related hypoventilation can have ominous prolonged hypopneas that last more than 30 to 70 seconds, causing arterial oxyhemoglobin desaturations to values less than 70% (**Fig. 5**). REM sleep is often absent and arousals or awakenings decreased in patients with NMD with severe sleep hypoventilation. A summary of the PSG findings in early, moderate, and severe sleep-related hypoventilation is shown in **Table 4**.

## WHEN TO START NOCTURNAL ASSISTED VENTILATION IN PATIENTS WITH NMD

Consider BPAP-S/T in patients with NMD after they become symptomatic (otherwise compliance is often poor, and many often deny symptoms) and in asymptomatic patients who have an FVC less than 50% of predicted, an MIP or sniff pressure that fails to generate less than -40 cm $H_2O$, and/or a waking $Paco_2$ more than 45 mm Hg (>6.0 kPa). The authors also screen patients with asymptomatic NMD for sleep hypoventilation who (1) have an FVC less than 60% with concomitant lung disease, excessive daytime sleepiness, are obese, and/or snore; (2) have scoliosis and an FVC less than 70% of predicted or an $FEV_1$ less than 65%[34]; and (3) any patients with NMD who are scheduled for scoliosis spinal stabilization surgeries. **Box 2** summarizes the Centers for Medicare and Medicaid Services' (CMS) guidelines for reimbursement of BPAP-S/T devices.

## TITRATING BPAP IN PATIENTS WITH NMD

The authors prefer to titrate BPAP during a comprehensive attended in-laboratory PSG in patients with NMD because they can then (1) manually adjust the device by determining the best ventilator mode (spontaneous [S], spontaneous-timed [S/T], and timed [T]) and by choosing the optimal IPAP and EPAP settings to deliver nocturnal ventilation that results in an adequate level of nocturnal $Paco_2$; (2) maximize patient comfort by adjusting inspiratory time; (3) (when supplemental oxygen seems necessary) assess the effect that this

---

**Table 3**
**A paucity of discrete respiratory events and sleep architecture abnormalities are common in patients with NMD with significant sleep-related central hypoventilation**

| Parameter | SDB | No SDB |
|---|---|---|
| Mean $SaO_2$ (%) | 93 | 97 |
| $SaO_2$ <90% of TST (%) | 25 | 0 |
| Nadir $SaO_2$ (%) | 80 | 92 |
| Mean $PtcCO_2$ (mm Hg) | 50 | 41 |
| $PtcCO_2$ >50 mm Hg (%TST) | 59 | 1 |
| RDI | 7/h | 1/h |
| Arousal index | 20/h | 12/h |

Mellies and colleagues (2003) found SDB in patients with myopathies resulted in a slight increase in arousal index but no disruption of sleep architecture: awake: 5 + 2%; stage 1: 5 + 3%; stage 2: 45 + 10%; slow wave sleep: 28 + 13%; REM sleep: 18 + 3%. Note the low respiratory disturbance index of 7/h of sleep even in the patients with severe sleep-related hypoventilation (mean nadir $SpO_2$ = 80%, 25% of TST with $SpO_2$ <90%, and 59% of TST with $PtcCO_2$ >50 mm Hg).

*Abbreviations:* $PtcCO_2$, transcutaneous $Pco_2$; RDI, respiratory disturbance index; TST, Total sleep time.

*Data from* Mellies U, Ragette R, Schwake C, et al. Daytime predictors of sleep disordered breathing in children and adolescents with neuromuscular disorders. Neuromuscul Disord 2003;13(2):123–8.

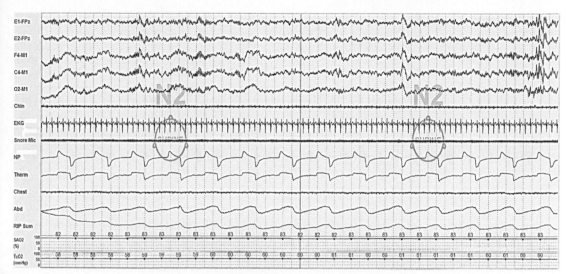

**Fig. 2.** 60-second epoch of PSG recorded during NREM 2 sleep in a 25-year-old man with congenital nemaline myopathy. The epoch shows sleep-related hypoventilation with a baseline SpO₂ of 82% to 83%, transcutaneous Pco₂ of 59 to 61 mm Hg, and a respiratory rate of 14 breaths per minute before BPAP was initiated.

may have on Paco₂ (levels of which may increase because of reductions in respiratory drive and abnormalities in ventilation/perfusion matching); (4) document the effects of BPAP on sleep quality, apneas, and hypopneas; (5) identify and treat patient-ventilator asynchrony; (6) document the effectiveness of NPPV settings in various body positions and sleep stages (often less effective in REM sleep and in the supine posture); and (7) change or adjust mask interfaces to maximize comfort and minimize leak.

When titrating BPAP in the laboratory, the authors monitor airflow, delivered pressure signals, mask leak, respiratory rate, pulse oximetry (SpO₂), transcutaneous Pco₂ (PtcCO₂), and intercostal EMG. Elevated PtcCO₂ indicates the need to increase IPAP (more pressure support), so as to achieve up to a 10 mm Hg reduction during the titration. Monitoring respiratory rate and intercostal EMG helps to assess if adequate respiratory muscle rest has been attained during the titration.

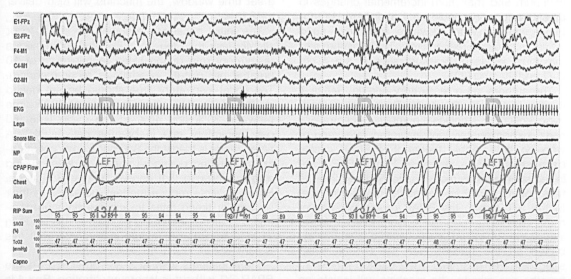

**Fig. 3.** Two-minute epoch of PSG recorded on a 15-year-old boy with DMD during REM sleep while titrating BPAP-S. Long central apneas are still occurring despite increasing BPAP. These apneas were eliminated by adding a backup rate.

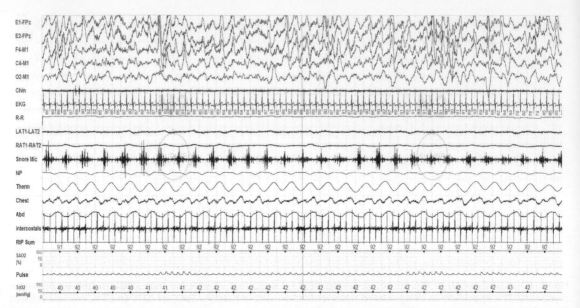

**Fig. 4.** A 60-second PSG epoch recorded in a 17-year-old patient during NREM sleep showing tachypnea with respiratory rates averaging 28 breaths per minute, SpO$_2$ 92%, and transcutaneous carbon dioxide (tCO$_2$) 42 mm Hg.

**Box 3** summarizes the authors' laboratory protocol for titrating BPAP, which accords with the protocol recommended by the AASM's practice guidelines for the adjustment of NPPV in stable chronic hypoventilation syndromes.[77] The AASM's practice guidelines call for starting IPAP and EPAP at 8 cm H$_2$O and 4 cm H$_2$O, respectively. The recommended maximum IPAP should be 30 cm H$_2$O for patients older than 12 years and 20 cm H$_2$O for those younger than 12 years; the minimum and maximum incremental changes in pressure support should be 1 and 2 cm H$_2$O for those younger than 12 years and those aged 12 years or older, respectively. The minimum and maximum levels of pressure support are 4 cm H$_2$O and 20 cm H$_2$O.

The authors set a respiratory rate (ie, S/T or T modes) in all patients with NMD who have central hypoventilation, significant numbers of central apneas, inappropriately low respiratory rates, and/or who do not reliably trigger IPAP/EPAP cycles because of muscle weakness. When BPAP is set in the spontaneous mode, patients determine the time spent in IPAP as well as the respiratory rate. In the S/T mode, the BPAP device will deliver a machine-triggered IPAP cycle if patients fail to initiate an IPAP/EPAP cycle within a time window based on the backup rate set by the sleep specialist. For example, if the backup rate is 10 breaths per minute, the machine will initiate an IPAP/EPAP cycle if patients do not breathe within 6 seconds. In the timed mode, BPAP delivers time-triggered breaths only; patients can take spontaneous breaths but these will not trigger an IPAP/EPAP cycle, and the rate at which breaths are delivered is set by the technologist (during the titration) or the sleep specialist (when the home unit is prescribed). Volume-assisted IPAP-EPAP devices automatically adjust the IPAP level against a fixed EPAP so as to deliver the amount of PS necessary to achieve a target tidal volume. If patients fail to initiate an IPAP/EPAP cycle within a set time window, the machine will also deliver a PS breath.

The initial backup rate should be equal to or slightly less than (eg, by 10%) the spontaneous respiratory rate during sleep (a minimum of 10 breaths per minute in adults is recommended). The initial inspiratory time should be set based on the respiratory rate to provide an IPAP time between 30% and 40% of the cycle time (60 per respiratory rate in breaths per minute). A timed mode is tried if the S/T mode does not stabilize respiration during all stages of sleep, using a rate similar to that chosen for the S/T mode. Some patients require modest increases in their backup or timed rates to achieve optimal respiration in sleep; the authors increase this value in 1- to 2-breaths-per-minute increments until this is achieved.

Many patients with ALS are prescribed home BPAP-S/T without in-laboratory titration. **Box 4** is a protocol for introducing and titrating BPAP-S/T in patients without PSG. IPAP is titrated at home

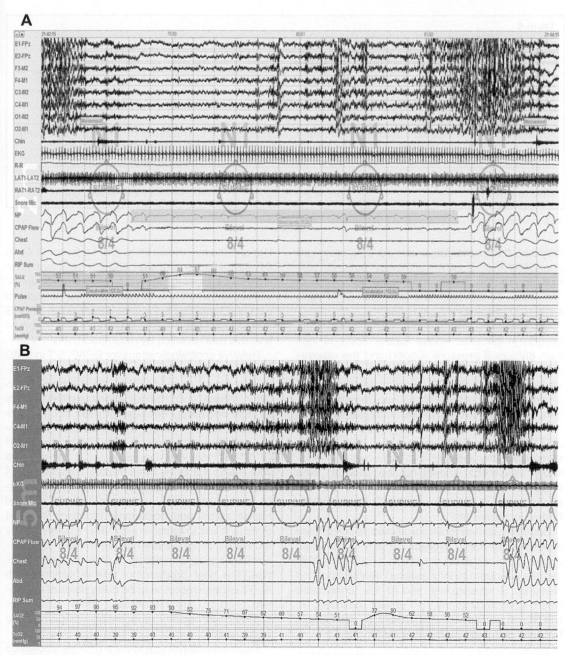

**Fig. 5.** (*A, B*) Note the long-lasting central apnea at the start of a BPAP S/T retitration in a patient with congenital nemaline myopathy. The initial setting of 8/4 cm $H_2O$ fails to produce significant airflow, indicating the need for increased IPAP.

and PSG confirmation sought based on whether the patients' subjective symptoms abate and daytime $Paco_2$ normalizes. In principle, the authors find this strategy unacceptable, but unfortunately it seems to be commonly used in the community, especially in patients with ALS. Prescribing BPAP-S/T without PSG titration is more likely to result in patients being left on suboptimal settings and at risk for patient-ventilator asynchrony.[78]

NPPV settings that are well tolerated when awake have been shown to be frequently associated with patient-ventilator asynchrony, ineffective respiratory efforts, and poor quality of nocturnal sleep.[78] Far too often, patients with ALS are empirically prescribed BPAP with IPAP that is too low and EPAP that is too high. Patients with ALS usually require IPAP of 14 to 18 cm $H_2O$ but rarely need (or tolerate) EPAP more than 4 cm $H_2O$ unless

**Table 4**
**Severity of PSG findings in patients with NMD**

|  | Early | Moderate | Severe |
|---|---|---|---|
| Mean $SpO_2$ | <96% | <94% | <92% |
| Mean $PetCO_2$ | Normal or ↓ | >45 mm Hg | >50 mm Hg |
| Respiratory rate | Tachypnea | Normal to ↑ | Normal |
| Arousals | Frequent arousals, ↑stage 1 | Frequent arousals and awakenings | Decreased arousals and awakenings Only awaken with prolonged desaturations |
| REM sleep | ↓ | Decreased to absent | Absent |
| Desaturations |  | REM desaturation | NREM and REM desaturation |

Abbreviation: $PetCO_2$, partial pressure of end-tidal carbon dioxide.

they also have obstructive apneas. A randomized controlled trial of BPAP-S/T in 92 patients with ALS found the mean IPAP was 15 cm $H_2O$ (maximum 24 cm $H_2O$) and the mean EPAP was 4 cm $H_2O$ (maximum 5 cm $H_2O$).[79]

On occasion, the authors add supplemental oxygen in patients whose awake $SpO_2$ is less than 88% or if pressure support and the respiratory rate during sleep is maximally optimized but an $SpO_2$ less than 90% remains for more than 5 minutes. The authors titrate supplemental oxygen beginning with 1 L/min, increase in increments of 1 L/min approximately every 15 minutes until adequate $SpO_2$ more than 90% is observed. Supplemental oxygen alone (without ventilatory assistance) should not be used to treat sleep-related hypoventilation unless it can be shown that it is not associated with unacceptable further increases in $Paco_2$.

Daytime assisted ventilation should be considered when waking $Paco_2$ exceeds 50 mm Hg or when awake oxyhemoglobin saturation is less than 92% despite adequate nightly assisted ventilation when sleeping. Tracheostomy should be considered when contraindications, or patient aversion, to NPPV are present or when NPPV is not feasible because of bulbar weakness or dysfunction.

## CLINICAL BENEFITS AND CHALLENGES OF ASSISTED NOCTURNAL VENTILATION IN NMD

Studies have shown that in patients with various NMDs, NPPV lessened daytime sleepiness and morning headache,[7] improved daytime and nighttime arterial blood gases,[80] improved sleep architecture,[11] decreased hospitalization rates,[7,80] and enhanced exercise capacity.[81] A prospective longitudinal study found that, in 30 patients (12 + 4 years of age) with various inherited NMDs, NPPV decreased arousals from sleep, lowered nocturnal transcutaneous $Pco_2$ (from a mean of 54 to 42 mm Hg) and diurnal arterial $Pco_2$ (from a mean of 48 to 41 mm Hg), and these effects persisted over a mean of 25 + 13 months.[12] Moreover, 3 nights' withdrawal of NPPV in 10 previously stable patients with NMD resulted in prompt deterioration of SDB and gas exchange returning to the pre-NPPV baseline; this was reversed by resumption of NPPV.

Relative contraindications for BPAP-S/T in NMD are severe dysphagia, inadequate family or caregiver support, or need for around-the-clock ventilation. Absolute contraindications are the inability to clear secretions because of peak cough flows that are too low (even with assistance), and/or the inability to fit or tolerate the NPPV interface.[82] BPAP-S/T use can be challenging for patients with NMD. Patients often report difficulty using BPAP because of air leaks, claustrophobia, excessive salivation, airway mucus accumulation, nasal bridge sores, and abdominal bloating. BPAP is difficult to use in patients with NMD who are poorly motivated or depressed or who have claustrophobia or severe limitation of limb or bulbar function. The best predictor of use in patients with ALS has been reported to be complaints of orthopnea and/or breathlessness when sitting or standing in water (suggesting diaphragmatic weakness).

Patient-ventilator asynchrony (PVA) is a common problem in patients with NMD prescribed NPPV, especially those in whom BPAP-S/T is prescribed empirically and without in-laboratory titration.[83] A recently published study found PVA events averaged 4.3 per hour in 18 patients with NMD who had in-laboratory titration. PVA was significantly more likely to occur (and go untreated) during subsequent home sleep studies. PVA at home was most often caused by air leaks. Automatic triggering was the most common cause of asynchrony, followed by ineffective inspiratory efforts and failure to trigger the transition from IPAP to EPAP. All types of PVA occurred more often in

**Box 2**
**Medicare guidelines for reimbursement for respiratory assist devices for NMD**

1. There are 2 types of bilevel positive pressure devices:
   a. BPAP device without a backup rate, BPAP-S (E0470)
   b. BPAP with a backup rate, BPAP-S/T (E0471)
2. To obtain BPAP-S/T for NMD, patients must fulfill criterion A, B, and C.
   a. *Criterion A:* Medical record documentation of an NMD by a qualified treating physician
      i. The treating physician must be one who is qualified by virtue of experience and training in noninvasive respiratory assistance to order and monitor the use of respiratory assist devices.
   b. *Criterion B:* need to meet B1, B2, or B3
      i. B1: $Paco_2$ greater than 45 mm Hg while awake and breathing patient's prescribed fraction of inspired oxygen ($F_{IO_2}$)
      ii. B2: Overnight pulse oximetry shows $SpO_2$ 88% or less for at least 5 consecutive minutes of nocturnal recording time while breathing prescribed $F_{IO_2}$ (2 hours minimum recording time)
      iii. B3 MIP less than 60 cm $H_2O$ or FVC less than 50% of predicted
   c. *Criterion C:* Chronic obstructive pulmonary disease does not contribute significantly to patients' pulmonary limitation.
3. If A, B, and C are met, then E0470 (BPAP device without backup) or E0471 (BPAP device with backup) will be covered by the CMS for the first 3 months of treatment. A formal sleep study is not needed to qualify for BPAP with or without a backup rate per the CMS.

BPAP devices with a backup rate (E0471) are a better long-term choice for patients with NMD. CMS guidelines for BPAP devices with a backup rate (E0741) include the following: (1) episodically low respiratory efforts (REM sleep) and tidal volume caused by muscle weakness or high work of breathing; (2) frequent central apneas at baseline or during NPPV titration/treatment; (3) inappropriately low respiratory rates; (4) respiratory muscle rest not achieved with maximum PS or maximum tolerated PS; and (5) adequate ventilation is not achieved with maximum PS (or maximum tolerated PS).

**Box 3**
**Titration of BPAP-S/T with PSG in patients with NMD**

- Perform careful mask fitting and discussion of the indications, treatment goals, and side effects of BPAP-S/T with patients (and caregivers), preferably before the night of the study.
- Begin with BPAP-S with IPAP at 8 cm $H_2O$, EPAP at 4 cm $H_2O$, and pressure relief (eg, bilevel with variable pressure relief), if available, at 3.
- Increase IPAP by 1 to 2 cm $H_2O$ for hypopneas, hypercapnia, hypoxia, or respiratory event–related arousals.
- Increase FPAP by 1 cm $H_2O$ for obstructive apneas.
- PS should be increased every 5 minutes if the tidal volume remains low (<6–8 mL/kg).
- If central apneas are noted, initiate backup rate at 10% less than the usual respiratory rate during REM sleep.
- When optimal titration is achieve, perform a trial of timed rate (typically at 10% less than the usual respiratory rate during REM sleep).
- The AASM recommended maximum IPAP pressure is 30 cm $H_2O$ for patients older than 12 years and 20 cm $H_2O$ for patients younger than 12 years.
- Most patients with NMD without obstructive sleep apnea cannot tolerate EPAP pressures greater than 4 to 5 cm $H_2O$.
- Use heated humidification.
- Use partial pressure of end-tidal carbon dioxide and $PtcCO_2$ during diagnostic PSG and $PtcCO_2$ during titration. Typically, it is not possible to achieve a decrease in $PtcCO_2$ of more than 10 mm Hg during sleep in the first night of titration.

NREM than in REM sleep. Automatic triggering and ineffective inspiratory efforts were more often associated with arousals than failure to transition to EPAP. Only 13% of arousals and awakenings were caused by PVA, but the investigators still concluded that PVA events of all types are often associated with arousals.

In-laboratory PSG monitoring facilitates the determination of the best ventilator settings, but subsequent home sleep studies may also help optimize NPPV treatment. Atkeson and colleagues[84] (2011) found patients with ALS empirically prescribed BPAP-S/T without in-laboratory

---

**Box 4**
**Protocol for introducing and titrating BPAP-S/T without PSG**

- Perform careful mask fitting and discussion of the indications, treatment goals, and side effects of BPAP-S/T with patients and care-givers, preferably before the night of the study.

- If patients have a component of OSA by history or physical examination, oximetry shows sawtooth pattern, or patients have difficulty tolerating NPPV, proceed to PSG titration.

- Begin BPAP-S/T with IPAP at 8 cm H2O; EPAP at 4 cm H2O; and pressure relief (eg, bilevel with variable pressure relief), if available, at 3 with a backup rate of 2 to 4 breaths per minute less than the spontaneous breathing rate awake.

- Encourage patients to use NPPV in office/clinic with close supervision for 30 to 60 minutes.

- Encourage patients to wear the mask and use the device awake until it feels comfortable enough to use it when sleeping.

- Gradually increase IPAP over days to weeks to
  ○ Normalize daytime $Paco_2$ measurements
  ○ Provide subjective relief of symptoms

- Follow-up at 1 week, 1 month, and 3 months for further adjustments.

- If sleep/wake complaints or abnormal daytime arterial blood gases remain, proceed to PSG titration.

---

PSG titration were likely to have PVA: mean asynchrony index 69 ± 46 per hour, mean asynchrony time as a percentage of the nocturnal recording time 17% ± 19%, mean nadir $SpO_2$ 85% ± 7%. The investigators argued that empiric prescriptions of BPAP-S/T are likely to be associated with ineffective nighttime gas exchange and in-laboratory PSG should be done to verify ventilator settings during sleep.

## ASSISTED NOCTURNAL VENTILATION SIGNIFICANTLY PROLONGS SURVIVAL IN NMD

Accumulating studies demonstrate that assisted nocturnal ventilation contributes to longer survival in patients with NMD once they develop hypoventilation.[1,3,40,85-87] The mean age of survival in males with DMD who used NPPV increased from 19 to 25 years in one study[88] and, in a more recent study, 39.6 years[40]; in patients with type 1 spinal

muscular atrophy, the age of survival increased from 10 ± 4 months to 65 ± 46 months.[89] A prospective randomized control trial in 48 patients with DMD with FVC less than 50% predicted and nocturnal hypercapnia ($PtcCO_2$ >45 mm Hg) randomized 26 patients to BPAP-S/T compared with 22 control patients who received no nocturnal ventilatory support.[8] The percentage of the night during which $PtcCO_2$ was more than 45 mm Hg decreased an average of 58% and the mean $SpO_2$ increased 3% in the BPAP group but not in the controls. Ninety percent of the (initially untreated) controls developed diurnal hypercapnia or respiratory complications and subsequently met criteria for starting NPPV after a mean of 8 ± 7 months. The investigators concluded that patients with DMD and nocturnal hypoventilation are likely to develop daytime hypercapnia and/or progressive symptoms within 2 years and may, therefore, benefit from NPPV before daytime hypercapnia develops. In a randomized control trial of BPAP in 92 patients with ALS, patients were randomly assigned to NPPV when they developed orthopnea along with MIP less than 60% of predicted or symptomatic hypercapnia.[79] BPAP-S/T improved survival and quality of life in those patients with ALS without severe bulbar dysfunction who used it for a mean of 9.3 h/d. BPAP-S/T improved sleep-related symptoms in those with severe bulbar dysfunction (who could only tolerate it a mean of 3.8 h/d) but provided no survival advantage. Studies in patients with DMD and ALS show no benefit of prophylactic use of BPAP-S/T as a strategy aiming to prevent respiratory decline or at improving long-term survival.

## IDENTIFY AND TREAT OTHER DISRUPTORS OF SLEEP IN PATIENTS WITH NMD

It is important to consider (and treat if possible) other disruptors of sleep in patients with NMD: (1) weakness, rigidity, reduced movement, or spasticity may result in decreased position shifts in sleep and lead to discomfort, pain, and disrupted sleep caused by pressure points; (2) nocturia, incomplete emptying or incontinence, constipation, painful defecation; and (3) abnormal body postures, splints, and sleeping frames may limit natural sleep postures.

Treatment strategies that may improve sleep quality for these individuals include the following: (1) using satin or nylon sheets or pajamas, which may make it easier to roll (or be turned) in bed; (2) facilitate the turning of oneself by tying a heavy belt or strap to bedposts or bed frame that can be grasped when necessary; (3) padding the bed with sheepskin or egg crate foam; (4) using a cervical collar or U-shaped travel neck pillow to support the neck when lying flat or reclining in bed or a lounge chair; (5) using long body pillows to prop the back for side sleeping or to prevent rolling backward; (6) propping pillows between the knees to decrease pressure discomfort and hip contractures; (7) tenting sheets and covers over a straight-back chair at the end of the bed to free the feet and legs; and (8) using bed garters to secure the edges of the blanket to the mattress.[90] A properly fitting wheelchair that encourages good posture (no slumping) is important because poor sitting postures favor progression of scoliosis and consequent pulmonary restrictive disease.

## STRUCTURED PROACTIVE FOLLOW-UP WITH SERIAL ADJUSTMENT OF ASSISTED VENTILATION: MANDATORY WHEN MANAGING SDB IN NMD

A structured proactive approach to respiratory management is crucial for prolonging life in patients with NMD. Serial monitoring of lung function is mandated for all patients with NMD once they are old enough to perform them (usually by 5–6 years of age).[30,31] Patients with progressive NMD should return for follow-up at least every 6 to 12 months to reevaluate their sleep/wake complaints, neurologic examination, waking arterial blood gases, and PFTs. As part of these visits, the authors review the compliance data from their NPPV device; confirm that the device is set at (and producing) the prescribed pressures, mode, and rate; assess for the presence of interface leak and comfort; and change or adjust the NPPV interface as necessary. If sleep/wake complaints develop or recur or there is worsening of their PFTs or arterial blood gases, the authors repeat the in-laboratory PSG titration.

The NICE published guidelines for respiratory management and NPPV in patients with ALS.[91] This document recommends the following: (1) respiratory assessment at or near the time of the initial diagnosis and repeated every 3 months; (2) at each visit, patients should be asked about sleep/wake complaints and examined for physical signs of ventilatory compromise; and (3) at each visit, measure $SpO_2$, FVC, and perform either sniff testing or MIP. **Fig. 1** summarizes assessment methods for noninvasive ventilation in ALS recommended by the NICE guidelines. Unfortunately, FVC, sniff testing, and MIP depend on a patient's voluntary effort and may be unreliable in patients who cannot perform the maneuver effectively. A facial mask can be used in patients who have facial weakness that prevents them from forming a tight lip seal around the mouthpiece. The

American Thoracic Society published a consensus statement in 2004 regarding respiratory care of patients with DMD; these are summarized in **Box 5**.[30]

Bach and colleagues (2011)[1] recently reported that aggressive use of mechanically assisted cough allowed many previously tracheostomized, mechanically ventilated patients with advanced DMD to be decannulated and converted to BPAP-S/T. Their management strategy for 101 patients with advanced DMD included the following: (1) nocturnal NPPV was initiated for symptomatic hypoventilation; (2) a pulse oximeter and mechanically assisted cough device were prescribed for home use when patients' maximum assisted cough peak flow decreased to less than 300 L/min; (3) patients were instructed to use NIV as often as

---

**Box 5**
**American Thoracic Society's recommendations for long-term management of respiration and ventilation in patients with DMD**

- Visit a physician specializing in pediatric sleep medicine every 6 months once wheelchair bound, FVC is less than 80% of predicted, or the child has reached 12 years of age.

- The quality of sleep and symptoms of SDB should be discussed at every patient encounter.

- The assessment of gas exchange during sleep is mandated for signs/symptoms of hypoventilation, a baseline FVC less than 40% of predicted and/or awake baseline blood or partial pressure of end-tidal carbon dioxide more than 45 mm Hg, an awake baseline $SpO_2$ less than 95% (at sea level), and/or an FVC less than 1.25 L in any teenager or older patient.

- Overnight PSG with $CO_2$ monitoring should be done at least annually once patients with DMD are wheelchair-bound.

- Perform a sitting FVC at least annually beginning at 6 years of age.

- Once ambulation is lost, perform a sitting FVC, MIP, maximum expiratory pressure, peak cough flow, $SpO_2$ and end-tidal (or arterial) $Pco_2$ while awake at least annually and every 6 months in patients who are nonambulatory and have any of the following: suspected hypoventilation, FVC less than 50% of predicted, and/or current use of assisted ventilation.

*Data from* Finder JD, Birnkrant D, Carl J, et al. Respiratory care of the patient with Duchenne muscular dystrophy: ATS consensus statement. Am J Respir Crit Care Med 2004;170(4):456–65.

necessary, or even continuously, and mechanically assisted cough until their $SpO_2$ returned to more than 95% during intercurrent respiratory infections or as otherwise needed; and (4) to use NIV when awake (continuously if needed) as their DMD advanced. Using these strategies, their patients initially required BPAP-S/T during sleep but later progressively extended their use of it during the day and eventually exhibited continuous use, day and night, for an average of $7 \pm 6$ years to a mean age of $30 \pm 6.1$ years. Fifty-six patients were still alive, using continuous NPPV, at the time of the report. They were also able to transition 39 previously tracheostomized, mechanically ventilated patients to BPAP-S/T coupled with aggressive use of devices that mechanically assisted cough. Sixty-seven patients died, with the cause of death thought to be cardiac in 52%, respiratory in 21%, and undetermined in 27%.

Retrospective studies have reported that adjustments of BPAP-S/T settings are commonly required when following patients with progressive NMD,[13,14] most often involving the need for increased pressure support. A retrospective review of 61 sleep studies recorded over a 12-month period in 45 children with NMD (median age, 8.3 years; 27 boys) found changes in sleep-related respiratory support were needed in 66% of the studies,[14] but none of the clinical parameters monitored predicted which of the children would require these adjustments.

Scoliosis commonly develops in patients with NMD, especially when they become wheelchair dependent. Lung capacity decreases with increasing kyphoscoliosis. When a patient's curve exceeds 35°, vital capacity is usually less than 40% predicted.[92] A large retrospective review found that prolonged ambulation reduced the risk of scoliosis development in 123 boys with DMD followed over a 10-year period.[93] Percent predicted FVC at 11 to 12 years of age was directly related to scoliosis severity. IVC decreased a mean of 4% of predicted for each 10° increase in the thoracic spine curvature. Ages at loss of ambulation and standing were inversely related to scoliosis severity at 17 years of age. Prednisone therapy seemed to be associated with a later onset of scoliosis but did not alter the severity of the scoliosis at 17 years. Prolonged mechanical ventilation (>72 hours) was needed in 15% of 46 consecutive patients with NMD following scoliosis surgery. Surgery to correct the scoliosis is often recommended when the curvature is progressing rapidly, when it has reached 35° to 50°, and before FVC has decreased to less than 30% of predicted.[94–96]

Another retrospective study reported the rate of respiratory decline was significantly slowed from a mean of 8% per year before surgery to 4% per year after posterior spinal fusion among 56 patients with DMD.[97] However, evidence for the benefits of scoliosis surgery in DMD are based largely on retrospective case series; there are no randomized controlled trials for its efficacy and benefits.[98] A recent study found no differences in survival, respiratory impairment, or sitting comfort among 123 patients with DMD and scoliosis, with or without scoliosis surgery, when assessed at 17 years of age.[96]

Mechanically assisted cough using devices, such as insufflator-exsufflators, are crucial for prolonging survival in patients with NMD with weak cough.[60,99,100] These devices are particularly useful in preventing hospitalization or tracheostomy in patients with peak cough expiratory flows of less than 160 L/min, especially when scoliosis prevents optimal use of manual strategies to assist in the clearance of respiratory secretions. Treatment of nocturnal hypoventilation with noninvasive ventilator support, along with augmenting cough and clearance of secretions, can significantly improve the quality of life and reduce morbidity and mortality.

## MALNUTRITION PREDICTS POORER SURVIVAL IN PATIENTS WITH DMD AND ALS

Malnutrition in NMD is to be avoided. The authors emphasize to patients with NMD (and their families) that food is medicine.[101,102] Malnutrition in NMD worsens lung function, impairs pulmonary immune function, and predisposes to lung infections.[102,103] Weight loss of more than 5% of body weight within 1 year after scoliosis surgery in 9 boys with DMD was associated with loss of self-feeding.[104] However, mild obesity may be protective in DMD. A cross-sectional study of patients with DMD showed that 54% of 13-year-old patients are obese and that 54% of 18-year-old patients are underweight; boys with DMD who have a body weight/age ratio of more than 151% at 13 years of age were more likely to become obese in late adolescence, but obesity prevented later underweight. The investigators recommended that milder degrees of obesity (weight/age ratios between 120%–150%) in DMD at 13 years of age may prevent more detrimental underweight when older. Reduction in body mass index predicts prognosis for survival in Japanese adults with ALS.[105] Malnutrition during the course of ALS was related to a shorter survival, and fat mass level was associated with a better outcome (relative risk was 0.9 for each 2.5 kg fat mass increment).[106]

## FUTURE DIRECTIONS FOR RESEARCH

New diagnostic methods and therapeutic strategies are being developed for patients with NMD. Piluso and colleagues[107] (2011) developed an NMD-Motor Chip that allows for faster analysis of DNA samples to facilitate molecular diagnosis of 245 genes involved in NMDs. Twenty percent of deaths in DMD are caused by cardiomyopathies. Lethal cardiac arrhythmias are common in DM1. Strain imaging, cardiac magnetic resonance imaging and proactive cardiotherapies are increasingly used to diagnose and manage cardiac pathologies in patients with DMD.[108–112] Transcutaneous neuromuscular electrostimulation of the biceps and quadriceps muscles twice daily was recently used to maintain muscle strength in 16 patients with sepsis who were mechanically ventilated for a mean of 13 days (range, 7–30 days).[113] Whether a similar strategy might be of benefit in patients with NMD may be worthy of investigation.

## REFERENCES

1. Bach JR, Martinez D. Duchenne muscular dystrophy: continuous noninvasive ventilatory support prolongs survival. Respir Care 2011;56(6):744–50.

2. Ishikawa Y, Bach JR. Physical medicine respiratory muscle aids to avert respiratory complications of pediatric chest wall and vertebral deformity and muscle dysfunction. Eur J Phys Rehabil Med 2010;46(4):581–97.

3. Eagle M, Bourke J, Bullock R, et al. Managing Duchenne muscular dystrophy–the additive effect of spinal surgery and home nocturnal ventilation in improving survival. Neuromuscul Disord 2007; 17(6):470–5.

4. Gordon PH, Salachas F, Lacomblez L, et al. Predicting survival of patients with amyotrophic lateral sclerosis at presentation: a 15-year experience. Neurodegener Dis 2012. [Epub ahead of print].

5. Hess DR. The growing role of noninvasive ventilation in patients requiring prolonged mechanical ventilation. Respir Care 2012;57(6):900–18 [discussion: 918–20].

6. Nabatame S, Taniike M, Sakai N, et al. Sleep disordered breathing in childhood-onset acid maltase deficiency. Brain Dev 2009;31(3):234–9.

7. Young HK, Lowe A, Fitzgerald DA, et al. Outcome of noninvasive ventilation in children with neuromuscular disease. Neurology 2007;68(3):198–201.

8. Ward S, Chatwin M, Heather S, et al. Randomised controlled trial of non-invasive ventilation (NIV) for nocturnal hypoventilation in neuromuscular and chest wall disease patients with daytime normocapnia. Thorax 2005;60(12):1019–24.

9. Suresh S, Wales P, Dakin C, et al. Sleep-related breathing disorder in Duchenne muscular dystrophy: disease spectrum in the paediatric population. J Paediatr Child Health 2005;41(9–10):500–3.

10. Edwards EA, Hsiao K, Nixon GM. Paediatric home ventilatory support: the Auckland experience. J Paediatr Child Health 2005;41(12):652–8.

11. Mellies U, Dohna-Schwake C, Stehling F, et al. Sleep disordered breathing in spinal muscular atrophy. Neuromuscul Disord 2004;14(12):797–803.

12. Mellies U, Ragette R, Dohna Schwake C, et al. Long-term noninvasive ventilation in children and adolescents with neuromuscular disorders. Eur Respir J 2003;22(4):631–6.

13. Guilleminault C, Philip P, Robinson A. Sleep and neuromuscular disease: bilevel positive airway pressure by nasal mask as a treatment for sleep disordered breathing in patients with neuromuscular disease. J Neurol Neurosurg Psychiatry 1998;65(2):225–32.

14. Tan E, Nixon GM, Edwards EA. Sleep studies frequently lead to changes in respiratory support in children. J Paediatr Child Health 2007;43(7-8):560–3.

15. Tagalakis AD, Dickson JG, Owen JS, et al. Correction of the neuropathogenic human apolipoprotein E4 (APOE4) gene to APOE3 in vitro using synthetic RNA/DNA oligonucleotides (chimeraplasts). J Mol Neurosci 2005;25(1):95–103.

16. Andersen PM, Abrahams S, Borasio GD, et al. EFNS guidelines on the clinical management of amyotrophic lateral sclerosis (MALS)–revised report of an EFNS task force. Eur J Neurol 2012; 19(3):360–75.

17. Iber C, Ancoli-Israel S, Chesson A, et al. The AASM manual for the scoring of sleep and associated events: rules, terminology and technical specifications. 1st edition. Westchester (IL): American Academy of Sleep Medicine; 2007.

18. Birnkrant DJ, Bushby KM, Amin RS, et al. The respiratory management of patients with Duchenne muscular dystrophy: a DMD care considerations working group specialty article. Pediatr Pulmonol 2010;45(8):739–48.

19. Kiyan E, Okumus G, Cuhadaroglu C, et al. Sleep apnea in adult myotonic dystrophy patients who have no excessive daytime sleepiness. Sleep Breath 2010;14(1):19–24.

20. Kawai H, Adachi K, Nishida Y, et al. Decrease in urinary excretion of 3-methylhistidine by patients with Duchenne muscular dystrophy during glucocorticoid treatment. J Neurol 1993;240(3):181–6.

21. Darras BT, Friedman NR. Metabolic myopathies: a clinical approach; part II. Pediatr Neurol 2000; 22(3):171–81.

22. Darras BT, Friedman NR. Metabolic myopathies: a clinical approach; part I. Pediatr Neurol 2000; 22(2):87–97.

23. Manni R, Piccolo G, Banfi P, et al. Respiratory patterns during sleep in mitochondrial myopathies with ophthalmoplegia. Eur Neurol 1991;31(1):12–7.

24. Tatsumi C, Takahashi M, Yorifuji S, et al. Mitochondrial encephalomyopathy with sleep apnea. Eur Neurol 1988;28(2):64–9.

25. Rimmer KP, Golar SD, Lee MA, et al. Myotonia of the respiratory muscles in myotonic dystrophy. Am Rev Respir Dis 1993;148(4 Pt 1):1018–22.

26. Yu H, Laberge L, Jaussent I, et al. Daytime sleepiness and REM sleep characteristics in myotonic dystrophy: a case-control study. Sleep 2011; 34(2):165–70.

27. Steier J, Jolley CJ, Seymour J, et al. Screening for sleep-disordered breathing in neuromuscular disease using a questionnaire for symptoms associated with diaphragm paralysis. Eur Respir J 2011;37(2):400–5.

28. Bertorini TE, Palmieri GM, Griffin JW, et al. Effect of chronic treatment with the calcium antagonist diltiazem in Duchenne muscular dystrophy. Neurology 1988;38(4):609–13.

29. Madsen KS, Miller JP, Province MA. The use of an extended baseline period in the evaluation of treatment in a longitudinal Duchenne muscular dystrophy trial. Stat Med 1986;5(3):231–41.

30. Finder JD, Birnkrant D, Carl J, et al. Respiratory care of the patient with Duchenne muscular dystrophy: ATS consensus statement. Am J Respir Crit Care Med 2004;170(4):456–65.

31. Myers SM, Challman TD, Bock GH. End-stage renal failure in Smith-Magenis syndrome. Am J Med Genet A 2007;143(16):1922–4.

32. Mellies U, Ragette R, Schwake C, et al. Daytime predictors of sleep disordered breathing in children and adolescents with neuromuscular disorders. Neuromuscul Disord 2003;13(2):123–8.

33. Dohna-Schwake C, Ragette R, Mellies U, et al. Respiratory function in congenital muscular dystrophy and limb girdle muscular dystrophy 2I. Neurology 2004; 62(3):513–4.

34. Katz SL, Gaboury I, Keilty K, et al. Nocturnal hypoventilation: predictors and outcomes in childhood progressive neuromuscular disease. Arch Dis Child 2010;95(12):998–1003.

35. Darras BT, Miller DT, Urion DK. Dystrophinopathies includes: Becker Muscular Dystrophy (BMD), DMD-Associated Dilated Cardiomyopathy, Duchenne Muscular Dystrophy (DMD). Gene Reviews (online). Available at: http://www.ncbi.nlm.nih.gov/books/NBK1119/. Accessed October 18, 2012.

36. Bushby K, Finkel R, Birnkrant DJ, et al. Diagnosis and management of Duchenne muscular dystrophy, part 2: implementation of multidisciplinary care. Lancet Neurol 2010;9(2):177–89.

37. Bushby K, Finkel R, Birnkrant DJ, et al. Diagnosis and management of Duchenne muscular dystrophy, part 1: diagnosis, and pharmacological and psychosocial management. Lancet Neurol 2010;9(1):77–93.

38. Hoffman EP, Brown RH Jr, Kunkel LM. Dystrophin: the protein product of the Duchenne muscular dystrophy locus. Cell 1987;51(6):919–28.

39. Tangorra A, Curatola G, Milani Comparetti M, et al. Susceptibility of erythrocyte membranes to treatment with L-alpha-lysophosphatidylcholine in Duchenne muscular dystrophy. Boll Soc Ital Biol Sper 1988; 64(5):477–84.

40. Ishikawa Y, Miura T, Aoyagi T, et al. Duchenne muscular dystrophy: survival by cardio-respiratory interventions. Neuromuscul Disord 2011;21(1):47–51.

41. Griggs RC, Moxley RT 3rd, Mendell JR, et al. Prednisone in Duchenne dystrophy. A randomized, controlled trial defining the time course and dose response. Clinical investigation of Duchenne dystrophy group. Arch Neurol 1991;48(4):383–8.

42. Beenakker EA, Fock JM, Van Tol MJ, et al. Intermittent prednisone therapy in Duchenne muscular dystrophy: a randomized controlled trial. Arch Neurol 2005;62(1):128–32.

43. McAdam LC, Mayo AL, Alman BA, et al. The Canadian experience with long-term deflazacort treatment in Duchenne muscular dystrophy. Acta Myol 2012;31(1):16–20.

44. King WM, Ruttencutter R, Nagaraja HN, et al. Orthopedic outcomes of long-term daily corticosteroid treatment in Duchenne muscular dystrophy. Neurology 2007;68(19):1607–13.

45. Biggar WD, Harris VA, Eliasoph L, et al. Long-term benefits of deflazacort treatment for boys with Duchenne muscular dystrophy in their second decade. Neuromuscul Disord 2006;16(4):249–55.

46. Houde S, Filiatrault M, Fournier A, et al. Deflazacort use in Duchenne muscular dystrophy: an 8-year follow-up. Pediatr Neurol 2008;38(3):200–6.

47. Moxley RT 3rd, Pandya S, Ciafaloni E, et al. Change in natural history of Duchenne muscular dystrophy with long-term corticosteroid treatment: implications for management. J Child Neurol 2010;25(9):1116–29.

48. Moxley RT 3rd, Ashwal S, Pandya S, et al. Practice parameter: corticosteroid treatment of Duchenne dystrophy: report of the Quality Standards Subcommittee of the American Academy of Neurology and the Practice Committee of the Child Neurology Society. Neurology 2005;64(1):13–20.

49. Andrews J. Amyotrophic lateral sclerosis: clinical management and research update. Curr Neurol Neurosci Rep 2009;9(1):59–68.

50. Jackson CE, Bryan WW. Amyotrophic lateral sclerosis. Semin Neurol 1998;18(1):27–39.

51. Chio A, Calvo A, Moglia C, et al. Non-invasive ventilation in amyotrophic lateral sclerosis: a 10 year population based study. J Neurol Neurosurg Psychiatry 2012;83(4):377–81.

52. Gordon PH, Salachas F, Bruneteau G, et al. Improving survival in a large French ALS center cohort. J Neurol 2012;259(9):1788–92.

53. O'Neill CL, Williams TL, Peel ET, et al. Non-invasive ventilation in motor neuron disease: an update of current UK practice. J Neurol Neurosurg Psychiatry 2012;83(4):371–6.

54. Achi EY, Rudnicki SA. ALS and frontotemporal dysfunction: a review. Neurol Res Int 2012;2012:806306.

55. Sriskandan N, Moody A, Howlett DC. Ultrasound-guided submandibular gland injection of botulinum toxin for hypersalivation in cerebral palsy. Br J Oral Maxillofac Surg 2010;48(1):58–60.

56. Strutt AM, Palcic J, Wager JG, et al. Cognition, behavior, and respiratory function in amyotrophic lateral sclerosis. ISRN Neurol 2012;2012:912123.

57. Chio A, Ilardi A, Cammarosano S, et al. Neurobehavioral dysfunction in ALS has a negative effect on outcome and use of PEG and NIV. Neurology 2012;78(14):1085–9.

58. Chio A, Calvo A, Ghiglione P, et al. Tracheostomy in amyotrophic lateral sclerosis: a 10-year population-based study in Italy. J Neurol Neurosurg Psychiatry 2010;81(10):1141–3.

59. Vianello A, Arcaro G, Palmieri A, et al. Survival and quality of life after tracheostomy for acute respiratory failure in patients with amyotrophic lateral sclerosis. J Crit Care 2011;26(3):329.e7–14.

60. Bach JR, Hon A. Amyotrophic lateral sclerosis: noninvasive ventilation, uncuffed tracheostomy tubes, and mechanically assisted coughing. Am J Phys Med Rehabil 2010;89(5):412–4.

61. Sancho J, Servera E, Banuls P, et al. Prolonging survival in amyotrophic lateral sclerosis: efficacy of noninvasive ventilation and uncuffed tracheostomy tubes. Am J Phys Med Rehabil 2010;89(5):407–11.

62. Lemoignan J, Ells C. Amyotrophic lateral sclerosis and assisted ventilation: how patients decide. Palliat Support Care 2010;8(2):207–13.

63. Dreyer PS, Felding M, Klitnaes CS, et al. Withdrawal of invasive home mechanical ventilation in patients with advanced amyotrophic lateral sclerosis: ten years of Danish experience. J Palliat Med 2012;15(2):205–9.

64. Berger JT. Preemptive use of palliative sedation and amyotrophic lateral sclerosis. J Pain Symptom Manage 2012;43(4):802–5.

65. Blackhall LJ. Amyotrophic lateral sclerosis and palliative care: where we are, and the road ahead. Muscle Nerve 2012;45(3):311–8.

66. Romigi A, Izzi F, Pisani V, et al. Sleep disorders in adult-onset myotonic dystrophy type 1: a controlled polysomnographic study. Eur J Neurol 2011;18(9):1139–45.

67. Pincherle A, Patruno V, Raimondi P, et al. Sleep breathing disorders in 40 Italian patients with myotonic dystrophy type 1. Neuromuscul Disord 2012;22(3):219–24.

68. Dauvilliers YA, Laberge L. Myotonic dystrophy type 1, daytime sleepiness and REM sleep dysregulation. Sleep Med Rev 2012;16(6):539–45.

69. Laberge L, Begin P, Montplaisir J, et al. Sleep complaints in patients with myotonic dystrophy. J Sleep Res 2004;13(1):95–100.

70. Gibbs JW 3rd, Ciafaloni E, Radtke RA. Excessive daytime somnolence and increased rapid eye movement pressure in myotonic dystrophy. Sleep 2002;25(6):662–5.

71. Avanzini A, Crossignani RM, Colombini A. Sleep apnea and respiratory dysfunction in congenital myotonic dystrophy. Minerva Pediatr 2001;53(3):221–5.

72. van der Meche FG, Bogaard JM, van der Sluys JC, et al. Daytime sleep in myotonic dystrophy is not caused by sleep apnoea. J Neurol Neurosurg Psychiatry 1994;57(5):626–8.

73. Wintzen AR, Lammers GJ, van Dijk JG. Does modafinil enhance activity of patients with myotonic dystrophy?: a double-blind placebo-controlled crossover study. J Neurol 2007;254(1):26–8.

74. Orlikowski D, Chevret S, Quera-Salva MA, et al. Modafinil for the treatment of hypersomnia associated with myotonic muscular dystrophy in adults: a multicenter, prospective, randomized, double-blind, placebo controlled, 4-week trial. Clin Ther 2009;31(8):1765–73.

75. Hilton-Jones D, Bowler M, Lochmueller H, et al. Modafinil for excessive daytime sleepiness in myotonic dystrophy type 1–the patients' perspective. Neuromuscul Disord 2012;22(7):597–603.

76. Ragette R, Mellies U, Schwake C, et al. Patterns and predictors of sleep disordered breathing in primary myopathies. Thorax 2002;57(8):724–8.

77. Berry RB, Chediak A, Brown LK, et al. Best clinical practices for the sleep center adjustment of noninvasive positive pressure ventilation (NPPV) in stable chronic alveolar hypoventilation syndromes. J Clin Sleep Med 2010;6(5):491–509.

78. Fanfulla F, Taurino AE, Lupo ND, et al. Effect of sleep on patient/ventilator asynchrony in patients undergoing chronic non-invasive mechanical ventilation. Respir Med 2007;101(8):1702–7.

79. Bourke SC, Tomlinson M, Williams TL, et al. Effects of non-invasive ventilation on survival and quality of life in patients with amyotrophic lateral sclerosis: a randomised controlled trial. Lancet Neurol 2006;5(2):140–7.

80. Bach JR, Robert D, Leger P, et al. Sleep fragmentation in kyphoscoliotic individuals with alveolar hypoventilation treated by NIPPV. Chest 1995;107(6):1552–8.

81. Fuschillo S, De Felice A, Gaudiosi C, et al. Nocturnal mechanical ventilation improves exercise capacity in kyphoscoliotic patients with respiratory impairment. Monaldi Arch Chest Dis 2003; 59(4):281–6.

82. Bach JR. Ventilator use by muscular dystrophy association patients. Arch Phys Med Rehabil 1992;73(2):179–83.

83. Crescimanno G, Canino M, Marrone O. Asynchronies and sleep disruption in neuromuscular patients under home noninvasive ventilation. Respir Med 2012;106(10):1478–85.

84. Atkeson AD, RoyChoudhury A, Harrington-Moroney G, et al. Patient-ventilator asynchrony with nocturnal noninvasive ventilation in ALS. Neurology 2011;77(6):549–55.

85. Kohler M, Clarenbach CF, Bahler C, et al. Disability and survival in Duchenne muscular dystrophy. J Neurol Neurosurg Psychiatry 2009;80(3): 320–5.

86. Jeppesen J, Green A, Steffensen BF, et al. The Duchenne muscular dystrophy population in Denmark, 1977-2001: prevalence, incidence and survival in relation to the introduction of ventilator use. Neuromuscul Disord 2003;13(10):804–12.

87. Eagle M, Baudouin SV, Chandler C, et al. Survival in Duchenne muscular dystrophy: improvements in life expectancy since 1967 and the impact of home nocturnal ventilation. Neuromuscul Disord 2002;12(10):926–9.

88. Dick DJ, Gardner-Medwin D, Gates PG, et al. A trial of flunarizine in the treatment of Duchenne muscular dystrophy. Muscle Nerve 1986;9(4):349–54.

89. van Hilten JJ, Kerkhof GA, van Dijk JG, et al. Disruption of sleep-wake rhythmicity and daytime sleepiness in myotonic dystrophy. J Neurol Sci 1993;114(1):68–75.

90. Siegel IM. Casey, patricia. A do-it-yourself-user's guide: 101 Hints to help-with-ease patients with neuromuscular diseases. 2nd edition. Tucson (AZ): Muscular Dystrophy Association; 2005.

91. (NICE) TNIfHaCE. Motor neurone disease: the use of non-invasive ventilation in the management of motor neurone disease Issued: NICE clinical guideline 105. NHS July 2010. Available at: http://guidance. nice.org.uk/CG105/NICEGuidance/pdf/English. Accessed September 6, 2012.

92. Smith AD, Koreska J, Moseley CF. Progression of scoliosis in Duchenne muscular dystrophy. J Bone Joint Surg Am 1989;71(7):1066–74.

93. Kinali M, Main M, Eliahoo J, et al. Predictive factors for the development of scoliosis in Duchenne muscular dystrophy. Eur J Paediatr Neurol 2007; 11(3):160–6.

94. Manzur AY, Kinali M, Muntoni F. Update on the management of Duchenne muscular dystrophy. Arch Dis Child 2008;93(11):986–90.

95. Ciafaloni E, Moxley RT. Treatment options for Duchenne muscular dystrophy. Curr Treat Options Neurol 2008;10(2):86–93.

96. Kinali M, Messina S, Mercuri E, et al. Management of scoliosis in Duchenne muscular dystrophy: a large 10-year retrospective study. Dev Med Child Neurol 2006;48(6):513–8.

97. Velasco MV, Colin AA, Zurakowski D, et al. Posterior spinal fusion for scoliosis in Duchenne muscular dystrophy diminishes the rate of respiratory decline. Spine (Phila Pa 1976) 2007;32(4):459–65.

98. Cheuk DK, Wong V, Wraige E, et al. Surgery for scoliosis in Duchenne muscular dystrophy. Cochrane Database Syst Rev 2007;(1):CD005375.

99. Miske LJ, Hickey EM, Kolb SM, et al. Use of the mechanical in-exsufflator in pediatric patients with neuromuscular disease and impaired cough. Chest 2004;125(4):1406–12.

100. Gomez-Merino E, Bach JR. Duchenne muscular dystrophy: prolongation of life by noninvasive ventilation and mechanically assisted coughing. Am J Phys Med Rehabil 2002;81(6):411–5.

101. Davoodi J, Markert CD, Voelker KA, et al. Nutrition strategies to improve physical capabilities in Duchenne muscular dystrophy. Phys Med Rehabil Clin N Am 2012;23(1):187–99 xii-xiii.

102. Davidson ZE, Truby H. A review of nutrition in Duchenne muscular dystrophy. J Hum Nutr Diet 2009;22(5):383–93.

103. Martin TR. The relationship between malnutrition and lung infections. Clin Chest Med 1987;8(3): 359–72.

104. Iannaccone ST, Owens H, Scott J, et al. Postoperative malnutrition in Duchenne muscular dystrophy. J Child Neurol 2003;18(1):17–20.

105. Shimizu T, Nagaoka U, Nakayama Y, et al. Reduction rate of body mass index predicts prognosis for survival in amyotrophic lateral sclerosis: a multicenter study in Japan. Amyotroph Lateral Scler 2012;13(4):363–6.

106. Marin B, Desport JC, Kajeu P, et al. Alteration of nutritional status at diagnosis is a prognostic factor for survival of amyotrophic lateral sclerosis patients. J Neurol Neurosurg Psychiatry 2011; 82(6):628–34.

107. Piluso G, Dionisi M, Del Vecchio Blanco F, et al. Motor chip: a comparative genomic hybridization microarray for copy-number mutations in 245 neuromuscular disorders. Clin Chem 2011 Nov; 57(11):1584–96.

108. Kaspar RW, Allen HD, Montanaro F. Current understanding and management of dilated cardiomyopathy in Duchenne and Becker muscular dystrophy. J Am Acad Nurse Pract 2009;21(5):241–9.

109. Hagenbuch SC, Gottliebson WM, Wansapura J, et al. Detection of progressive cardiac dysfunction

by serial evaluation of circumferential strain in patients with Duchenne muscular dystrophy. Am J Cardiol 2010;105(10):1451–5.

110. Mazur W, Hor KN, Germann JT, et al. Patterns of left ventricular remodeling in patients with Duchenne Muscular Dystrophy: a cardiacMRI study of ventricular geometry, global function, and strain. Int J Cardiovasc Imaging 2012;28(1):99–107.

111. Otto RK, Ferguson MR, Friedman SD, et al. Cardiac MRI in muscular dystrophy: an overview and future directions. Phys Med Rehabil Clin N Am 2012; 23(1):123–32, xi–xii.

112. Spurney CF. Cardiomyopathy of Duchenne muscular dystrophy: current understanding and future directions. Muscle Nerve 2011;44(1):8–19.

113. Rodriguez PO, Setten M, Maskin LP, et al. Muscle weakness in septic patients requiring mechanical ventilation: protective effect of transcutaneous neuromuscular electrical stimulation. J Crit Care 2012;27(3):319.e1–e8.

# Congenital Disorders Affecting Sleep

Stamatia Alexiou, MD*, Lee J. Brooks, MD

## KEYWORDS

- Obstructive sleep apnea • Micrognathia • Craniosynostosis • Pierre Robin sequence
- Achondroplasia • Trisomy 21 • CHARGE syndrome • Mucopolysaccharidoses

## KEY POINTS

- Many congenital disorders result in an increased risk for sleep-disordered breathing.
- Genetic syndromes affecting sleep can be classified into 1 of 4 categories: those producing micrognathia, those producing midface hypoplasia, disorders of neuromuscular control, and miscellaneous disorders.
- It is important to have a high index of suspicion for sleep-disordered breathing in these patients; overnight polysomnography is important to diagnose and confirm the severity of the abnormality and track the response to treatment.
- Treatment should be directed at correcting or improving the underlying abnormality.

## MICROGNATHIA

Congenital disorders resulting in micrognathia predispose the patient to sleep-disordered breathing, owing to their increased risk of upper airway obstruction (Table 1).

### Treacher-Collins Syndrome

Treacher-Collins syndrome (TCS) is an autosomal dominant disorder caused by a mutation in the *TCOF1* gene in the region of 5q32-33.2 that codes for a nucleolar phosphoprotein (treacle).[1,2] Mutations in *POLR1D* and *POLR1C* may also contribute to the etiology of this syndrome.[3] Sixty percent of the cases represent new mutations. There is wide variability in expression, but the characteristic findings include mandibular hypoplasia (78% of cases), often with malar hypoplasia (81%), antimongoloid slanting palpebral fissures (89%), malformed auricles (77%), and coloboma of the eyelid. Conductive deafness is present in 40% of patients. Mental deficiency is reported in only 5% of cases.[4]

The small jaw and malar hypoplasia place these patients at risk for obstructive sleep apnea (OSA). The prevalence of OSA in patients with TCS ranges from 46% to 95%. In a cohort study of 35 patients with TCS, 46% (54% of children; 41% of adults) had OSA as determined by ambulatory polysomnography.[5] In a Norwegian study of 19 patients with TCS, OSA was found in 95% of patients who underwent laboratory polysomnography.[6] Symptom scores are not helpful in determining the presence of OSA in patients with TCS.[7] Both the Brouillette score for children and the Epworth Sleepiness Scale (ESS) for adults had low sensitivity, and poor positive and negative predictive values; the investigators suggested that all patients with the syndrome should undergo evaluation by polysomnography.

Mandibular distraction may be very effective in treating OSA in some patients and may prevent the need for tracheostomy.[8,9] Nasal continuous positive airway pressure (CPAP) can also been used as a bridge[10] pending an increase in the posterior airway space with mandibular growth.

Division of Pediatric Pulmonology and Sleep Medicine, Children's Hospital of Philadelphia, 34th Street and Civic Center Boulevard, Philadelphia, PA 19104, USA
* Corresponding author.
E-mail address: alexious1@email.chop.edu

Sleep Med Clin 7 (2012) 689–702
http://dx.doi.org/10.1016/j.jsmc.2012.10.002
1556-407X/12/$ – see front matter Published by Elsevier Inc.

**Table 1**
Classification of congenital disorders affecting breathing during sleep

| Micrognathia | Midface Hypoplasia | Abnormal Respiratory Control | Multifactorial and Miscellaneous Disorders |
|---|---|---|---|
| Pierre Robin sequence | Achondroplasia | Arnold-Chiari malformation | Mucopolysaccharidoses |
| Treacher-Collins syndrome | Crouzon syndrome | Prader-Willi syndrome | Down syndrome |
| | Apert syndrome | | Sickle cell anemia |
| | Pfeiffer syndrome | | CHARGE syndrome |
| | Smith-Magenis syndrome | | |

## Pierre Robin Sequence

The Robin sequence, consisting of micrognathia and posterior displacement of the tongue and soft palate, may occur singly or in association with other malformations, such as trisomy 18, Stickler syndrome, velocardiofacial/DiGeorge syndrome, or cerebro-costo-mandibular syndrome.[11] The initiating defect is the presence of micrognathia or retrognathia at the same time that the palatal shelves are fusing, which occurs between 9 and 11 weeks of gestation. This defect prevents the tongue from settling into the oral cavity and away from the base of the skull. As a result, it remains retrodisplaced between the palatal shelves, impairing fusion and resulting in a U-shaped cleft palate. Eighty-three percent of patients have complete or incomplete cleft palate. This posterior displacement of the tongue is not only a risk factor for airway obstruction, but may also impair the action of the genioglossus, an important dilating muscle of the upper airway.[12] Three-fourths of the patients are symptomatic at birth[13]; up to 83% develop significant airway obstruction within 6 weeks, contributing to morbidity as high as 30%.[4]

Significant hypoxemia may be present without clinically apparent symptoms,[6] but oximetry alone does not provide adequate assessment because obstructive episodes without desaturation will not be detected.[14] Therefore, full polysomnography is recommended.[4,14,15] In a retrospective study of 33 infants who were identified as having Robin sequence,[16] 13 underwent polysomnography within the first year of life, 11 of whom (85%) had OSA with a mean Respiratory Disturbance Index (RDI; calculated as the average number of episodes of apnea, hypopnea, and event-related arousals per hour of sleep) of 40.4. Half of the children with an RDI greater than 10 did not snore, suggesting that snoring should not be used as an indicator for the presence or severity of OSA. Fifteen percent of the patients in one series had gastroesophageal reflux contributing to the frequency and severity of respiratory events[14]; esophageal pH monitoring during polysomnography should be considered in any patient with symptoms suggestive of gastroesophageal reflux or who fails to thrive despite apparently appropriate treatment of their airway obstruction. Untreated OSA can exacerbate feeding difficulties, so early identification and airway intervention may also help lower the incidence of failure to thrive in these infants.

Treatment of OSA in patients with Robin sequence depends on the severity of the obstruction and the presence of associated abnormalities. In a study of 74 infants with Robin sequence,[17] 36 were managed with prone positioning alone and 13 with nasopharyngeal intubation. There have been several studies suggesting that CPAP can successfully be used in patients with Robin sequence[18–20] resulting in a significantly decreased work of breathing as measured by breathing patterns, respiratory efforts, and transcutaneous carbon dioxide pressures (**Fig. 1**).

In severe cases or when conservative management fails, surgical intervention may be required to maintain a patent airway. Several cephalometric-based studies have suggested that the hypoplastic mandible fails to "catch up" and overcome the intrinsic disruption.[21–23] Because of its complications and long-term commitment, the goal of management in infants with Pierre Robin sequence is often to avoid tracheostomy; however, it remains the gold standard for bypassing upper airway obstruction. In a retrospective study of 61 infants with Robin sequence,[24] 25 required tracheostomy. At a mean 4-year follow-up, 52% had tracheostomy-specific complications including tracheitis, pneumonia, and wound breakdown and infection. Other complications included developmental delay and organ dysfunction. Several studies have suggested mandibular distraction

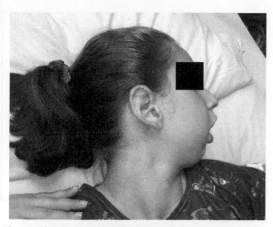

**Fig. 1.** This 8-year-old girl with Pierre Robin sequence and obstructive sleep apnea has been successfully treated with 12/6 cm $H_2O$ bllevel positive airway pressure since age 3 years pending mandibular advancement surgery.

osteogenesis as an alternative. Although this procedure addresses the underlying issue in patients with Pierre Robin, the patients may be required to undergo up to 3 separate surgical procedures.[25] Glossopexy and subperiosteal floor-of-mouth release may also serve as alternative interventions; however, the need for adjunctive procedures and lack of long-term data make them less popular.

Although the obstruction may improve clinically with some of the aforementioned interventions, some degree of micrognathia often persists, which can contribute to OSA later in life. Sixty-five percent of 20 teenagers and young adults with Robin sequence who responded to a questionnaire reported chronic snoring.[26] Eight of the patients agreed to polysomnographic, electrocardiographic, echocardiographic, and cephalometric evaluation. These patients had more respiratory events during sleep and lower oxyhemoglobin saturation than did controls, and all patients had right ventricular end-diastolic dimensions greater than the 50th percentile for weight.[26]

## CRANIOSYNOSTOSIS SYNDROMES

Craniosynostosis, the premature fusion of cranial sutures, results in midface hypoplasia and a shortened anteroposterior diameter of the skull. Upper airway narrowing contributes to OSA.

### Fibroblast Growth Factor Receptor Defects

Mutations in the fibroblast growth factor receptor (FGFR) 2 genes, which map to chromosome 10q25-q26, are responsible for Apert, Crouzon, and Pfeiffer syndromes. These syndromes may be genetically heterogeneous, with some cases of Pfeiffer syndrome due to FGFR1 mapping to chromosome 8p11.22-p12, and some cases of Crouzon syndrome due to mutations in FGFR3 mapping to 4p16.3, the gene for achondroplasia. All are autosomal dominant, but the majority of cases represent fresh mutations.[4] Common features of these syndromes include craniosynostosis, which limits anterior-posterior growth of the cranium, producing maxillary hypoplasia. Cleft palate and mental retardation may also be associated.[27]

The prevalence of OSA in these patients ranges from 24% to 88%.[28,29] Abnormalities of the cartilaginous structures, including the lower respiratory tree, may lead to other abnormalities in managing the airway.[29,30] Eleven of 12 patients reported by Mixter and colleagues[29] had laryngomalacla and/or tracheomalacia. The trachea and mainstem bronchi may also be firm, without rings but rather a full cartilaginous sleeve.[29,30]

In contrast to children with Robin sequence, patients with Apert, Crouzon, and Pfeiffer syndromes may have worsening of their OSA with growth. As the maxillary complex fails to grow, the mandible and other structures grow at a normal rate, resulting in further narrowing of the nasopharyngeal airway.[31] Serial polysomnography is required to define the nature and extent of sleep-disordered breathing, as well as the response to treatment. As with normal children,[32] not all patients with a clinical history suggestive of sleep apnea had confirmation on polysomnography.[29]

Midface advancement by LeFort osteotomy has been described as "very effective in relieving apnea,"[33] but Mixter and colleagues[29] found little polysomnographic improvement following the procedure. An improved technique, halo distraction of the LeFort III osteotomy, is able to provide more significant maxillary advancement than the conventional LeFort osteotomy. It eliminated sleep apnea in most patients, and was not associated with long-term effects on sleep or mastication.[34] Tracheostomy has been suggested in young patients with severe OSA,[33] but the high prevalence of tracheobronchial abnormalities can lead to severe complications[29]; careful observation postoperatively is imperative. The tracheobronchial anatomy should be defined by bronchoscopy before surgery if tracheotomy is contemplated.

Hui and colleagues[35] described 2 brothers with Crouzon syndrome and severe OSA in whom application of nasal CPAP, 8 to 9 cm $H_2O$, resulted in marked improvement in polysomnography as well as catch-up growth. Nasal CPAP is probably the safest treatment for OSA pending surgical repair,[29,35] but particular skill and experience with children are necessary to obtain compliance.[36]

If the patient is obese, a weight-loss program should be instituted in addition to medical and surgical management.

Although patients with Smith-Magenis syndrome (SMS) also manifest midfacial hypoplasia, this entity is cytogenetically distinct from the better known FGFR mutations. It was first described in 1982 and has an estimated prevalence of 1 in 25,000 births.[37] Common features include brachycephaly with characteristic features including: midface hypoplasia; short stature; brachydactyly; infantile hypotonia and failure to thrive; speech delay with or without associated hearing loss; peripheral neuropathy; variable degrees of mental retardation; and behavioral problems including sleep disturbance.[38]

Virtually all patients with this disorder manifest a 2 to 9 megabase deletion of 17p11.2. One of the genes affected by this deletion is RAI1, which has been shown to result in a disrupted circadian rhythm.[39–41] By measuring the urine concentration of a melatonin surrogate, 6-sulfatoxymelatonin (aMT6), Boone and colleagues[40] found that patients with SMS had the lowest concentration of aMT6 in their first morning void, suggesting the lack of physiologic increase in melatonin throughout the night. These patients may benefit from treatment with a $\beta$1-adrenergic antagonist to suppress melatonin secretion in the morning, and supplemental melatonin in the evening to normalize their circadian rhythms.[42]

The midface hypoplasia and hypotonia also put SMS patients at risk for sleep-disordered breathing. More than two-thirds of patients in a questionnaire study of 39 individuals reported snoring and daytime sleepiness.[38] Leoni and colleagues[43] described a 2-year-old boy with SMS who had rapid eye movement (REM) hypoventilation without hypopneas or apneas on polysomnography after presenting with frequent oxyhemoglobin desaturations while sleeping.

## Achondroplasia

Achondroplasia is an autosomal dominant skeletal dysplasia, primarily of endochondral bone. It occurs with a frequency of 1 in 15,000 births. Virtually all cases demonstrate the same single base-pair substitution in the gene encoding FGFR3, located at 4p16.3. About 90% of the cases represent a fresh mutation, often associated with older paternal age.[4] Defective endochondral ossification results in small stature with disproportionate shortening of the proximal limbs, short flared ribs, megalocephaly, and midface hypoplasia (Fig. 2).

These patients are at risk for several types of respiratory complications. Their abnormal rib

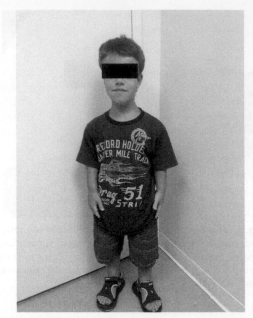

Fig. 2. This 11-year-old boy with achondroplasia presented with a history of snoring and restless sleep at age 6 years. His apnea-hypopnea index (AHI) was 16.2, which normalized to 0.2 with 8 cm $H_2O$ continuous positive airway pressure (CPAP).

cage results in low functional residual capacity that may cause airway closure, atelectasis, hypoxemia, and/or alveolar hypoventilation.[44] The abnormal skull base can result in spinal cord compression and central apnea,[45] which may produce sudden unexpected death,[46] but OSA is the most common respiratory complication. Waters and colleagues[47] described 20 patients with achondroplasia; all had a history of snoring, and 75% had more than 5 apneas per hour of sleep documented on polysomnography. A similar prevalence of OSA was found in other studies.[48,49]

Guidelines from the American Academy of Pediatrics advise that there should be a low threshold for evaluation by polysomnography if OSA is suspected.[50,51] A recent study showed that even in the first few months of life, infants with achondroplasia have increased apneic events and a decreased arousal response, possibly contributing to this population's increased risk for unexplained sudden death.[52] Twenty-eight of the 30 (93%) children studied by Julliand and colleagues[53] had an abnormal polysomnogram; 26 (87%) had an apnea-hypopnea index (number of apneas and hypopneas per hour of sleep) of 5 or more. An adenotonsillectomy was performed or nasal CPAP was used in 20 of the 28 patients with OSA, with a follow-up polysomnogram showing improved respiratory and arousal indices and improved oxygen saturation.

Seventeen of the 88 children studied by Mogayzel and colleagues[54] had at least one obstructive apnea per hour of sleep, but there were more frequent episodes of hypoxemia that might represent hypopnea. Therefore, all patients with achondroplasia warrant a thorough pulmonary evaluation, and overnight polysomnography with measurement of exhaled $CO_2$ to evaluate central and obstructive apnea and hypoventilation.[44] Electrocardiography and echocardiography may be needed to evaluate for pulmonary hypertension.[55] Pulmonary function testing is helpful in patients old enough to cooperate. Although there seems to be no relationship between foramen magnum stenosis and sleep-disordered breathing,[49,53,56] patients with respiratory problems that are not caused by OSA, restrictive pulmonary disease, or other primary pulmonary system disorders should undergo imaging of the brainstem; some of these patients may benefit from cervical cord decompression.[45,57]

CPAP is often the first line of treatment of OSA in patients with achondroplasia.[48,54,58] If CPAP fails to resolve the obstruction, an adenotonsillectomy may be considered; however, one study showed that it was effective in only 3 of 10 patients.[48] This result is not surprising, given the complex anatomic and physiologic factors that interact to produce OSA in these patients.

## ABNORMAL RESPIRATORY CONTROL

Compression of the brainstem can affect the respiratory drive, leading to altered ventilation and increased floppiness of the upper airway from impaired innervation of pharyngeal and laryngeal muscles.

### Arnold-Chiari Malformation

Arnold-Chiari malformation is a congenital malformation of the hindbrain, characterized by a downward elongation of the brainstem and cerebellum into the cervical portion of the spinal cord. It is commonly associated with spina bifida.[59] The exact mechanism of the malformation is unclear; one family has been reported with an autosomal dominant inheritance,[60] but teratogenic mechanisms have also been implicated. Patients with a Chiari II malformation also have myelomeningocele or hydrocephalus; patients with a Chiari I malformation have the brainstem malformation alone. Patients with either malformation may present with signs and symptoms of damage to the cerebellum, medulla, and lower cranial nerves. These symptoms may include oculomotor disturbance, syncope, torticollis, paralysis, or even sudden death.[61] Compression of the brainstem

may cause central apnea by reducing central response to hypercapnia or affecting peripheral response to hypoxia by compromising ninth cranial nerve afferents from the carotid body.[62] OSA may result from abductor vocal cord paralysis[63] or a decrease in pharyngeal muscle dilator response[64] caused by compression of the ninth or tenth cranial nerve.

Three of 11 patients described by Dure and colleagues[61] had apnea, but there was no differentiation between central and obstructive events. A larger, earlier study did not describe any respiratory symptoms in 71 patients with type I Arnold-Chiari malformation, although they noted that 14% of patients had "respiratory depression...-most marked at night" following posterior fossa decompression, and 1 additional patient died 36 hours postoperatively during an episode of sleep apnea.[65] Waters and colleagues[66] found that 17 of 83 patients with Arnold-Chiari malformation had had posterior fossa decompression and 8 had adenoidectomy and/or tonsillectomy before the study.

In one study of 46 patients, sleep apnea was present in 70% of those with Chiari I malformation and in 50% of those with Chiari II.[67] In a recent case report,[68] a 14-year-old boy was referred for polysomnography after a 2-year history of somnambulism and frequent nighttime awakenings. He had had an adenotonsillectomy at age 10 for suspected sleep apnea. The polysomnography showed a markedly elevated apnea-hypopnea index of 67, and a cine-magnetic resonance imaging study was performed to determine his level of obstruction. He was found to have a Chiari I malformation. Two weeks after a posterior fossa craniectomy and decompression surgery, there was complete resolution of his parasomnias, and a polysomnogram 8 weeks later showed improvement of his sleep apnea.

There have been multiple case reports of central apnea in patients with Arnold-Chiari malformation[69–71] that resolved with posterior fossa decompression. There are now reports suggesting that obstructive sleep apnea may also benefit from neurosurgery, confirmed by polysomnography.[72,73] The patient reported by Doherty and colleagues[64] showed improvement in his OSA 3 months following decompression, but this worsened within 2 years and he suddenly died in his sleep 3 years after surgery. Another patient required tracheostomy when his vocal cord abductor paralysis did not resolve after posterior fossa decompression.[63] Milerad and colleagues[74] described 2 infants who clinically responded well to acetazolamide as a respiratory stimulant, although 1 of them still has frequent mixed and OSAs during sleep. Nasal

CPAP has been successfully been used in some patients.[75]

## Prader-Willi Syndrome

Prader-Willi syndrome (PWS) is characterized by infantile hypotonia, obesity, hypogonadism, and mild to moderate mental retardation. It occurs in about 1 in 15,000 births. Approximately 70% of affected individuals have a deletion of the long arm of chromosome 15 at q11q13. The syndrome only occurs if the deletion is in the paternal chromosome; a deletion in the same region of the maternally derived chromosome 15 results in Angelman syndrome.[4] In another 20% of cases, there is inheritance of both copies of chromosome 15 from the mother (maternal uniparental disomy).[76]

In one study, 76% of patients with genetically confirmed PWS had sleep disorders,[77] but excessive somnolence was "almost universal" in a report of older patients with the syndrome.[78] These patients are at risk for both central and obstructive apneas because of their obesity, hypotonia, and an elevated hypercapneic arousal threshold[79] owing to underlying hypothalamic dysfunction.[80] Ventilatory failure with cor pulmonale has been reported as a cause of death.[78]

The prevalence of OSA in PWS patients is reported to be between 10% and 50%.[81–83] Although some individuals may have severe OSA,[84] the mean apnea-hypopnea index is often less than 10.[85,86] Hypopneas and hypoventilation may be even more prevalent than obstructive events. The number of hypopneas and degree of oxyhemoglobin saturation are related to the level of obesity,[81,85] and may be compounded by a restrictive pulmonary defect and/or decreased chemoreceptor sensitivity.[79,87–89] These respiratory events may result in sleep fragmentation and excessive daytime sleepiness.[80,83] Patients with PWS may have a primary sleep disorder, as some studies have demonstrated a high prevalence of sleep-onset REM independent of respiratory events,[79,81] but this has not been a universal finding.[81,82,86]

Early identification of sleep-disordered breathing can facilitate early therapeutic intervention, which may prevent or delay the onset of cor pulmonale. Weight control is extremely difficult in these patients.[90,91] Treatment with growth hormone can help facilitate weight loss and improve learning, behavior, and cognition.[92–94] It has also shown to increase ventilatory responsiveness to hypercapnia or hypoxemia during wakefulness,[94,95] but not during sleep.[96] Those being treated with growth hormone should continue to be monitored for OSA because there may be worsening of sleep-disordered breathing, especially in the first

6 weeks after beginning treatment.[95] There are also reports of an increased risk of sudden death in patients being treated with growth hormone in the setting of a respiratory infection.[95,97] Individual case reports have described treating hypoventilation with progesterone,[98] and treating OSA with nasal CPAP.[84] Smith and colleagues[99] described 4 patients with PWS with snoring, daytime somnolence, and nocturnal hypoxemia with respiratory failure, who were successfully treated with nocturnal CPAP.

## MULTIFACTORIAL AND MISCELLANEOUS

In some cases, OSA is not the result of a single anatomic or central abnormality, but a combination of both. Other underlying causes may include enzyme deficiencies and hematologic abnormalities.

## Mucopolysaccharidoses

The mucopolysaccharidoses are a group of metabolic diseases caused by a deficiency of enzymes normally responsible for mucopolysaccharide degradation. The first one of these disorders to be described was Hunter syndrome, an X-linked recessive disorder whose primary defect is a deficiency of iduronate sulfatase. The gene for Hunter syndrome has been mapped to Xq27-q28.[4] Hurler syndrome was described in 1912, 2 years after Hunter's report, and this disorder consists of a deficiency of $\alpha$-L-iduronidase (IDUA), which is responsible for the degradation of the glycosaminoglycans, heparin sulfate and dermatan sulfate. Inheritance is autosomal recessive, and the IDUA gene has been mapped to chromosome 4p16.3. Different mutations of the gene can lead to milder phenotypes, such as Scheie syndrome (mild) or Hurler-Scheie syndrome (intermediate). The 3 together are classified mucopolysaccharidoses I.

Although these disorders share biochemical and clinical similarities, their phenotypic distinctions, natural histories, and prognoses depend in large part on the specific organ system in which, and to what degree, glycosaminoglycan catabolites accumulate.[100] Boys with Hunter syndrome have coarse facial features, macrocephaly, and macroglossia, with a declining growth rate and mental and neurologic deterioration. Patients with Hurler syndrome can have, in addition, hazy corneas and a more rapid onset of features.[4]

Sleep problems are common across all subtypes, with an overall prevalence of 66%.[101] The patients are at risk for airway obstruction caused by cervical spine instability as well as macroglossia, a deformed pharynx, and a short, thick neck. Thickening of the epiglottis, tonsillar and adenoidal tissues, and tracheal narrowing occur as a result of mucopolysaccharide accumulation.[4] Semenza and Pyeritz[100] described the respiratory complications of 21 patients with mucopolysaccharidosis, representing 21% of the 98 patients with mucopolysaccharidoses followed at the time at Johns Hopkins Hospital. All patients had varying degrees of bony involvement that potentially affected respiratory function, including scoliosis, hyperkyphosis, thoracolumbar gibbus, and/or lumbar hyperlordosis. Eighteen of the 21 patients had a narrow upper airway. Nine patients underwent overnight polysomnography, and OSA was confirmed in 8 of those 9. Thus, the prevalence of OSA in patients with mucopolysaccharidosis is somewhere between 89% (8 of 9) and 8% (8 of 98). None of the patients had central apnea. Belani and colleagues[102] described clinical OSA in 50% of 30 patients with mucopolysaccharidosis, although not all patients underwent polysomnography.

Its complex, multifactorial pathophysiology makes OSA difficult to treat in patients with mucopolysaccharidosis. Continued deposition of mucopolysaccharides in the airway and pharynx can result in progression of obstructive events after treatment. Removal of the tonsils and/or adenoids was not particularly helpful in the 4 patients described by Shapiro and colleagues,[103] and 3 went on to require tracheostomies. Even this procedure may not be sufficient because more than 1 in 5 patients may have tracheomalacia and/or tracheal narrowing.[102] Adachi and Chole[104] described 2 children with Hurler syndrome who had continued upper airway obstruction despite tracheostomy, and required repeated laser excision of mucopolysaccharide deposits from the trachea. Bone marrow transplantation resulted in marked improvement in symptoms suggestive of OSA in all children who underwent this therapy, but no polysomnographic data were reported.[102] Nasal CPAP may also prove useful in these patients.

The most promising therapy is direct replacement of the deficient enzyme. Kakkis and colleagues[105] treated 10 patients with mucopolysaccharidosis I with recombinant $\alpha$-L-iduronidase for 1 year. Nine of the 10 had airway obstruction at baseline, and 7 had apnea documented on polysomnography. Six patients had required treatment with adenotonsillectomy, CPAP, or tracheostomy. Following the year of enzyme replacement therapy, 8 of the 10 patients reported their breathing had improved, and there was overall a 61% decrease in the number of apneas and hypopneas per night.[105]

## Down Syndrome

Down syndrome is the most common pattern of malformation in humans, occurring in 1 in 660

newborns. First described in 1866, the syndrome is the result of trisomy or mosaic trisomy for all or part of chromosome 21. Older maternal age is an important risk factor; the syndrome occurs in 1 in 50 births to mothers older than 45 years, but in only 1 in 1500 births to mothers between 15 and 29 years old.

The patients tend to be hypotonic with mental deficiencies. About 40% have congenital cardiac lesions, including endocardial cushion defect, ventricular septal defect, and patent ductus arteriosus, among others.[4] Patients are at increased risk for OSA because of their craniofacial structure (maxillary hypoplasia, small nose with low nasal bridge), likely compounded by poor neuromuscular activation of the pharynx owing to hypotonia and/or mental deficiencies. These patients also have an 11-fold increase in the incidence of lingual tonsillar hypertrophy when compared with control subjects.[106] Respiratory difficulties may be compounded by spinal cord compression caused by atlantoaxial instability.

Sleep-disordered breathing is common in patients with Down syndrome (**Figs. 3** and **4**). One-third of the patients studied by Stebbens and colleagues[107] had upper airway obstruction identified by a questionnaire and/or limited recordings during sleep. More than three-fourths of the 53 patients studied by Marcus and colleagues[108] had abnormal nap polysomnograms. Twenty-four

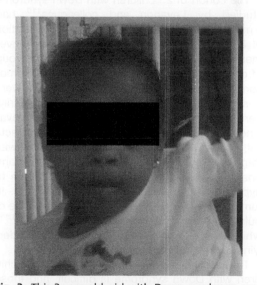

**Fig. 3.** This 3-year-old girl with Down syndrome presented at age 19 months with minimal snoring but tonsils that extended to the uvula. Her AHI at baseline was 5.3 with oxyhemoglobin desaturation as low as 83%. There was minimal improvement with an adenotonsillectomy, and she is now being treated with 4 cm $H_2O$ nasal CPAP.

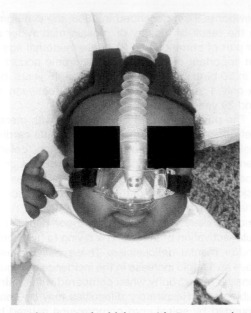

**Fig. 4.** This 9-month-old boy with Down syndrome had severe obstructive sleep apnea (AHI 57.5). He is being treated successfully with 5 cm $H_2O$ CPAP, which he tolerates extremely well.

children had obstructive apnea. However, hypoventilation was the most common abnormality, found in 35 children. The hypoventilation may be a result of pulmonary hypoplasia[109] and/or decreased respiratory drive.

The cohort of 23 children with Down syndrome studied by Levanon and colleagues[110] had a mean RDI of 2.3, with a mean minimal saturation of 87.5% and frequent arousals and leg movements, all significantly worse than a control group of children with primary snoring without chromosomal abnormalities. Both of these studies were designed to detect obstructive events primarily; Ferri and colleagues[111] reported a higher prevalence of central respiratory events in subjects with Down syndrome than a control group with fragile X syndrome. Thus, both central and obstructive respiratory events may contribute to hypoxemia in patients with Down syndrome. In turn this may contribute to the high prevalence of pulmonary hypertension in these children,[98,112] which seems to be out of proportion to any underlying congenital cardiac abnormalities.

Treatment of sleep-disordered breathing in children with Down syndrome is difficult, and those children with the lowest level of neurophysiologic functioning seem to have the poorest response to all treatments.[113] Respiratory stimulants, such as medroxyprogesterone or protriptyline, may be helpful in some patients,[114] especially those in whom hypoventilation is the predominant feature.

Adenotonsillectomy usually results in improvement but may not completely normalize OSA.[108,115] Patients with Down syndrome are 5 times more likely to have respiratory complications following tonsillectomy or adenotonsillectomy, and should be monitored closely.[116] More extensive pharyngeal surgery has been suggested, ranging from uvulopalatopharyngoplasty, tongue reduction, and/or maxillary or midface advancement.[117,118] Tracheostomy may be preferred over CPAP in some instances, because of concerns that pressures applied by the interface may result in midface hypoplasia.[119] There are now studies suggesting that some patients may eventually outgrow their OSA[120,121] although the risk of recurrence is high.[122]

### Sickle Cell Disease

Sickle cell anemia results when valine is substituted for glutamic acid at the sixth position of the β chain of hemoglobin. When this hemoglobin is deoxygenated, interactions between adjacent molecules result in the formation of highly ordered molecular polymers that elongate to form filamentous structures, which in turn aggregate into rigid, crystal-like rods.[123] Patients with sickle cell disease suffer from chronic hemolytic disease resulting from premature destruction of brittle, poorly deformable erythrocytes.

These erythrocytes can occlude the microvessels, resulting in chronic pain that may result in hospitalization. Occlusion of the vessels in other end organs can result in stroke, hepatic crisis, priapism, acute renal infarction, and acute chest syndrome. Although the occurrence of pain is often without precipitates, several factors have been recognized to contribute to the development of pain in selected patients, including cold exposure, acute respiratory illness, exercise, dehydration, and psychological stress. Factors promoting hypoxemia and/or vascular spasm might be logically expected to promote vaso-occlusive events.

Hemoglobin desaturation is common during sleep; normal individuals may experience hemoglobin desaturations owing to hypoventilation and upper airway obstruction.[124] However, patients with sickle cell disease may be at an additional risk for OSA because of reduced upper airway size from compensatory hyperplasia of the tonsils and adenoids following splenic infarction.[125–127] Wittig and colleagues[126] reported and increased incidence of snoring in patients with sickle cell disease in comparison with their unaffected siblings. A temporal relationship between desaturation during sleep and painful crises has been observed.[128] Samuels and colleagues[129] reported that 36% of patients with sickle cell disease had upper airway obstruction. Sixteen of the 18 patients underwent adenotonsillectomy, and all had an improvement in clinical signs and symptoms after surgery. Data on vaso-occlusive episodes were not reported. Castele and colleagues[130] reported on 7 adult patients with sickle cell disease and frequent vaso-occlusive crises whose oxyhemoglobin saturation decreased during sleep. OSA has been implicated as a precipitating event of stroke in sickle cell patients,[8] and has been correlated with an increased incidence of vaso-occlusive crises.[127,131,132]

Despite these suggestive clinical observations and an intellectually attractive pathophysiology, a relationship between nocturnal hypoxemia and sickle cell complications has not been convincingly demonstrated. Maddern and colleagues[125] estimated the prevalence of OSA syndrome in patients with sickle cell disease to be 5%, similar to that of the general population. There was no difference in the sleep architecture, oxyhemoglobin saturation, or the number of respiratory events of children with mild sickle cell disease (no painful crises in the preceding year) when compared with children with severe disease (2 or more hospitalizations for painful crises in the preceding year).[133] Needleman and colleagues[134] found no relationship between obstructive apneas and mean nocturnal oxyhemoglobin saturation. Despite the lack of convincing group data, the effects of nocturnal hypoxemia can be devastating to individual patients with sickle cell disease.[131,135]

Screening by history and physical examination may not predict the presence of OSA.[129] Daytime oxyhemoglobin saturation was the best predictor of nocturnal hypoxemia.[134] It seems reasonable to routinely measure daytime oxyhemoglobin saturation of patients with sickle cell disease, followed if necessary by pulmonary function testing and polysomnography to determine the presence and cause of any nocturnal desaturations. In this way, treatment can be directed at the underlying cause: OSA, hypoventilation, or pulmonary infarction.

### CHARGE Syndrome

First described by Hall in 1979, CHARGE syndrome can be diagnosed clinically based on the constellation of findings: **C**oloboma of the eye, **H**eart defects, choanal **A**tresia, **R**etardation of growth and/or development, **G**enitourinary abnormalities, and **E**ar abnormalities.[136] Although the incidence is estimated to be about 1 in 8500,[137] many patients are not diagnosed until after 5 years of age.[138] The genetic cause of

CHARGE syndrome has been identified to be *Chromodomain helicase* DNA-*binding protein-7* (CHD-7) located at chromosome 8q12.1. Since its discovery, studies have shown that the mutation exists in approximately two-thirds of individuals with the syndrome.[139,140] Cranial nerve abnormalities include involvement of cranial nerve V (weak chewing/sucking), cranial nerve VII (facial palsy), cranial nerve VIII (sensorineural hearing loss and balance/vestibular problems), and cranial nerve IX/X (swallowing problems).[141]

Fifty-eight percent of children with CHARGE syndrome have sleep disturbances, with sleep breathing disorders, disorders initiating and maintaining sleep, and sleep-wake transition disorders being most common.[142] The same study hypothesized that choanal atresia, cleft palate, and otitis media are associated with sleep disturbances in CHARGE syndrome.

Thirty-three of 51 patients with CHARGE syndrome had OSA as diagnosed by parental questionnaires. Treatments included adenotonsillectomy, CPAP, and/or tracheostomy.[143] Because sleep disturbances can exacerbate behavioral problems in these children, early identification and treatment is imperative.

## SUMMARY

Genetic syndromes can affect breathing during sleep through effects on the bony anatomy of the skull and face, soft tissue of the airway, and/or neuromuscular control of the pharynx. Awareness of these potential complications should lead to quicker diagnosis and improved therapy.

## REFERENCES

1. Treacher Collins Syndrome Collaborative Group: positional cloning of a gene involved in the pathogenesis of Treacher Collins Syndrome. Nat Genet 1996;12(2):130–6.
2. Wise CA, Chiang LC, Paznekas WA, et al. TCOF1 gene encodes a putative nuclear phosphoprotein that exhibits mutations in Treacher Collins syndrome throughout its coding region. Proc Natl Acad Sci U S A 1997;94(7):3110–5.
3. Dauwerse JG, Dixon J, Seland S, et al. Mutations in genes encoding subunits of RNA polymerases I and III cause Treacher Collins syndrome. Nat Genet 2011;43(1):20–2.
4. Jones KL. Smith's recognizable patterns of human malformation. Philadelphia: W.B. Saunders; 1997. p. 250–251, 234–235, 416–421, 346–351, 202–205, 450–471, 8–13.
5. Plomp RG, Bredero-Boelhouwer HH, Joosten KF, et al. Obstructive sleep apnoea in Treacher Collins

syndrome: prevalence, severity and cause. Int J Oral Maxillofac Surg 2012;41(6):696–701.

6. Akre H, Øverland B, Åsten P, et al. Obstructive sleep apnea in Treacher Collins syndrome. Eur Arch Otorhinolaryngol 2012;269(1):331–7.

7. Plomp RG, Joosten KF, Wolvius EB, et al. Screening for obstructive sleep apnea in Treacher-Collins syndrome. Laryngoscope 2012;122(4):930–4.

8. Miloro M. Mandibular distraction osteogenesis for pediatric airway management. J Oral Maxillofac Surg 2010;68(7):1512–23.

9. Genecov DG, Barceló CR, Steinberg D, et al. Clinical experience with the application of distraction osteogenesis for airway obstruction. J Craniofac Surg 2009;20(Suppl 2):1817–21.

10. Miller SD, Glynn SF, Kiely JL, et al. The role of nasal CPAP in obstructive sleep apnoea syndrome due to mandibular hypoplasia. Respirology 2010; 15(2):377–9.

11. Plotz FB, Van Essen AJ, Bosschaart AN, et al. Cerebro-costo-mandibular syndrome. Am J Med Genet 1996;62:286–92.

12. Sher AE. Mechanics of airway obstruction in Robin sequence: implications for treatment. Cleft Palate Craniofac J 1992;29(3):224–31.

13. Monroe CW, Ogo K. Treatment of micrognathia in the neonatal period. Plast Reconstr Surg 1972; 50(4):317–25.

14. Bull MJ, Givan DC, Sadove AM, et al. Improved outcome in Pierre Robin sequence: effect of multidisciplinary evaluation and management. Pediatrics 1990;86(2):294–301.

15. Freed GF, Pearlman MA, Brown AS, et al. Polysomnographic indications for surgical intervention Pierre Robin sequence: acute airway management and follow up studies after repair and takedown of tongue lip adhesion. Cleft Palate J 1988;25(2): 151–5.

16. Anderson IC, Sedaghat AR, McGinley BM, et al. Prevalence and severity of obstructive sleep apnea and snoring in infants with Pierre Robin sequence. Cleft Palate Craniofac J 2011;48(5):614–8.

17. Meyer AC, Lidsky ME, Sampson DE, et al. Airway interventions in children with Pierre Robin sequence. Otolaryngol Head Neck Surg 2008; 138(6):782–7.

18. Leboulanger N, Picard A, Soupre V, et al. Physiologic and clinical benefits of noninvasive ventilation in infants with Pierre Robin sequence. Pediatrics 2010;126(5):e1056–63.

19. Essouri S, Nicot F, Clement A, et al. Noninvasive positive pressure ventilation in infants with upper airway obstruction: comparison of continuous and bilevel positive pressure. Intensive Care Med 2005;31(4):574–80.

20. Fauroux B, Leboulanger N, Roger G, et al. Noninvasive positive-pressure ventilation avoids recannulation and facilitates early weaning from tracheotomy in children. Pediatr Crit Care Med 2010;11(1):31–7.

21. Krimmel M, Kluba S, Breidt M, et al. Three-dimensional assessment of facial development in children with Pierre Robin sequence. J Craniofac Surg 2009;20:2055–60.

22. Suri S, Ross RB, Tompson BD. Craniofacial morphology and adolescent facial growth in Pierre Robin sequence. Am J Orthod Dentofacial Orthop 2010;137:763–74.

23. Daskalogiannakis J, Ross RB, Tompson BD. The mandibular catch-up growth controversy in Pierre Robin sequence. Am J Orthod Dentofacial Orthop 2001;120:280–5.

24. Han KD, Seruya M, Oh AK, et al. "Natural" decannulation in patients with Robin sequence and severe airway obstruction. Ann Otol Rhinol Laryngol 2012; 121(1):44–50.

25. Jarrahy R. Controversies in the management of neonatal micrognathia: to distract or not to distract, that is the question. J Craniofac Surg 2012;23(1): 243–9.

26. Spier S, Rivlin J, Rowe RD, et al. Sleep in Pierre Robin syndrome. Chest 1986;90(5):711–5.

27. Kaplan LC. Clinical assessment and multi specialty management of Apert syndrome. Clin Plast Surg 1991;18:217–25.

28. Kakitsuba N, Sadaoka T, Motoyama S, et al. Sleep apnea and sleep-related breathing disorders in patients with craniofacial synostosis. Acta Otolaryngol Suppl 1994;517:6–10.

29. Mixter RC, David DJ, Perloff WH, et al. Obstructive sleep apnea in Apert's and Pfeiffer's syndromes: more than a craniofacial abnormality. Plast Reconstr Surg 1990;86(3):457–63.

30. Cohen MM Jr, Kreiborg S. Upper and lower airway compromise in the Apert syndrome. Am J Med Genet 1992;44(1):90–3.

31. McGill T. Otolaryngologic aspects of Apert syndrome. Clin Plast Surg 1991;18(2):309–13.

32. Suen JS, Arnold JE, Brooks LJ. Adenotonsillectomy for treatment of obstructive sleep apnea in children. Arch Otolaryngol Head Neck Surg 1995; 121(5):525–30.

33. Tajima S, Imai K. Obstructive sleep apnea attack in complex craniosynostosis. Acta Otolaryngol Suppl 1994;517:17–20.

34. Fearon J. Halo distraction of the Le Fort III in syndromic craniosynostosis: a long-term assessment. Plast Reconstr Surg 2005;115(6):1524–36.

35. Hui S, Wing YK, Kew J, et al. Obstructive sleep apnea syndrome in a family with Crouzon's syndrome. Sleep 1998;21(3):298–303.

36. Brooks LJ, Crooks RL, Sleeper GP. Compliance with nasal CPAP by children with obstructive sleep apnea [abstract]. Am Rev Respir Dis 1992;445:A556.

37. Greenberg F, Guzzetta V, Montes de Oca-Luna R, et al. Molecular analysis of the Smith-Magenis syndrome: a possible contiguous-gene syndrome associated with del(17)(p11.2). Am J Hum Genet 1991;49(6):1207–18.

38. Smith AC, Dykens E, Greenberg F. Sleep disturbance in Smith-Magenis syndrome (del 17 p11.2). Am J Med Genet 1998;81(2):186–91.

39. Williams SR, Zies D, Mullegama SV, et al. Smith-Magenis syndrome results in disruption of CLOCK gene transcription and reveals an integral role for RAI1 in the maintenance of circadian rhythmicity. Am J Hum Genet 2012;90(6):941–9.

40. Boone PM, Reiter RJ, Glaze DG, et al. Abnormal circadian rhythm of melatonin in Smith-Magenis syndrome patients with RAI1 point mutations. Am J Med Genet A 2011;155A(8):2024–7.

41. Potocki L, Shaw CJ, Stankiewicz P, et al. Variability in clinical phenotype despite common chromosomal deletion in Smith-Magenis syndrome [del(17) (p11.2p11.2)]. Genet Med 2003;5(6):430–4.

42. Carpizo R, Martínez A, Mediavilla D, et al. Smith-Magenis syndrome: a case report of improved sleep after treatment with beta1-adrenergic antagonists and melatonin. J Pediatr 2006;149:409–11.

43. Leoni C, Cesarini L, Dittoni S, et al. Hypoventilation in REM sleep in a case of 17p11.2 deletion (Smith-Magenis syndrome). Am J Med Genet A 2010; 152A(3):708–12.

44. Stokes DC, Phillips JA, Leonard CO, et al. Respiratory complications of achondroplasia. J Pediatr 1983;102(4):534–41.

45. Fremion AS, Garg BP, Kalsbeck J. Apnea as the sole manifestation of cord compression in achondroplasia. J Pediatr 1984;104(3):398–401.

46. Pauli RM, Scott CI, Wassman ER Jr, et al. Apnea and sudden unexpected death in infants with achondroplasia. J Pediatr 1984;104(3):342–8.

47. Waters KA, Everett F, Sillence D, et al. Breathing abnormalities in sleep in achondroplasia. Arch Dis Child 1993;69(2):191–6.

48. Waters KA, Everett F, Sillence DO, et al. Treatment of obstructive sleep apnea in achondroplasia: evaluation of sleep, breathing, and somatosensory-evoked potentials. Am J Med Genet 1995;59(4):460–6.

49. Zucconi M, Weber G, Castronovo V, et al. Sleep and upper airway obstruction in children with achondroplasia. J Pediatr 1996;129(5):743–9.

50. Trotter TL, Hall JG. American Academy of Pediatrics Committee on Genetics. Health supervision for children with achondroplasia. Pediatrics 2005; 116(3):771–83.

51. Wright MJ, Irving MD. Clinical management of achondroplasia. Arch Dis Child 2012;97(2):129–34.

52. Ednick M, Tinkle BT, Phromchairak J, et al. Sleep-related respiratory abnormalities and arousal pattern in achondroplasia during early infancy. J Pediatr 2009;155(4):510–5.

53. Julliand S, Boulé M, Baujat G, et al. Lung function, diagnosis, and treatment of sleep-disordered breathing in children with achondroplasia. Am J Med Genet A 2012;158A(8):1987–93.

54. Mogayzel PJ Jr, Carroll JL, Loughlin GM, et al. Sleep-disordered breathing in children with achondroplasia. J Pediatr 1998;132(4):667–71.

55. Schiller O, Schwartz M, Bruckheimer E, et al. Pulmonary hypertension in an infant with achondroplasia. Pediatr Neurosurg 2008;44(4):341–3.

56. Afsharpaiman S, Sillence DO, Sheikhvatan M, et al. Respiratory events and obstructive sleep apnea in children with achondroplasia: investigation and treatment outcomes. Sleep Breath 2011;15(4):755–61.

57. Reid CS, Pyeritz RE, Kopits SE, et al. Cervicomedullary cord compression in young children with achondroplasia: value of comprehensive neurologic and respiratory evaluation. Basic Life Sci 1988;48:199–206.

58. Schlüter B, De Sousa G, Trowitzsch E, et al. Diagnostics and management of sleep-related respiratory disturbances in children with skeletal dysplasia caused by FGFR3 mutations (achondroplasia and hypochondroplasia). Georgian Med News 2011;(196–197):63–72.

59. Greer M. Arnold-Chiari malformation. In: Rowland LP, editor. Merritt's textbook of neurology. Baltimore (MD): Williams & Wilkins; 1995. p. 528–32.

60. Coria F, Quintana F, Rebollo M, et al. Occipital dysplasia and Chiari type I deformity in a family. Clinical and radiological study of three generations. J Neurol Sci 1983;62(1–3):147–58.

61. Dure LS, Percy AK, Cheek WR, et al. Chiari type I malformation in children. J Pediatr 1989;115(4):573–6.

62. Keefover R, Sam M, Bodensteiner J, et al. Hypersomnolence and pure central sleep apnea associated with the Chiari I malformation. J Child Neurol 1995;10(1):65–7.

63. Ruff ME, Oakes WJ, Fisher SR, et al. Sleep apnea and vocal cord paralysis secondary to type I Chiari malformation. Pediatrics 1987;80(2):231–4.

64. Doherty J, Spence DP, Young C, et al. Obstructive sleep apnoea with Arnold-Chiari malformation. Thorax 1995;50(6):690–1.

65. Paul KS, Lye RH, Strang FA, et al. Arnold-Chiari malformation. Review of 71 cases. J Neurosurg 1983;58(2):183–7.

66. Waters KA, Forbes P, Morielli A, et al. Sleep-disordered breathing in children with myelomeningocele. J Pediatr 1998;132(4):672–81.

67. Dauvilliers Y, Stal V, Abril B, et al. Chiari malformation and sleep related breathing disorders. J Neurol Neurosurg Psychiatry 2007;78:1344–8.

68. Daftary AS, Walker JM, Farney RJ. NREM sleep parasomnia associated with Chiari I malformation. J Clin Sleep Med 2011;7(5):526–9.

69. Spence J, Pasterkamp H, McDonald PJ. Isolated central sleep apnea in type I Chiari malformation: improvement after surgery. Pediatr Pulmonol 2010;45(11):1141–4.

70. Botelho RV, Bittencourt LR, Rotta JM, et al. The effects of posterior fossa decompressive surgery in adult patients with Chiari malformation and sleep apnea. J Neurosurg 2010;112(4):800–7.

71. Gagnadoux F, Meslier N, Svab I, et al. Sleep-disordered breathing in patients with Chiari malformation: improvement after surgery. Neurology 2006; 66(1):136–8.

72. Tran K, Hukins CA. Obstructive and central sleep apnoea in Arnold-Chiari malformation: resolution following surgical decompression. Sleep Breath 2011;15(3):611–3.

73. Luigetti M, Losurdo A, Dittoni S, et al. Improvement of obstructive sleep apneas caused by hydrocephalus associated with Chiari malformation Type II following surgery. J Neurosurg Pediatr 2010;6(4): 336–9.

74. Milerad J, Lagercrantz H, Johnson P. Obstructive sleep apnea in Arnold-Chiari malformation treated with acetazolamide. Acta Paediatr 1992;81(8):609–12.

75. Marcus CL, Ward SL, Mallory GB, et al. Use of nasal continuous positive airway pressure as treatment of childhood obstructive sleep apnea. J Pediatr 1995; 127(1):88–94.

76. Mascari MJ, Gottlieb W, Rogan PK, et al. The frequency of uniparental disomy in Prader-Willi syndrome. Implications for molecular diagnosis. N Engl J Med 1992;326(24):1599–607.

77. Gunay-Aygun M, Schwartz S, Heeger S, et al. The changing purpose of Prader-Willi syndrome clinical diagnostic criteria and proposed revised criteria. Pediatrics 2001;108:E92.

78. Laurance BM, Brito A, Wilkinson J. Prader-Willi Syndrome after age 15 years. Arch Dis Child 1981;56(3):181–6.

79. Livingston FR, Arens R, Bailey SL, et al. Hypercapnic arousal responses in Prader-Willi syndrome. Chest 1995;108:1627–31.

80. Hertz G, Cataletto M, Feinsilver SH, et al. Sleep and breathing patterns in patients with Prader Willi syndrome (PWS): effects of age and gender. Sleep 1993;16(4):366–71.

81. Brooks LJ, Owens RP. Sleep and breathing patterns in patients with Prader-Willi syndrome. Sleep Research 1992;21:258.

82. Clift S, Dahlitz M, Parkes JD. Sleep apnoea in the Prader-Willi syndrome. J Sleep Res 1994;3(2):121–6.

83. Camfferman D, McEvoy RD, O'Donoghue F, et al. Prader Willi syndrome and excessive daytime sleepiness. Sleep Med Rev 2008;12(1):65–75.

84. Sforza E, Krieger J, Geisert J, et al. Sleep and breathing abnormalities in a case of Prader-Willi syndrome. The effects of acute continuous positive airway pressure treatment. Acta Paediatr Scand 1991;80(1):80–5.

85. Hertz G, Cataletto M, Feinsilver SH, et al. Developmental trends of sleep-disordered breathing in Prader-Willi syndrome: the role of obesity. Am J Med Genet 1995;56(2):188–90.

86. Kaplan J, Fredrickson PA, Richardson JW. Sleep and breathing in patients with the Prader-Willi syndrome. Mayo Clin Proc 1991;66(11):1124–6.

87. Arens R, Gozal D, Omlin KJ, et al. Hypoxic and hypercapnic ventilatory responses in Prader-Willi syndrome. J Appl Physiol 1994;77(5):2224–30.

88. Gozal D, Arens R, Omlin KJ, et al. Absent peripheral chemosensitivity in Prader-Willi syndrome. J Appl Physiol 1994;77(5):2231–6.

89. Orenstein DM, Boat TF, Owens RP, et al. The obesity hypoventilation syndrome in children with the Prader-Willi syndrome: a possible role for familial decreased response to carbon dioxide. J Pediatr 1980;97(5):765–7.

90. Bray GA, Dahms WT, Swerdloff RS, et al. The Prader-Willi syndrome: a study of 40 patients and a review of the literature. Medicine 1983;62(2):59–80.

91. Donaldson MD, Chu CE, Cooke A, et al. The Prader-Willi syndrome. Arch Dis Child 1994;70(1): 58–63.

92. Lindgren AC, Hagenas L, Muller J, et al. Growth hormone treatment of children with Prader-Willi syndrome affects linear growth and body composition favourably. Acta Paediatr 1998;87:28–31.

93. Carrel AL, Myers SE, Whitman BY, et al. Growth hormone improves body composition, fat utilization, physical strength and agility, and growth in Prader-Willi syndrome: a controlled study. J Pediatr 1999;134:215–21.

94. Haqq AM, Stadler DD, Jackson RH, et al. Effects of growth hormone on pulmonary function, sleep quality, behavior, cognition, growth velocity, body composition, and resting energy expenditure in Prader-Willi syndrome. J Clin Endocrinol Metab 2003;88:2206–12.

95. Miller J, Silverstein J, Shuster J, et al. Short-term effects of growth hormone on sleep abnormalities in Prader-Willi syndrome. J Clin Endocrinol Metab 2006;91(2):413–7.

96. Katz-Salamon M, Lindgren AC, Cohen G. The effect of growth hormone on sleep-related cardio-respiratory control in Prader-Willi syndrome. Acta Paediatr 2012;101(6):643–8.

97. Festen DA, de Weerd AW, van den Bossche RA, et al. Sleep-related breathing disorders in prepubertal children with Prader-Willi syndrome and effects of growth hormone treatment. J Clin Endocrinol Metab 2006;91(12):4911–5.

98. Orenstein DM, Boat TF, Stern RC, et al. Progesterone treatment of the obesity hypoventilation syndrome in a child. J Pediatr 1977;90(3):477–9.

99. Smith IE, King MA, Siklos PW, et al. Treatment of ventilatory failure in the Prader-Willi syndrome. Eur Respir J 1998;11(5):1150–2.

100. Semenza GL, Pyeritz RE. Respiratory complications of mucopolysaccharide storage disorders. Medicine 1988;67(4):209–19.

101. Bax MC, Colville GA. Behaviour in mucopolysaccharide disorders. Arch Dis Child 1995;73(1):77–81.

102. Belani KG, Krivit W, Carpenter BL, et al. Children with mucopolysaccharidosis: perioperative care, morbidity, mortality, and new findings. J Pediatr Surg 1993;28(3):403–8.

103. Shapiro J, Strome M, Crocker AC. Airway obstruction and sleep apnea in Hurler and Hunter syndromes. Ann Otol Rhinol Laryngol 1985;94(5 Pt 1): 458–61.

104. Adachi K, Chole RA. Management of tracheal lesions in Hurler syndrome. Arch Otolaryngol Head Neck Surg 1990;116(10):1205–7.

105. Kakkis ED, Muenzer J, Tiller GE, et al. Enzyme-replacement therapy in mucopolysaccharidosis I. N Engl J Med 2001;344(3):182–8.

106. Rosen D. Management of obstructive sleep apnea associated with Down syndrome and other craniofacial dysmorphologies. Curr Opin Pulm Med 2011; 17(6):431–6.

107. Stebbens VA, Dennis J, Samuels MP, et al. Sleep related upper airway obstruction in a cohort with Down's syndrome. Arch Dis Child 1991;66(11). 1333–8.

108. Marcus CL, Keens TG, Bautista DB, et al. Obstructive sleep apnea in children with Down syndrome. Pediatrics 1991;88(1):132–9.

109. Cooney TP, Thurlbeck WM. Pulmonary hypoplasia in Down's syndrome. N Engl J Med 1982;307(19): 1170–3.

110. Levanon A, Tarasiuk A, Tal A. Sleep characteristics in children with Down syndrome. J Pediatr 1999; 134(6):755–60.

111. Ferri R, Curzi-Dascalova L, Del Gracco S, et al. Respiratory patterns during sleep in Down's syndrome: importance of central apnoeas. J Sleep Res 1997;6(2):134–41.

112. Loughlin GM, Wynne JW, Victorica BE. Sleep apnea as a possible cause of pulmonary hypertension in Down syndrome. J Pediatr 1981;98(3):435–7.

113. Brooks LJ, Bacevice AM, Beebe A, et al. Relationship between neuropsychological function and success of treatment for OSA in children with Down syndrome [abstract]. Am J Respir Crit Care Med 1997;155:A710.

114. Clark RW, Schmidt HS, Schuller DE. Sleep-induced ventilatory dysfunction in Down's syndrome. Arch Intern Med 1980;140(1):45–50.

115. Shete MM, Stocks RM, Sebelik ME, et al. Effects of adeno-tonsillectomy on polysomnography patterns in Down syndrome children with obstructive sleep apnea: a comparative study with children without Down syndrome. Int J Pediatr Otorhinolaryngol 2010;74(3):241–4.

116. Goldstein NA, Armfield DR, Kingsley LA, et al. Postoperative complications after tonsillectomy and adenoidectomy in children with Down syndrome. Arch Otolaryngol Head Neck Surg 1998;124(2):171–6.

117. Lefaivre JF, Cohen SR, Burstein FD, et al. Down syndrome: identification and surgical management of obstructive sleep apnea. Plast Reconstr Surg 1997;99(3):629–37.

118. Donaldson JD, Redmond WM. Surgical management of obstructive sleep apnea in children with Down syndrome. J Otolaryngol 1988;17(7):398–403.

119. Li KK, Riley RW, Guilleminault C. An unreported risk in the use of home nasal continuous positive airway pressure and home nasal ventilation in children. Chest 2000;117:916–8.

120. Rosen D. Some infants with Down syndrome spontaneously outgrow their obstructive sleep apnea. Clin Pediatr (Phila) 2010;49(11):1068–71.

121. Downey R, Perkin RM, MacQuarrie J. Nasal continuous positive airway pressure use in children with obstructive sleep apnea younger than 2 years of age. Chest 2000;117:1608–12.

122. Ng DK, Hui HN, Chan CH, et al. Obstructive sleep apnoea in children with Down syndrome. Singapore Med J 2006;47:774–9.

123. Honig GR. Hemoglobin disorders. In: Behrman RE, Kliegman RM, Nelson WE, et al, editors. Nelson textbook of pediatrics. Philadelphia: W.B. Saunders; 1992. p. 1246–54.

124. Block AJ, Boysen PG, Wynne JW, et al. Sleep apnea, hypopnea and oxygen desaturation in normal subjects. N Engl J Med 1979;300(10):513–7.

125. Maddern BR, Reed HT, Ohene-Frempong K, et al. Obstructive sleep apnea syndrome in sickle cell disease. Ann Otol Rhinol Laryngol 1989;98(3):174–8.

126. Wittig RM, Roth T, Keenum AJ, et al. Snoring, daytime sleepiness, and sickle cell anemia. Am J Dis Child 1988;142(6):589.

127. Strauss T, Sin S, Marcus CL, et al. Upper airway lymphoid tissue size in children with sickle cell disease. Chest 2012;142(1):94–100.

128. Scharf MB, Lobel JS, Caldwell E, et al. Nocturnal oxygen desaturation in patients with sickle cell anemia. JAMA 1983;249(13):1753–5.

129. Samuels MP, Stebbens VA, Davies SC, et al. Sleep related upper airway obstruction and hypoxaemia in sickle cell disease. Arch Dis Child 1992;67(7): 925–9.

130. Castele RJ, Strohl KP, Chester CS, et al. Oxygen saturation with sleep in patients with sickle cell disease. Arch Intern Med 1986;146(4):722–5.

131. Sidman JD, Fry TL. Exacerbation of sickle cell disease by obstructive sleep apnea. Arch Otolaryngol Head Neck Surg 1988;114(8):916–7.

132. Buck J, Davies SC. Surgery in sickle cell disease. Hematol Oncol Clin North Am 2005;19(5):897–902.

133. Brooks LJ, Koziol SM, Chiarucci KM, et al. Does sleep-disordered breathing contribute to the clinical severity of sickle cell anemia? J Pediatr Hematol Oncol 1996;18(2):135–9.

134. Needleman JP, Franco ME, Varlotta L, et al. Mechanisms of nocturnal oxyhemoglobin desaturation in children and adolescents with sickle cell disease. Pediatr Pulmonol 1999;28(6):418–22.

135. Robertson PL, Aldrich MS, Hanash SM, et al. Stroke associated with obstructive sleep apnea in a child with sickle cell anemia. Ann Neurol 1988;23(6):614–6.

136. Hall BD. Choanal atresia and associated multiple anomalies. J Pediatr 1979;95(3):395–8.

137. Issekutz KA, Graham JM Jr, Prasad C, et al. An epidemiological analysis of CHARGE syndrome: preliminary results from a Canadian study. Am J Med Genet A 2005;133A(3):309–17.

138. Blake KD, Salem-Hartshorne N, Daoud MA, et al. Adolescent and adult issues in CHARGE syndrome. Clin Pediatr 2005;44(2):151–9.

139. Janssen N, Bergman JE, Swertz MA, et al. Mutation update on the CHD7 gene involved in CHARGE syndrome. Hum Mutat 2012;33(8):1149–60.

140. Zentner GE, Layman WS, Martin DM, et al. Molecular and phenotypic aspects of CHD7 mutation in CHARGE syndrome. Am J Med Genet A 2010;152A(3):674–86.

141. Blake KD, Hartshorne TS, Lawand C, et al. Cranial nerve manifestations in CHARGE syndrome. Am J Med Genet A 2008;146A(5):585–92.

142. Hartshorne TS, Heussler HS, Dailor AN, et al. Sleep disturbances in CHARGE syndrome: types and relationships with behavior and caregiver well-being. Dev Med Child Neurol 2009;51(2):143–50.

143. Trider CL, Corsten G, Morrison D, et al. Understanding obstructive sleep apnea in children with CHARGE syndrome. Int J Pediatr Otorhinolaryngol 2012;76(7):947–53.

# Sleep Derangements in Central Nervous System Infections

Gilbert Seda, MD, PhD, Teofilo Lee-Chiong, MD,
John Harrington, MD, MPH*

## KEYWORDS

- Narcolepsy • Insomnia • Central nervous system infections • Parasomnias • Sleeping sickness
- HIV

## KEY POINTS

- Different infectious pathogens can alter sleep, either resulting from systemic inflammation, autoimmune responses, direct CNS injury, or adverse reaction to pharmacologic therapy.
- Many reports involved a handful of cases, thus making recommendations regarding diagnosis or therapy difficult.
- A thorough clinical history aided by appropriate testing is necessary, and prompt therapy may improve outcomes.

## INTRODUCTION

There is a bidirectional interaction between the peripheral immune system and the central nervous system (CNS). The response of the immune system and CNS to infectious pathogens manifests in several ways, including altered thermoregulation with the development of fever, increased catabolic activity and suppression of appetite, increased respiratory drive, changes in cardiovascular function, and altered neuronal activity.[1] In addition, infections of the CNS result in profound changes in sleep architecture and quality; these changes in sleep differ among the various infectious agents.

## SLEEP ARCHITECTURE

Animal studies investigating the effects of sepsis on sleep have demonstrated sleep fragmentation and changes in non–rapid eye movement (NREM) and rapid eye movement (REM) sleep. Lancel and colleagues[2] investigated the role of sepsis on sleep

duration, electroencephalographic (EEG) patterns, and brain temperature in rats. After lipopolysacchride was administered intraperitoneally, brain temperature increased, REM sleep decreased, and NREM episodes shortened during the initial 12 hours. The number and duration of NREM and REM episodes increased during the subsequent 12-hour period. In another study, Baracchi and colleagues,[3] using a rat sepsis model consisting of cecal ligation and puncture, found that onset of sepsis was accompanied by an increase in NREM sleep during the dark period and suppression of REM sleep in the first 24 hours after surgery. REM sleep subsequently increased; however, sleep remained fragmented. One hypothesis explaining these EEG changes in sleep suggests that fever is an adaptive response of the CNS, and that REM sleep reduction and NREM sleep fragmentation serve to conserve heat.

The global and local regulation of sleep and wakefulness is altered by CNS infections. Sleep fragmentation and hyperarousal can result in insomnia, whereas increased cytokine production

Disclaimer: The views expressed in this presentation are those of the author and do not necessarily reflect the official policy or position of the Department of the Navy, Department of Defense, or the United States government.

Division of Pulmonary Sciences and Critical Care Medicine, National Jewish Health, University of Colorado, 1400 Jackson Street, Suite A02, Denver, CO 80206–2761, USA

* Corresponding author.

E-mail address: harringtonj@njhealth.org

Sleep Med Clin 7 (2012) 703–711

http://dx.doi.org/10.1016/j.jsmc.2012.10.003

or destruction of sleep-wake promoting neurons can result in hypersomnia or insomnia. For instance, individuals can develop central hypersomnia caused by postinfectious autoimmune processes by the interaction between innate genetic susceptibility and exposure to specific pathogens as is seen in some cases of narcolepsy.[4] Likewise, infection with HIV can give rise to insomnia, daytime fatigue, and depression. One study found that HIV-seropositive persons with insomnia had longer sleep-onset latency (SOL), decreased sleep efficiency (SE), and decreased REM sleep compared with their HIV-seronegative counterparts.[5]

CNS infections can affect the brainstem respiratory centers resulting in abnormal breathing patterns during sleep. These respiratory aberrations are a consequence of direct injury to the brainstem, release of inflammatory cytokines, or metabolic changes related to the disease process itself. Risk of obstructive sleep apnea (OSA) is increased in HIV because of the development of lipodystrophy, weight gain, or dyslipidemia, or as a result of active antiretroviral therapy.[6] Furthermore, there are case reports of patients with encephalitis who develop alterations in respiration during sleep, including central or obstructive apneas, caused by immune-mediated destruction of the medulla.[7] Finally, there are rare reports of encephalitis related to use of nasal continuous positive airway pressure devices.[8]

Alterations in circadian rhythms have been described in some CNS infections. Patients afflicted with African sleeping sickness can exhibit disorganization and reversal of their 24-hour sleep-wake cycles, including daytime sleeping episodes and nighttime waking periods.[9]

Movement disorders during sleep and parasomnias also can be seen. One case report described the development of REM sleep behavior disorder after acute encephalitis.[10] Movement disorders observed with CNS infections include periodic limb movements during sleep, motor spasms, and the opsoclonus-myoclonus syndrome. Periodic limb movements during sleep have been reported in patients with postpolio syndrome and are believed to be caused by dysfunction of the surviving spinal cord neurons or abnormal dopamine production.[11] Stiff person syndrome, a neurologic condition characterized by waxing and waning muscle rigidity and spasms, is generally considered an autoimmune disease. Although sleep can relieve muscle stiffness associated with this disorder, spasms can reemerge during sleep stage transitions or during arousals.[12] Opsoclonus-myoclonus syndrome is a rare paraneoplastic syndrome commonly seen in children

with neuroblastoma or adults with small cell lung cancer; it is also seen in association with infections with *Streptococcus*, influenza, hepatitis C, HIV, *Mycoplasma pneumoniae*, varicella zoster virus, Epstein-Barr virus, Coxsackie virus, and enterovirus.[13]

Other consequences of CNS infections that can disturb sleep include febrile seizures, complex partial seizures, periodic sharp wave complexes, focal temporal or lateralized polymorphic delta activity, and postencephalitic epilepsy. New-onset seizures are frequent manifestations of HIV infection and often result in long-term morbidity.[14,15] Partial complex seizures have been seen in association with neurosyphillis.[16] Periodic lateralized epileptiform discharges are EEG abnormalities that consist of repetitive spike or sharp wave discharges, either focal or lateralized over one hemisphere, and recur at nearly fixed time intervals. These periodic lateralized epileptiform discharges have been reported in patients with mycoplasma encephalitis or HIV infection, and are believed to possess epileptogenic potential.[17,18]

CNS infections commonly associated with alteration in sleep are narcolepsy, HIV, African sleeping sickness, encephalitis, and meningitis.

## NARCOLEPSY

Narcolepsy is a disease caused by significant loss of hypothalamic neurons containing the neuropeptide hypocretin. Approximately 90% of patients with narcolepsy have decreased levels of this neurotransmitter. Narcolepsy is commonly associated with human leukocyte antigen (HLA) subtypes DQB1*0602 and DR2/DRB1*1501, and this association with certain HLA subtypes led some investigators to hypothesize that certain cases of narcolepsy might be related to autoimmune destruction of hypocretin neurons. Supporting this pathophysiologic model is the development of the disorder with recent streptococcal infection, H1N1 viral vaccination or infection, and anti-TRIB2 antibodies.[19]

### Poststreptococcal Infection and Narcolepsy

Group A streptococcus can induce an autoimmune reaction involving the cardiovascular, musculoskeletal, and CNS systems. In rheumatic fever, molecular mimicry between streptococcal and selected cardiac antigens triggers an autoimmune process that results in cardiac valvular damage. A similar process can occur in the CNS where poststreptococcal sequelae include movement disorders (eg, Sydenham chorea, tics, dystonia, and parkinsonism) and psychiatric disorders, such as pediatric autoimmune neuropsychiatric disorders associated with streptococcal infections (PANDAS).[20]

Evidence suggests that streptococcal throat infection might be a risk factor for narcolepsy-cataplexy in genetically susceptible individuals. However, investigations into the connection between streptococcal infection and narcolepsy-cataplexy have yielded conflicting results. Because antibody titers subsequently return to normal levels after acute streptococcal infections, it is possible that the former might be within normal limits by the time narcolepsy is diagnosed.[21] In a retrospective case-control study, Aran and colleagues[22] noted that antistreptococcal antibody titers were higher in patients with DQB1*0602 confirmed, low hypocretin-1 narcolepsy compared with age-matched controls (anti–streptolysin O [ASO] >200 IU in 34.5% vs 18.5%; odds ratio [OR] = 2.3; $P$ = .0003). Interestingly, ASO titers were higher in patients whose onset of narcolepsy was within 3 years. In another retrospective study reviewing 51 cases of childhood narcolepsy-cataplexy, streptococcal-positive throat infections were found in 20% of cases within 6 months of the onset of narcolepsy.[23] Finally, a population-based control study determined that 90% of 45 patients with DQB1*0602-confirmed narcolepsy reported a history of streptococcal throat infection (adjusted OR = 5.2; 95% confidence interval, 1.16–16.8), and that those who reported having a streptococcal throat infection before age 21 years had 5.4 times greater risk of developing narcolepsy.[24] These studies offer some indirect evidence that post-streptococcal autoimmunity might play a pathogenetic role in a subset of individuals with narcolepsy.

## Post-H1N1 Narcolepsy-Cataplexy

In August 2010, the Swedish Medical Product agency first reported, with six cases, the possibility that narcolepsy could be an adverse effect of the H1N1 flu vaccine. Finland reported an additional 14 cases that were linked to the Pandemrix vaccine that, unlike the H1N1 agent in the United States, contained the adjuvant AS03. Montpellier, France (six cases), Montreal, Canada (four cases), and Stanford University, United States (four cases) added to the number of reports after vaccination or H1N1 infections. Sixteen cases had narcolepsy-cataplexy and were HLA-DQB1*0602–positive. In 10 cases, cerebrospinal fluid (CSF) hypocretin-1 levels were significantly below the normal range (ie, <110 pg/mL), and multiple sleep latency test results were abnormal and consistent with a diagnosis of narcolepsy (mean SOL <8 minutes and ≥2 sleep-onset REM periods) in 11 cases. Post-streptococcal ASO titers were elevated in 11

cases. None of the post-H1N1 cases were anti-Tribbles homolog 2 (Trib2) positive. Of the 14 postvaccination cases, 3 were vaccinated without the adjuvant and 11 received the adjuvanted agent. Furthermore, onset of narcolepsy occurred within 2 to 8 weeks in 9 of 14 postvaccination cases.[25]

Two studies were conducted in Finland to determine the association between the Pandemrix influenza vaccine and narcolepsy. A retrospective cohort study of 67 confirmed cases of narcolepsy from January 2009 to December 2010 found a narcolepsy incidence of 9 per 100,000 in the AS03-adjuvanted Pandemrix versus 0.7 per 100,000 in the unvaccinated groups.[26] Moreover, a study investigating the incidence of narcolepsy between the years 2002 and 2010 found an increase from 0.31 to 5.3 cases per 100,000. Incidence of narcolepsy increased 17-fold during the time the Pandemrix influenza vaccine was being used.[27] It is possible that exposure to the Pandemrix vaccination in genetically susceptible persons was responsible for the significantly higher incidence of narcolepsy during this period.

Dauvilliers and colleagues[25] proposed several hypotheses to explain the association between the H1N1 vaccine and the development of narcolepsy. One explanation is molecular mimicry where similarities between H1N1 antigens and hypocretin peptides result in cross-activation of autoreactive T or B lymphocytes. Use of the adjuvant vaccine or recent H1N1 infection results in heightened immune responses; the latter may, in turn, compromise the blood-brain barrier, allowing autoantibodies to target hypocretin cells. High ASO titers after H1N1 vaccination can act as nonspecific immune triggers that activate dormant autoreactive T lymphocytes. However, the evidence supporting a link between narcolepsy and H1N1 vaccination has its limitations: a large proportion of the population administered the H1N1 vaccine did not develop narcolepsy. Thus, there may simply be a temporal association, rather can causation, between vaccination and narcolepsy.

## Anti-TRIB2 Antibodies in Narcolepsy

To screen for hypocretin-coexpressed peptides that may be targets of an autoimmune attack in narcolepsy, Cvetkovic-Lopes and colleagues[28] engineered a transgenic mouse model. They demonstrated that the Trib2 transcript is highly expressed in hypocretin-producing neurons. Among 119 European patients with narcolepsy with cataplexy, 14% had elevated anti-Trib2 autoantibodies. Furthermore, Trib2 titers were elevated during the first 2 years of the onset of narcolepsy.

Kawashima and colleagues[29] investigated anti-Trib2 and ASO antibodies in 90 patients with narcolepsy plus cataplexy, 57 narcolepsy without cataplexy, and 156 age-matched controls. Anti-Trib2 antibodies were present in 25% HLA-DQB1*0602–positive cases with cataplexy but were generally negative in those without cataplexy (3.5%) and in control subjects (4.5%). Interestingly, anti-Trib2 positivity and increased ASO antibody titers were observed in 39 cases of DQB1*0602-positive recent-onset narcolepsy. Anti-Trib2 autoantibodies were rarely found in cases without cataplexy or with more distant onset. Toyoda and colleagues[30] compared anti-Trib2 antibodies in 88 Japanese patients with narcolepsy-cataplexy, 18 narcolepsy without cataplexy, 11 idiopathic hypersomnia with long sleep time, and in 87 healthy control subjects. Anti-Trib2 positivity was significantly higher in narcolepsy-cataplexy (26.1%) compared with narcolepsy without cataplexy (5.6%), idiopathic hypersomnia (0%), or control subjects (2.3%).

What mechanisms might be responsible for the proposed autoimmune processes occurring in narcolepsy-cataplexy? Lim and Scammell[31] suggested several possible explanations. First, it is possible that because of high Trib2 transcripts in hypocretin cells, anti-Trib2 antibodies can destroy these neurons. It has been argued, however, that Trib2 is widely expressed throughout brain and yet other cell groups are relatively preserved. Second, anti-Trib2 antibodies may be a consequence rather than the inciting cause of hypocretin cell destruction, the latter releasing intracellular Trib2 leading to the formation of autoantibodies. If the latter is true, then the cause of the initial destruction of hypocretin neurons is an altogether unrelated process, such as a direct infection of the lateral hypothalamus by a neurotropic virus, or a neurodegenerative process. Finally, anti-Trib2 antibodies may have no association with hypocretin neuronal injury, and an inflammatory response injuring hypocretin neurons may independently produce anti-Trib2 antibodies.

## HIV INFECTION

Sleep disturbances are prevalent and distressing symptoms experienced by patients with HIV infection. Sleep problems are reported by 30% to 100% of adults in this population. In HIV infection, poor sleep quality has been correlated with disease progression, opportunistic infections, encephalopathy, changes in immune status, antiretroviral therapy, psychosocial stress, social and occupational functioning, and poor sleep hygiene. Psychological comorbidity is the most important

risk factor for the development of insomnia in this population. Other significant risk factors include cognitive impairment, therapy with efavirenz, and an AIDS-defining illness.[32]

It is estimated that 73% of HIV-positive adults have insomnia, defined as nonrestorative sleep, poor sleep quality, difficulty initiating sleep, difficulty maintaining sleep, or early morning awakenings. Patients with HIV complain of daytime fatigue, depression, cognitive impairment, and diminished quality of life. In the Women's Interagency HIV Study, infected women were 17% more likely to endorse insomnia symptoms than noninfected women (OR = 1.17; 95% confidence interval, 1.04–1.34; $P<.05$).[33] Prevalence of insomnia was higher (26%) among women in the 31- to 40-year age group.

Low and colleagues[34] conducted an investigation to determine the cause of fatigue, a chronic symptom in patients with HIV, and the relationship between fatigue and insomnia. Using the Piper Fatigue Scale as their dependent variable, they performed a regression analysis using the Insomnia Severity Index, Hospital Anxiety and Depression Scale, and Hamilton Depression Rating Scale. Greater fatigue severity was associated with insomnia severity, and depression contributed to insomnia and fatigue. Pence and colleagues[35] demonstrated that HIV-related fatigue scales moderately correlated with poor quality of nighttime sleep as measured by the Pittsburgh Sleep Quality Index (PSQI) ($P = .46$). In one study, 73% of HIV-seropositive respondents were classified as having a sleep disturbance by the PSQI test, but only 33% had documented sleep problems charted in their medical records; using multivariate analysis, the best predictors of insomnia were cognitive impairment (OR = 1.4) and depression (OR = 1.2).[36] Salahuddin and colleagues,[37] in a longitudinal study, also found a correlation between poor nighttime sleep and intensity of fatigue.

Insomnia in patients with HIV may be affected by a variety of factors, including the systemic infection itself or comorbid conditions, and medications used to treat AIDS or opportunistic infections.[38] Therefore, appropriate treatment of insomnia in HIV-seropositive patients should be individualized, preferably using a combination of nonpharmacologic and pharmacologic interventions. Nonpharmacologic therapies for insomnia include sleep hygiene, stimulus control, and sleep restriction; although these techniques have not been specifically studied in this patient group, there is no reason to suspect that treatment responses in patients with HIV should differ from other populations.[39] In a pilot study involving HIV-seropositive women in which the effect of a sleep hygiene educational intervention was evaluated by self-report and actigraphy, subjects who reported sleep initiation difficulties (SOL ≥30 minutes) or poor nighttime sleep (wakefulness during the night >30%) had significant improvements in sleep measures. However, objective measures of nighttime sleep did not substantially change in the group as a whole.[40] In another report, reducing caffeine intake by 90% or more for 30 days in HIV-positive patients resulted in 35% improvement in sleep quality compared with control subjects (P<.001).[41] Finally, 5 weeks of individualized acupuncture therapy significantly improved sleep activity as assessed by actigraphy and subjective sleep quality as measured by PSQI.[42]

Sleep architecture is frequently abnormal in HIV-infected patients. A prospective longitudinal study found the following symptoms in more than half of patients with HIV: lack of energy (65%); drowsy feeling (57%); and difficulty sleeping (56%).[43] Patients with HIV who have higher self-reports of pain reported greater sleep disturbances.[44] Changes in sleep architecture associated with HIV infection include increases in SOL, percentage of slow wave sleep, stage N1 sleep shifts, percentage of N2 sleep, duration of REM sleep, and frequency of arousals.[45] Cyclic alternating pattern rate is also increased.[46] In contrast to HIV-seronegative controls, patients with HIV demonstrated reverse-direction phase coupling of delta frequency EEG amplitude and growth hormone secretion, suggesting aberrations in sleep physiology.[47] Sleep impairment in patients with HIV infection is also correlated with anxiety or depression.[48] Depression resulting from poor sleep quality could reduce medication regimen adherence, which may be particularly problematic in this patient population.[42]

Worse sleep quality may be related to impaired functional status, longer duration of HIV disease, pain, fatigue, and stress.[49,50] In one report, increased levels of psychological distress were associated with significantly lowered T-cytotoxic/suppressor (CD3+CD8+) cell counts.[51] There are several causes for pain in patients with HIV infection, including Kaposi's sarcoma, arthritides, myopathies, and neuropathies.[39]

Highly active antiretroviral therapy can be associated with sleep disturbances. Administration of efavirenz, a nucleoside reverse transcriptase inhibitor, frequently results in poor sleep quality, more severe anxiety, and increased reports of unusual dreams.[52] The major late-emergent neuropsychiatric adverse reactions among patients receiving at least 3 months of efavirenz were mostly related to sleep, such as abnormal dreams (24.7%),

nocturnal waking (19.6%), and difficulty falling asleep (17.8%).[53] Patients have reported increased dream recollection and morning sluggishness. Sleep architecture may be altered with prolongation of SOL, reduction in stage N2 sleep, increase in slow wave sleep, and a modest increase in REM sleep.[54] Additionally, patients with HIV with insomnia taking efavirenz also had reduced SE, decreased REM sleep, and increased frequency of daytime napping. Reductions in SE have been correlated with plasma concentrations of efavirenz.[55] One study examining the long-term effects of efavirenz treatment found the bad dreams persisted at 3 years of therapy.[56]

Poor quality of sleep has been shown to correlate with low medication adherence.[57] Other factors that are associated with poor quality of sleep and medication nonadherence are symptoms of depression, suicidal ideation, unemployment, use of illicit drugs, history of incarceration, and increased viral load.[58]

OSA may be independently associated with HIV-infection. Risk factors for development of OSA in patients with HIV positivity include adenotonsillar hypertrophy, dyslipidemia, insulin resistance, diabetes, lipodystropy, and systemic inflammation. In a group of asymptomatic patients with HIV infection, adenotonsillar hypertrophy, a feature of HIV disease, was the only consistent risk factor for OSA.[59] Additionally, OSA can arise from the use of antiretroviral therapy as a result of weight gain and lipodystrophy. A report consisting of 12 HIV-infected subjects with OSA noted that 11 were overweight or obese, 11 had neck circumference of greater than or equal to 40 cm, and 7 had lipodystrophy.[60]

## SLEEPING SICKNESS

Human African trypanosomiasis, also known as sleeping sickness, is caused by infection with Trypanosoma brucei (Tb). There are two distinguishable types: Tb gambiense or West African form, and Tb rhodesiense or Eastern African variant occurring west or east of the Rift valley, respectively. The Gambian form is characterized by a slow progression of the disease lasting months to years, whereas the Rhodesian form has a more rapid progression ranging from weeks to months. Sleeping sickness consists of two stages. The initial hemolymphatic stage is characterized by fever, cervical adenopathy, and cardiac arrhythmias. This is followed by a terminal meningoencephalitic stage in which infected patients present with progressive hypersomnolence, sensory deficits, and abnormal reflexes. Altered consciousness, cachexia, coma, and eventually death develop in untreated patients. Reversal of sleep-wake periods may occur. The disorder is diagnosed by identifying the offending pathogens in blood, bone marrow, lymph node aspirates, or CSF.[9]

Experimental studies with rodents infected with *Trypanosoma* demonstrated that parasites do not penetrate the blood-brain barrier in the initial stage of infection but rather are localized to the choroid plexus, circumventricular organs, and peripheral nerve root ganglia where inflammatory products from the trypanosomes and cytokines are released into the CSF and, from there, diffuse into surrounding tissues.[61] Alterations in the circadian release of cortisol, prolactin, growth hormone, and plasma renin has been described.[62] Interestingly, the physiologic secretion of melatonin by the pineal gland seems to be preserved.[63] Alterations in sleep are believed to result from activation of inflammatory mediators, such as interferon-$\gamma$ and tumor necrosis factor-$\alpha$.[61,64]

Polysomnographic features consist of paucity of vertex sharp waves, sleep spindles, and K complexes. Shortened REM sleep latency or sleep-onset REM periods may be present as is dysregulation of the 24-hour distribution of sleep and wakefulness and disappearance of diurnal rhythm with disease progression. Disruption of the sleep-wake cycle is partially reversible with antiparasitic therapy in some patients.[65] Treatment consists of antiparasitic medications (eg, pentamidine, suramin, melasoprol, or eflornithine) and drug selection is primarily based on disease stage and pathogen.[66]

## MENINGITIS AND ENCEPHALITIS

The Romanian psychiatrist and neurologist, Constantin Von Economo, first described sleep disturbances associated with encephalitis in 1917. During an encephalitis epidemic from 1917 to the late 1920s, he described a syndrome known as encephalitis lethargica, which is characterized by high fever, sore throat, headache, lethargy, double vision, delayed physical and mental responsiveness, catatonia, and sleep inversion similar to African sleeping sickness.[67] Damage to the ventrolateral preoptic area resulted in severe insomnia, whereas damage to the posterior hypothalamus resulted in hypersomnia. Subsequent investigations have suggested that patient's may have developed autoimmune encephalitis secondary to a poststreptococcal infection as in Sydenham chorea and PANDAS. There is also some evidence that patients with encephalitis lethargica have autoantibodies that bind to neurons in the basal ganglia and midbrain.[68] Another possibility is that

encephalitis lethargic represents an autoimmune reaction to the Spanish influenza virus.[69]

It is well known that many patients with bacterial and viral meningitis experience long-term neurologic and neuropsychological sequelae, including deficits in attention, learning, and short-term memory. Schmidt and colleagues[70] investigated the long-term effects on sleep in patients with bacterial and viral meningitis. They administered two standardized questionnaires (ie, PSQI and Schlaffragebogen B) to 86 adults who had viral or bacterial meningitis during the previous year and to healthy age-matched volunteers. Subjects with prior meningitis had abnormal mean PSQI total scores; they described reduced sleep quality and less restful sleep compared with healthy control subjects.

Changes in sleep architecture are common in patients with encephalitis. A study investigating chronic neurologic abnormalities related to Lyme disease found that 89% of 27 patients reported disturbed sleep.[71] Pardasani and colleagues,[72] who conducted a case control study involving 43 patients with tuberculous meningitis and age- and gender-matched normal healthy control subjects, observed that the former had greater sleep time ($P<.0005$), more daytime sleep episodes ($P<.0005$), less nocturnal sleep ($P<.0005$), and more frequent ($P = .019$) and longer awakenings ($P<.0005$) than healthy control subjects.

Sleep-related breathing disorders have been reported in patients with meningitis or encephalitis. There are two case reports of failure of automatic control of ventilation (acquired Ondine curse), one involving an 8-year-old boy with viral brainstem encephalitis[73] and another of a 48-year-old man with *Listeria monocytogenes* encephalitis.[74] Kurz and colleagues[75] reported a case of central apneas developing in an infant with enterovirus-associated meningoencephalitis. Pneumococcal meningitis in a 9-year-old boy resulted in medullary lesions with impairment in respiratory rhythmogenesis; polysomnography revealed oxygen desaturation, decreased respiratory rate, and an irregular respiratory pattern during REM and NREM sleep.[76] There are case reports of transient OSA associated with cryptococcal meningoencephalitis and viral encephalitis.[77,78] White and colleagues[71] observed a case of sleep apnea and nocturnal hypoventilation associated with Western equine encephalitis that improved over several months. McCarthy and colleagues[79] reported a case of a child with parainfluenza encephalitis who had central apneas and periodic breathing. Central apneas were noted in a patient with medullary lesions caused by *Listeria* rhomboencephalitis.[80] There are rare cases of patients developing bacterial meningitis after initiation of nasal continuous positive airway pressure therapy.[8]

Extreme spindles are diffuse, continuous high-voltage frontocentral, 8- to 15-Hz spindles. There are two case reports of extreme spindles associated with *M pneumoniae* encephalitis.[81,82] A study investigating the enterovirus 71 (EV71) outbreak in Taiwan in 1998 found that myoclonus with sleep disturbance was the most important early sign of EV71 CNS infection.[83] There is also a case report of a 40-year-old woman who developed REM behavior disorder after an acute inflammatory rhomboencephalitis; on T1-weighted magnetic resonance imaging, she had small hypodenisities on the right pontine tegmentum and right dorsal medulla. Her REM sleep behavior disorder did not response to clonazepam but improved with melatonin.[10]

## SUMMARY

Different infectious pathogens can alter sleep, either resulting from systemic inflammation, auto-immune responses, direct CNS injury, or adverse reaction to pharmacologic therapy. Many reports involved a handful of cases, thus making recommendations regarding diagnosis or therapy difficult. A thorough clinical history aided by appropriate testing is necessary, and prompt therapy may improve outcomes.

## REFERENCES

1. Opp MR, Imeri L. Sleep as a behavioral model of neuro-immune interactions. Acta Neurobiol Exp (Wars) 1999;59:45–53.

2. Lancel M, Crönlein J, Müller-Preuss P, et al. Lipopolysaccharide increases EEG delta activity within non-REM sleep and disrupts sleep continuity in rats. Am J Phys 1995;268:R1310–8.

3. Baracchi F, Ingiosi AM, Raymond RM Jr, et al. Sepsis-induced alterations in sleep of rats. Am J Physiol Regul Integr Comp Physiol 2011;301: R1467–78.

4. Kornum BR, Faraco J, Mignot E. Narcolepsy with hypocretin/orexin deficiency, infections and autoimmunity of the brain. Curr Opin Neurobiol 2011;21:897–903.

5. Low Y, Goforth HW, Omonuwa T, et al. Comparison of polysomnographic data in age-, sex- and axis I psychiatric diagnosis matched HIV-seropositive and HIV-seronegative insomnia patients. Clin Neurophysiol 2012. http://dx.doi.org/10.1016/j.clinph.2012.05.004.

6. Dorey-Stein Z, Amorosa VK, Kostman JR, et al. Severe weight gain, lipodystrophy, dyslipidemia, and obstructive sleep apnea in a human immunodeficiency virus-infected patient following highly active

antiretroviral therapy. J Cardiometab Syndr 2008;3: 111–4.

7. Thalhofer S, Dorow P. Celtral sleep apnea. Respiration 1997;64:2–9.

8. Kuzniar TJ, Gruber B, Mutlu GM. Cerebrospinal fluid leak and meningitis associated with nasal continuous positive airway pressure therapy. Chest 2005; 128:1882–4.

9. Lundkvist GB, Kristensson K, Bentivoglio M. Why trypanosomes cause sleeping sickness. Physiology (Bethesda) 2004;19:198–206.

10. Limousin N, Dehais C, Gout O, et al. A brainstem inflammatory lesion causing REM sleep behavior disorder and sleepwalking (parasomnia overlap disorder). Sleep Med 2009;10:1059–62.

11. Van Kralingen KW, Ivanyi B, Van Keimpema AR, et al. Sleep complaints in postpolio syndrome. Arch Phys Med Rehabil 1996;77:609–11.

12. Ehler E, Latta J, Mandysová P, et al. Stiff-person syndrome following tick-borne meningoencephalitis. Acta Medica (Hradec Kralove) 2011;54:170–4.

13. Gorman MP. Update on diagnosis, treatment, and prognosis in opsoclonus-myoclonus-ataxia syndrome. Curr Opin Pediatr 2010;22:745–50.

14. Sardar P, Bandyopadhyay D, Roy D, et al. Non tuberculous mycobacteria and toxoplasma co-infection of the central nervous system in a patient with AIDS. Braz J Infect Dis 2009;13:449–51.

15. Sellner J, Trinka E. Seizures and epilepsy in herpes simplex virus encephalitis. current concepts and future directions of pathogenesis and management. J Neurol 2012;259(10):2019–30.

16. Anghinah R, Camargo EC, Braga NI, et al. Generalized periodic EEG activity in two cases of neurosyphilis. Arq Neuropsiquiatr 2006;64:122–4.

17. Hulihan JF, Bebin EM, Westmoreland BF. Bilateral periodic lateralized epileptiform discharges in mycoplasma encephalitis. Pediatr Neurol 1992;8:292–4.

18. Cury RF, Wichert-Ana L, Sakamoto AC, et al. Focal nonconvulsive status epilepticus associated to PLEDs and intense focal hyperemia in an AIDS patient. Seizure 2004;13:358–61.

19. Michael J, Sateia. editor. International classification of sleep disorders. 2nd edition. Diagnostic and coding manual. Westchester (IL): American Academy of Sleep Medicine; 2005.

20. Dale RC. Post-streptococcal autoimmune disorders of the central nervous system. Dev Med Child Neurol 2005;47:785–91.

21. Longstreth WT Jr, Ton TG, Koepsell TD. Narcolepsy and streptococcal infections. Sleep 2009;32:1548.

22. Aran A, Lin L, Nevsimalova S, et al. Elevated anti-streptococcal antibodies in patients with recent narcolepsy onset. Sleep 2009;32:979–83.

23. Aran A, Einen M, Lin L, et al. Clinical and therapeutic aspects of childhood narcolepsy-cataplexy: a retrospective study of 51 children. Sleep 2010;33:1457–64.

24. Koepsell TD, Longstreth WT, Ton TG. Medical exposures in youth and the frequency of narcolepsy with cataplexy: a population-based case-control study in genetically predisposed people. J Sleep Res 2010; 19:80–6.

25. Dauvilliers Y, Montplaisir J, Cochen V, et al. Post-H1N1 narcolepsy-cataplexy. Sleep 2010;33: 1428–30.

26. Nohynek H, Jokinen J, Partinen M, et al. AS03 adjuvanted AH1N1 vaccine associated with an abrupt increase in the incidence of childhood narcolepsy in Finland. PLoS One 2012;7:e33536.

27. Partinen M, Saarenpää-Heikkilä O, Ilveskoski I, et al. Increased incidence and clinical picture of childhood narcolepsy following the 2009 H1N1 pandemic vaccination campaign in Finland. PLoS One 2012;7: e33723.

28. Cvetkovic-Lopes V, Bayer L, Dorsaz S, et al. Elevated Tribbles homolog 2-specific antibody levels in narcolepsy patients. J Clin Invest 2010; 120:713–9.

29. Kawashima M, Lin L, Tanaka S, et al. Anti-Tribbles homolog 2 (TRIB2) autoantibodies in narcolepsy are associated with recent onset of cataplexy. Sleep 2010;33:869–74.

30. Toyoda H, Tanaka S, Miyagawa T, et al. Anti-Tribbles homolog 2 autoantibodies in Japanese patients with narcolepsy. Sleep 2010;33:875–8.

31. Lim AS, Scammell TE. The trouble with Tribbles: do antibodies against TRIB2 cause narcolepsy? Sleep 2010;33:857–8.

32. Reid S, Dwyer J. Insomnia in HIV infection: a systematic review of prevalence, correlates, and management. Pyschosom Med 2005;67:260–9.

33. Jean-Louis G, Weber KM, Aouizerat BE, et al. Insomnia symptoms and HIV infection among participants in the Women's Interagency HIV Study. Sleep 2012;35:131–7.

34. Low Y, Preud'homme X, Goforth HW, et al. The association of fatigue with depression and insomnia in HIV-seropositive patients: a pilot study. Sleep 2011;34:1723–6.

35. Pence BW, Barroso J, Leserman J, et al. Measuring fatigue in people living with HIV/AIDS: psychometric characteristics of the HIV-related fatigue scale. AIDS Care 2008;20:829–37.

36. Rubinstein ML, Selwyn PA. High prevalence of insomnia in an outpatient population with HIV infection. J Acquir Immune Defic Syndr Hum Retrovirol 1998;19:260–5.

37. Salahuddin N, Barroso J, Leserman J, et al. Daytime sleepiness, nighttime sleep quality, stressful life events, and HIV-related fatigue. J Assoc Nurses AIDS Care 2009;20:6–13.

38. Omonuwa TS, Goforth HW, Preud'homme X, et al. The pharmacologic management of insomnia in patients with HIV. J Clin Sleep Med 2009;5:251–62.

39. Reid S, McGrathl L. HIV/AIDS. Sleep Med Clin 2007; 2:51–8.

40. Hudson AL, Portillo CJ, Lee KA. Sleep disturbances in women with HIV or AIDS: efficacy of a tailored sleep promotion intervention. Nurse Res 2008;57: 360–6.

41. Dreher HM. The effect of caffeine reduction on sleep quality and well-being in persons with HIV. J Psychosom Res 2003;54:191–8.

42. Phillips KD, Moneyham L, Murdaugh C, et al. Sleep disturbance and depression as barriers to adherence. Clin Nurs Res 2005;14:273–93.

43. Lee KA, Gay C, Portillo CJ, et al. Symptom experience in HIV-infected adults: a function of demographic and clinical characteristics. J Pain Symptom Manage 2009;38:882–93.

44. Aouizerat BE, Miaskowski CA, Gay C, et al. Risk factors and symptoms associated with pain in HIV-infected adults. J Assoc Nurses AIDS Care 2010; 21:125–33.

45. Norman SE, Chediak AD, Kiel M, et al. Sleep disturbances in HIV-infected homosexual men. AIDS 1990;4:775–81.

46. Ferini-Strambi L, Oldani A, Tirloni G, et al. Slow wave sleep and cyclic alternating pattern (CAP) in HIV-infected asymptomatic men. Sleep 1995;18:446–50.

47. Darko DF, Mitler MM, Miller JC. Growth hormone, fatigue, poor sleep, and disability in HIV infection. Neuroendocrinology 1998;67:317–24.

48. Junqueira P, Bellucci S, Rossini S, et al. Women living with HIV/AIDS: sleep impairment, anxiety and depression symptoms. Arq Neuropsiquiatr 2008; 66:817–20.

49. Nokes KM, Kendrew J. Correlates of sleep quality in persons with HIV disease. J Assoc Nurses AIDS Care 2001;12(1):17–22.

50. Robbins JL, Phillips KD, Dudgeon WD, et al. Physiological and psychological correlates of sleep in HIV infection. Clin Nurs Res 2004;13:33–52.

51. Cruess DG, Antoni MH, Gonzalez J, et al. Sleep disturbance mediates the association between psychological distress and immune status among HIV-positive men and women on combination antiretroviral therapy. J Psychosom Res 2003;54:185–9.

52. Rihs TA, Begley K, Smith DE, et al. Efavirenz and chronic neuropsychiatric symptoms: a cross-sectional case control study. HIV Med 2006;7:544–8.

53. Lochet P, Peyrière H, Lotthé A, et al. Long-term assessment of neuropsychiatric adverse reactions associated with efavirenz. HIV Med 2003;4:62–6.

54. Moyle G, Fletcher C, Brown H, et al. Changes in sleep quality and brain wave patterns following initiation of an efavirenz-containing triple antiretroviral regimen. HIV Med 2006;7:243–7.

55. Gallego L, Barreiro P, Del Río R, et al. Analyzing sleep abnormalities in HIV-infected patients treated with Efavirenz. Clin Infect Dis 2004;38:430–2.

56. Clifford DB, Evans S, Yang Y, et al. Long-term impact of efavirenz on neuropsychological performance and symptoms in HIV-infected individuals (ACTG 5097s). HIV Clin Trials 2009;10:343–55.

57. Gay C, Portillo CJ, Kelly R, et al. Self-reported medication adherence and symptom experience in adults with HIV. J Assoc Nurses AIDS Care 2011; 22:257–68.

58. Saberi P, Neilands TB, Johnson MO. Quality of sleep: associations with antiretroviral nonadherence. AIDS Patient Care STDS 2011;25:517–24.

59. Epstein LJ, Strollo PJ Jr, Donegan RB, et al. Obstructive sleep apnea in patients with human immunodeficiency virus (HIV) disease. Sleep 1995; 18:368–76.

60. Lo Re V, Schutte-Rodin S, Kostman JR. Obstructive sleep apnoea among HIV patients. Int J STD AIDS 2006;17:614–20.

61. Kristensson K, Mhlanga JD, Bentivoglio M. Parasites and the brain: neuroinvasion, immunopathogenesis and neuronal dysfunctions. Curr Top Microbiol Immunol 2002;265:227–57.

62. Radomski MW, Buguet A, Bogui P, et al. Disruptions in the secretion of cortisol, prolactin, and certain cytokines in human African trypanosomiasis patients. Bull Soc Pathol Exot 1994;87:376–9.

63. Claustrat B, Buguet A, Geoffriau M, et al. Plasma melatonin rhythm is maintained in human African trypanosomiasis. Neuroendocrinology 1998;68:64–70.

64. Paludan SR. Synergistic action of pro-inflammatory agents: cellular and molecular aspects. J Leukoc Biol 2000;67:18–25.

65. Buguet A, Bisser S, Josenando T, et al. Sleep structure: a new diagnostic tool for stage determination in sleeping sickness. Acta Trop 2005;93:107–17.

66. Bruun R, Blum J, Chappuis F, et al. Human African trypanosomiasis. Lancet 2010;375:148–59.

67. Berry RB. Neurobiology of sleep. Fundaments of sleep medicine: expert consult. Philadelphia: WB Saunders; 2011. p. 91–100.

68. Dale RC, Church AJ, Surtees RA, et al. Encephalitis lethargica syndrome: 20 new cases and evidence of basal ganglia autoimmunity. Brain 2004;127:21–33.

69. Vilensky JA, Foley P, Gilman S. Children and encephalitis lethargica: a historical review. Pediatr Neurol 2007;37:79–84.

70. Schmidt H, Cohrs S, Heinemann T, et al. Sleep disorders are long-term sequelae of both bacterial and viral meningitis. J Neurol Neurosurg Psychiatry 2006;77:554–8.

71. White DP, Miller F, Erickson RW. Sleep apnea and nocturnal hypoventilation after western equine encephalitis. Am Rev Respir Dis 1983;127:132–3.

72. Pardasani V, Shukla G, Singh S, et al. Abnormal sleep-wake cycles in patients with tuberculous meningitis: a case-control study. J Neurol Sci 2008; 269:126–32.

73. Giangaspero F, Schiavina M, Sturani C, et al. Failure of automatic control of ventilation (Ondine's curse) associated with viral encephalitis of the brainstem: a clinicopathologic study of one case. Clin Neuropathol 1988;7:234–7.

74. Jensen TH, Hansen PB, Brodersen P. Ondine's curse in listeria monocytogenes brain stem encephalitis. Acta Neurol Scand 1988;77:505–6.

75. Kurz H, Jakelj J, Aberle SW, et al. Long central apnea as the chief symptom of aseptic meningoencephalitis in a 6-week-old infant. Wien Klin Wochenschr 1999;111:294–7.

76. Hasegawa T, Kohyama J, Kohji T, et al. Impairment of respiratory rhythmogenesis and sequelae of bacterial meningitis. Pediatr Neurol 1995;12:357–60.

77. Buyse B, Gysbrechts C, Michiels E, et al. Temporary obstructive apnoea syndrome attributed to cryptococcus (meningo) encephalitis. Respir Med 1996; 90:571–4.

78. Dyken ME, Yamada T, Berger HA. Transient obstructive sleep apnea and asystole in association with presumed viral encephalopathy. Neurology 2003; 60:1692–4.

79. McCarthy VP, Zimmerman AW, Miller CA. Central nervous system manifestations of parainfluenza virus type 3 infections in childhood. Pediatr Neurol 1990;6:197–201.

80. Milhaud D, Bernardin G, Roger PM, et al. Central apnea with consciousness impairment due to *Listeria* rhombencephalitis sequelae. Rev Neurol (Paris) 1999;155:152–4 [in French].

81. Heatwole CR, Berg MJ, Henry JC, et al. Extreme spindles: a distinctive EEG pattern in mycoplasma pneumoniae encephalitis. Neurology 2005;64: 1096–7.

82. Akaboshi S, Koeda T, Houdou S. Transient extreme spindles in a case of subacute mycoplasma pneumoniae encephalitis. Acta Paediatr Jpn 1998;40: 479–82.

83. Liu CC, Tseng HW, Wang SM, et al. An outbreak of enterovirus 71 infection in Taiwan, 1998: epidemiologic and clinical manifestations. J Clin Virol 2000; 17:23–30.

# Index

*Note:* Page numbers of article titles are in **boldface** type.

## A

Acetazolamide, for Arnold-Chiari malformation, 693–694

Achondroplasia, 692–693

Actigraphy, 585
    for circadian sleep disorders, 615
    for hypersomnia, 614
    for insomnia, 590

Acupuncture, for insomnia, 592

Adaptive servo-ventilation, for central sleep apnea, 602

African trypanosomiasis, 707–708

Amplitude, in chronobiology, 656

Amyotrophic lateral sclerosis, 590, 671–672

Anticoagulants, chronopharmacology of, 663

Antiepileptic medications, effects on sleep, 623–624

Antihistamines, proconvulsant effects of, 620

Antihypertensive agents, chronopharmacology of, 663

Antiretroviral therapy, sleep disorders due to, 707

Anxiety
    in spinal cord injury, 648–649
    in traumatic brain injury, 614–615

Apert syndrome, 691–692

Arnold-Chiari malformation, 693–694

Arrhythmias, obstructive sleep apnea/stroke relationship to, 600

Atherosclerosis, obstructive sleep apnea/stroke relationship to, 600

Atrial fibrillation, obstructive sleep apnea/stroke relationship to, 600

Autoset continuous positive airway pressure, for obstructive sleep apnea, 601

## B

Becker muscular dystrophy, 670–671

Benzodiazepines, for insomnia, 592, 603

Berger, Johannes, as sleep medicine pioneer, 577

Berlin Sleep Questionnaire, for Parkinson disease, 637

Bilevel positive airway pressure (BPAP), for neuromuscular diseases, 674–682

Biologic rhythms. *See also* Chronobiology; Circadian rhythm sleep disorders.
    definition of, 655

Blepharospasm, 640

Blood pressure swings, obstructive sleep apnea/ stroke relationship to, 599

Body temperature disruptions, in spinal cord injury, 646–647

Brain injury, traumatic. *See* Traumatic brain injury.

Brainstem, compression of, sleep disorders in, 693–694

Breathing disorders, types of, 579

Bright light therapy, for insomnia, 592

## C

Cabergoline, for periodic leg movements, 636

Cancer, chronobiology of, 659

Carbamazepine, effects on sleep, 623

Cataplexy, from influenza vaccine, 705

Central nervous system infections, **703–711**
    encephalitis, 708–709
    HIV, 704, 706–707
    meningitis, 708–709
    narcolepsy in, 704–706
    sleep architecture in, 703–704
    sleeping sickness, 707–708

Central sleep apnea
    definition of, 598
    in achondroplasia, 692–693
    in Arnold-Chiari malformation, 693–694
    in Down syndrome, 696
    in encephalitis, 708
    pathophysiology of, 598
    stroke and, 601–602

Cerebellar ataxia, movement disorders in, 644

Cerebral blood flow, reduction of, obstructive sleep apnea/stroke relationship to, 599–600

Cerebro-costo-mandibular syndrome, 690

Cervical dystonia, 639–640

CHARGE syndrome, 697

Cheyne-Stokes respiration, in stroke, 601–602

Chorea, 638–639

Chronobiology, **655–666**. *See also* Circadian rhythm sleep disorders.
    circadian time structure in
        chronotypes in, 656–658
        disruption of, 658–659
        medication response and, 662–663
        mental performance and, 659–661
        physical performance and, 659–661
        re-entraining of, 661
        severity of disease and, 661–662
    essentials of, 655–658
    sleep-wake cycles and, 658

**United States Postal Service**

## Statement of Ownership, Management, and Circulation
(All Periodicals Publications Except Requestor Publications)

| 1. Publication Title | 2. Publication Number | | | | | | | | 3. Filing Date |
|---|---|---|---|---|---|---|---|---|---|
| Sleep Medicine Clinics | 0 | 2 | 5 | - | 0 | 5 | 3 | | 9/14/12 |

| 4. Issue Frequency | 5. Number of Issues Published Annually | 6. Annual Subscription Price |
|---|---|---|
| Mar, Jun, Sep, Dec | 4 | $174.00 |

7. Complete Mailing Address of Known Office of Publication (*Not printer*) (*Street, city, county, state, and ZIP+4®*)

Elsevier Inc.
360 Park Avenue South
New York, NY 10010-1710

Contact Person
Stephen R. Bushing

Telephone (*Include area code*)
215-239-3688

8. Complete Mailing Address of Headquarters or General Business Office of Publisher (*Not printer*)

Elsevier Inc., 360 Park Avenue South, New York, NY 10010-1710

9. Full Names and Complete Mailing Addresses of Publisher, Editor, and Managing Editor (*Do not leave blank*)

Publisher (*Name and complete mailing address*)

Kim Murphy, Elsevier, Inc., 1600 John F. Kennedy Blvd. Suite 1800, Philadelphia, PA 19103-2899

Editor (*Name and complete mailing address*)

Katie Hartner, Elsevier, Inc., 1600 John F. Kennedy Blvd. Suite 1800, Philadelphia, PA 19103-2899

Managing Editor (*Name and complete mailing address*)

Sarah Barth, Elsevier, Inc., 1600 John F. Kennedy Blvd. Suite 1800, Philadelphia, PA 19103-2899

10. Owner (*Do not leave blank. If the publication is owned by a corporation, give the name and address of the corporation immediately followed by the names and addresses of all stockholders owning or holding 1 percent or more of the total amount of stock. If not owned by a corporation, give the names and addresses of the individual owners. If owned by a partnership or other unincorporated firm, give its name and address as well as those of each individual owner. If the publication is published by a nonprofit organization, give its name and address.*)

| Full Name | Complete Mailing Address |
|---|---|
| Wholly owned subsidiary of | 1600 John F. Kennedy Blvd., Ste. 1830 |
| Reed/Elsevier, US holdings | Philadelphia, PA 19103-2899 |

11. Known Bondholders, Mortgagees, and Other Security Holders Owning or Holding 1 Percent or More of Total Amount of Bonds, Mortgages, or Other Securities. If none, check box ☐ None

| Full Name | Complete Mailing Address |
|---|---|
| N/A | |

12. Tax Status (*For completion by nonprofit organizations authorized to mail at nonprofit rates*) (*Check one*)
The purpose, function, and nonprofit status of this organization and the exempt status for federal income tax purposes:
☐ Has Not Changed During Preceding 12 Months
☐ Has Changed During Preceding 12 Months (*Publisher must submit explanation of change with this statement*)

PS Form 3526, September 2007 (Page 1 of 3 (Instructions Page 3)) PSN 7530-01-000-9931 PRIVACY NOTICE: See our Privacy policy in www.usps.com

---

| 13. Publication Title | 14. Issue Date for Circulation Data Below |
|---|---|
| Sleep Medicine Clinics | September 2012 |

| 15. Extent and Nature of Circulation | | Average No. Copies Each Issue During Preceding 12 Months | No. Copies of Single Issue Published Nearest to Filing Date |
|---|---|---|---|
| a. Total Number of Copies (*Net press run*) | | 617 | 601 |
| b. Paid Circulation (By Mail and Outside the Mail) | (1) Mailed Outside-County Paid Subscriptions Stated on PS Form 3541. (*Include paid distribution above nominal rate, advertiser's proof copies, and exchange copies*) | 419 | 411 |
| | (2) Mailed In-County Paid Subscriptions Stated on PS Form 3541 (*Include paid distribution above nominal rate, advertiser's proof copies, and exchange copies*) | | |
| | (3) Paid Distribution Outside the Mails Including Sales Through Dealers and Carriers, Street Vendors, Counter Sales, and Other Paid Distribution Outside USPS® | 27 | 29 |
| | (4) Paid Distribution by Other Classes Mailed Through the USPS (e.g. First-Class Mail®) | | |
| c. Total Paid Distribution (*Sum of 15f (1), (2), (3), and (4)*) ▲ | | 446 | 440 |
| d. Free or Nominal Rate Distribution (By Mail and Outside the Mail) | (1) Free or Nominal Rate Outside-County Copies Included on PS Form 3541 | 54 | 46 |
| | (2) Free or Nominal Rate In-County Copies Included on PS Form 3541 | | |
| | (3) Free or Nominal Rate Copies Mailed at Other Classes Through the USPS (e.g. First-Class Mail) | | |
| | (4) Free or Nominal Rate Distribution Outside the Mail (Carriers or other means) | | |
| e. Total Free or Nominal Rate Distribution (Sum of 15d (1), (2), (3) and (4) | | 54 | 46 |
| f. Total Distribution (Sum of 15c and 15e) ▲ | | 500 | 486 |
| g. Copies not Distributed (See instructions to publishers #4 (page #3)) | | 117 | 115 |
| h. Total (Sum of 15f and g) ▲ | | 617 | 601 |
| i. Percent Paid (15c divided by 15f times 100) | | 89.20% | 90.53& |

16. Publication of Statement of Ownership

If the publication is a general publication, publication of this statement is required. Will be printed in the **December 2012** issue of this publication.

☐ Publication not required.

17. Signature and Title of Editor, Publisher, Business Manager, or Owner

*Stephen R. Bushing* — Inventory Distribution Coordinator

Date September 14, 2012

Stephen R. Bushing – Inventory Distribution Coordinator

I certify that all information furnished on this form is true and complete. I understand that anyone who furnishes false or misleading information on this form or who omits material or information requested on the form may be subject to criminal sanctions (including fines and imprisonment) and/or civil sanctions (including civil penalties).

PS Form 3526, September 2007 (Page 2 of 3)

# Moving?

## Make sure your subscription moves with you!

To notify us of your new address, find your **Clinics Account Number** (located on your mailing label above your name), and contact customer service at:

**Email: journalscustomerservice-usa@elsevier.com**

**800-654-2452** (subscribers in the U.S. & Canada)
**314-447-8871** (subscribers outside of the U.S. & Canada)

**Fax number: 314-447-8029**

**Elsevier Health Sciences Division**
**Subscription Customer Service**
**3251 Riverport Lane**
**Maryland Heights, MO 63043**

*To ensure uninterrupted delivery of your subscription, please notify us at least 4 weeks in advance of move.

Printed and bound by CPI Group (UK) Ltd, Croydon, CR0 4YY

03/10/2024

01040347-0008